Thieme Dissector

Second Edition

Volume II

Abdomen and Lower Limb

T0313941

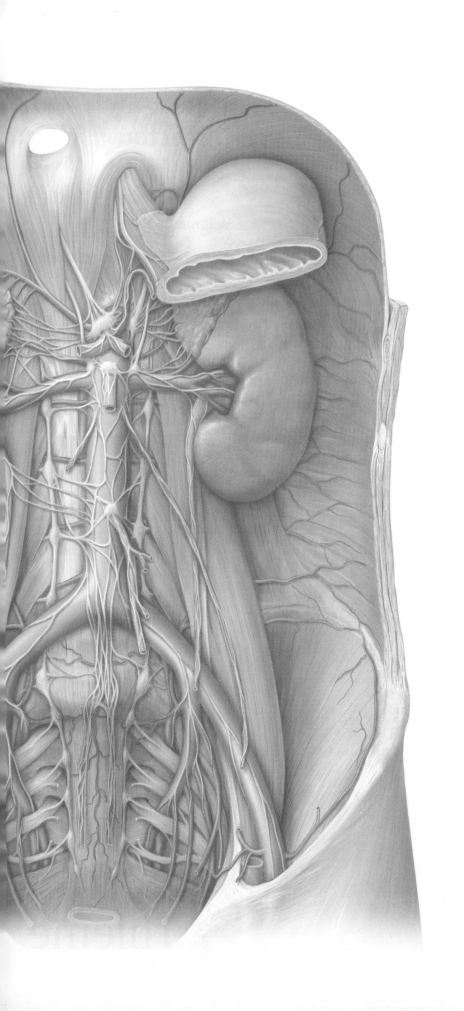

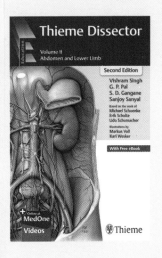

Access your free e-book now!

With three easy steps, unlock free access to your e-book on MedOne, Thieme's online platform.

1. Note your personal access code below. Once this code is activated, your printed book can no longer be returned.

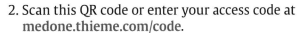

Important Notes

- The personal access code is disabled once the e-book is first activated. Use of this product is restricted to the buyer or, for library copies, authorized users.

- Sharing passwords is not permitted. The publisher has the right to take legal steps for violations.

- Access to online material is solely provided to the buyer for private use. Commercial use is not permitted.

2. Scan this QR code or enter your access code at medone.thieme.com/code.

3. Set up a username on MedOne and sign in to activate your e-book on most phones, tablets, or PCs.

Quick Access

After you successfully register and activate your code, you can find your book and additional online media at medone.thieme.com/9789392819179 or with this QR code.

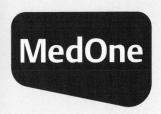

Medical information how and when you need it.

Thieme
Dissector

Second Edition

Volume II

Abdomen and Lower Limb

Vishram Singh, MBBS, MS, PhD (hc), MICPS, FASI, FIMSA
Adjunct Professor
Department of Anatomy
KMC, Manipal Academy of Higher Education
Mangalore, Karnataka, India;
Editor-in-Chief
Journal of the Anatomical Society of India;
Member, Federative International Committee for Scientific Publications (FICSP)
International Federation of Association on Anatomists (IFAA)
Geneva, Switzerland

G. P. Pal, MBBS, MS, DSc, FASI, FAMS, FNASc, FASc, Bhatnagar Laureate
Director Professor
Department of Anatomy
Index Medical College;
Emeritus Professor
MGM Medical College
Indore, Madhya Pradesh, India

S. D. Gangane, MBBS, MS, FAIMS
Professor and Head
Department of Anatomy
Terna Medical College
Navi Mumbai, Maharashtra, India

Sanjoy Sanyal MBBS, MS, MSc, ADPHA
Provost and Dean
Professor and Department Chair Anatomical Sciences
Richmond Gabriel University College of Medicine
St. Vincent and the Grenadines
Canada

Based on the work of
Michael Schuenke
Erik Schulte
Udo Schumacher

Illustrations by
Markus Voll
Karl Wesker

Thieme
Delhi • Stuttgart • New York • Rio de Janeiro

Publishing Director: Ritu Sharma
Senior Development Editor: Dr. Nidhi Srivastava
Director-Editorial Services: Rachna Sinha
Project Manager: Aishwarya Panday
National Sales Manager: Bishwajit Kumar Mishra
Managing Director & CEO: Ajit Kohli

Thieme Medical and Scientific Publishers Private Limited.
A - 12, Second Floor, Sector - 2, Noida - 201 301,
Uttar Pradesh, India, +911204556600
Email: customerservice@thieme.in
www.thieme.in

Cover design: Thieme Publishing Group
Cover image source: Voll M and Wesker K

Illustrations by Voll M and Wesker K. From: Schuenke M,
Schulte E, Schumacher U, THIEME Atlas of Anatomy.

Page make-up by RECTO Graphics, India

Printed in India

First Reprint, 2022
Second Reprint, 2023
Third Reprint, 2023

ISBN: 978-93-92819-17-9
Also available as an e-book:
eISBN (PDF): 978-93-92819-22-3
eISBN (ePub): 978-93-92819-24-7

Important note: Medicine is an ever-changing science undergoing continual development. Research and clinical experience are continually expanding our knowledge, in particular, our knowledge of proper treatment and drug therapy. Insofar as this book mentions any dosage or application, readers may rest assured that the authors, editors, and publishers have made every effort to ensure that such references are in accordance with **the state of knowledge at the time of production of the book**.

Nevertheless, this does not involve, imply, or express any guarantee or responsibility on the part of the publishers in respect to any dosage instructions and forms of applications stated in the book. **Every user is requested to examine carefully** the manufacturers' leaflets accompanying each drug and to check, if necessary, in consultation with a physician or specialist, whether the dosage schedules mentioned therein or the contraindications stated by the manufacturers differ from the statements made in the present book. Such examination is particularly important with drugs that are either rarely used or have been newly released in the market. Every dosage schedule or every form of application used is entirely at the user's own risk and responsibility. The authors and publishers request every user to report to the publishers any discrepancies or inaccuracies noticed. If errors in this work are found after publication, errata will be posted at www.thieme.com on the product description page.

Some of the product names, patents, and registered designs referred to in this book are in fact registered trademarks or proprietary names even though specific reference to this fact is not always made in the text. Therefore, the appearance of a name without designation as proprietary is not to be construed as a representation by the publisher that it is in the public domain.

Thieme addresses people of all gender identities equally. We encourage our authors to use gender-neutral or gender-equal expressions wherever the context allows.

To my students, past and present.

Vishram Singh

To my grandson, Yatharth.

G. P. Pal

To my family and colleagues, for their support;
my patients and students, for teaching me to learn from them;
the willed body-donors, for their silent altruism to medical science.

Sanjoy Sanyal

Contents

Video Contents   ix

Note from the Authors   xi

About the Authors   xv

Contributors to Volume II   xvii

1. Introduction and an Overview of the Bones of the Lower Limb   1

2. Anterior and Medial Compartments of the Thigh   13

3. Gluteal Region   29

4. Posterior Compartment of the Thigh and Popliteal Fossa   37

5. Anterior and Lateral Compartments of the Leg and Dorsum of the Foot   45

6. Posterior Compartment of the Leg   55

7. Sole of the Foot   63

8. Joints of the Lower Limb   77

9. Introduction and Overview of the Bones of the Abdomen   97

10. Anterior Abdominal Wall   103

11. Male External Genitalia   123

12. Loin   135

13. Abdominal Cavity and Peritoneum   139

14. Abdominal Part of Esophagus, Stomach, Celiac Trunk, and Spleen   151

15. Duodenum, Pancreas, and Portal Vein   163

16. Small and Large Intestines   173

17. Liver and Biliary System   187

18. Kidney, Ureter, and Suprarenal Gland   197

19. Diaphragm and Posterior Abdominal Wall   209

20. Introduction to Pelvis and Perineum   229

21. Pelvic Viscera   235

22. Rectum and Anal Canal   247

23. Uterus, Vagina, and Ovary   253

24. Pelvic Wall   261

25. Perineum   275

26. Joints of the Pelvis   289

Appendix   293

Index   295

Video Contents

Video 2.1	Muscles of anterior compartment of thigh	16
Video 2.2	Femoral nerve	18
Video 2.3	Fascia lata	20
Video 2.4	Adductor brevis	21
Video 2.5	Femoral triangle and adductor canal	26
Video 3.1	Gluteal region—Part 1	31
Video 3.2	Gluteal region—Part 2	34
Video 3.3	Gluteal muscles	34
Video 4.1	Hamstring muscles	39
Video 4.2	Hamstring muscles and sciatic nerve	39
Video 4.3	Popliteal fossa—Part 1	42
Video 4.4	Popliteal fossa—Part 2	42
Video 5.1	Tendons on dorsum of foot	48
Video 5.2	Anterior compartment of leg	50
Video 5.3	Anterior lateral aspect of leg and dorsum of foot	53
Video 6.1	Posterior aspect of leg—Part 1	56
Video 6.2	Posterior aspect of leg—Part 2	59
Video 6.3	Posterior aspect of leg—Part 3	59
Video 7.1	Sole of foot aponeurosis muscle layers and plantar nerves	64
Video 8.1	Knee—Part 1	84
Video 8.2	Knee—Part 2	84
Video 8.3	Ankle joint/Talocrural joint (movements and axis)	90
Video 8.4	Joints of foot	94
Video 10.1	Abdominal wall—flat muscles, rectus sheath, and linea alba	111
Video 10.2	Abdominal wall—rectus muscles, posterior rectus sheath, and vessels	116
Video 11.1	Spermatic cord and testis	124
Video 11.2	Testis, epididymis, spermatic cord, ductus deferens, and clinical aspects	124
Video 11.3	Male genital organs—structural configuration	130
Video 13.1	Peritoneal cavity—greater sac, lesser sac, and greater omentum	144
Video 13.2	Peritoneal cavity—Foramen of Winslow	147

Video 14.1   Overview of abdominal organs   151

Video 14.2   Abdominal viscera—an overview   153

Video 15.1   Duodenum: parts, relations, and vasculature   165

Video 15.2   Pancreas   166

Video 15.3   Portal vein   170

Video 16.1   Small intestine and its mesentery   173

Video 16.2   Superior mesenteric artery and its distribution   174

Video 16.3   Distribution of Inferior mesenteric artery in hindgut—
              high-definition clinical demonstration   178

Video 16.4   Large intestine   181

Video 17.1   Liver in situ   190

Video 17.2   Gallbladder and extrahepatic biliary apparatus   193

Video 18.1   Kidney   197

Video 18.2   Renal pelvis and ureter   206

Video 18.3   Locations of Suprarenal glands   206

Video 19.1   Posterior abdominal wall   210

Video 19.2   Lumbar plexus   211

Video 21.1   Urinary bladder: Parts, ligaments, and vessels   236

Video 21.2   Urinary bladder, UV junction, and trigone   238

Video 21.3   Bladder neck, trigone, and prostatic urethra   238

Video 21.4   Pelvic part of ureter, bladder of urinary relations, and
              trigone of urinary bladder   238

Video 22.1   Ampulla of ductus deferens, seminal vesicle, rectum,
              and pelvic vessels   249

Video 22.2   Ischioanal fossa, Alcock's canal, and sciatic foramen   251

Video 23.1   Layers of uterine wall   254

Video 23.2   Female pelvic organs with endopelvic fascia and pelvic vessels   256

Video 23.3   Bony pelvis male vs. female: obstetric fractures   256

Video 24.1   Bony pelvis inlet–outlet and diameters   262

Video 25.1   Neurovascular structure of male perineum   279

Note from the Authors

There was a long-felt need of a good dissection manual for first-year undergraduate medical students undertaking the anatomy course. Anatomy is the foundation of all medical subjects, and hence, its thorough knowledge is essential for all students aspiring to become good doctors, especially in surgical fields.

The best *modus operandi* to learn anatomy is through dissection. Recently, due to information explosion in the medical field, the health sciences curricula have markedly reduced the time allocation for studying and teaching anatomy; yet it is realized by all that the gross structure of the human body, including its three-dimensional conceptualization, must be understood thoroughly before proceeding further to learn medicine.

Therefore, we have made a sincere effort to meet all the needs of the students in creating this three-volume set of dissection manuals. They not only delineate instructions for students to perform perfect dissection but also provide gross anatomy descriptions, supplemented by clinical correlations of gross structures studied during dissection. The textual descriptions are complemented by numerous colored illustrations that will help students recognize significant structures with more precision. To further enhance understanding, the content of the volumes is organized in sections like (a) Learning Objectives, (b) Surface Landmarks, (c) Dissection and Identification, (d) Description of Gross Anatomy, and (e) Clinical Notes. Laced with all these features, we hope that these volumes will be useful not only for medical and dental students but also for teachers of anatomy. The value of these volumes is further enhanced by providing videos at relevant places.

As educators of anatomy, we have tried our best to make these manuals easy for learning. We highly appreciate the contribution of Prof. Poonam Kharb and Mr. D. Krishna Chaitanya in Volume II and Prof. Shabana M. Borate in Volume I. For further improvements, we would sincerely welcome comments and suggestions from all students and teachers.

The second edition of this dissection manual is thoroughly updated with new line diagrams, X-ray pictures, and CT and MRI scans.

All dissection steps are supplemented by dissection videos in all the three volumes for easy understanding of gross and clinical anatomy by the students.

Vishram Singh, MBBS, MS, PhD (hc), MICPS, FASI, FIMSA

The medical curriculum in India requires basic anatomy, along with some other basic subjects, to be taught to students in the first year of the course. This often leads to an information overload for them. For some students, the situation is made even more difficult due to linguistic limitations and late admissions. As a result, there has long been a pressing need for comprehensive teaching resources that create thorough understanding of these courses in a short time span. Specifically for anatomy, one cannot stress enough on the value of a complete and detailed dissection manual that explains basic concepts in a simple and lucid manner, without duplication of facts or unnecessary complexities.

In Volume III, every care has been taken to describe all steps involved in the dissection of the head, neck, and brain in a stepwise manner that is easy to understand for the beginners. Several high-quality illustrations have been used to explain each step. They help show the dissections with a great amount of detailing and clarity. To make the discourse interesting, relevant clinical conditions have also been presented under separate sections called "Clinical Notes."

Producing a book with hundreds of illustrations is a joint effort by the author and the publisher in a true sense.

I strongly believe that this book will be an invaluable learning resource for students and teachers of anatomy in medical and dental courses.

G. P. Pal, MBBS, MS, DSc, FASI, FAMS, FNASc, FASc, Bhatnagar Laureate

Cadaveric dissection is an integral part of teaching anatomy in medical schools. It offers an unmatched firsthand experience of exploring the structure of organs and their relationship with each other. *Thieme Dissector* provides a complete account of dissection of human body through a set of three volumes.

The first volume deals with the upper limb and thorax. The introduction of this volume gives general information about preservation of cadaver, instruments required for dissection, and anatomical terms, followed by a discussion on basic tissues of the body. This is followed by 10 chapters on upper limb and 5 chapters on thorax. Each chapter begins with "Learning Objectives," followed by an introduction to the topic, dissection steps with description of the relevant structures, and clinical notes.

To facilitate understanding of the subject, photographs of actual dissected parts and real dissection videos have been provided. Access to these videos will help and enrich students' learning process.

My heartfelt gratitude to Dr. Shabana M. Borate, Associate Professor, Department of Anatomy, at Grant Government Medical College and Sir J. J. Group of Hospitals, Mumbai, Maharashtra, India, Dr. Sachin Yadav, Assistant Professor at Grant Government Medical College and Sir J. J. Group of Hospitals, Mumbai, Maharashtra, India, and Dr. Shilpa Domkundwar, Professor and Head, Department of Radiodiagnosis, Grant Government Medical College and Sir J. J. Group of Hospitals, Mumbai, Maharashtra, India, for their untiring efforts in preparation of this volume. I am grateful to the entire team of Thieme Publishers for their constant support, and special thanks to Dr. Vishram Singh sir, who has been the guiding force for all of us in preparation of the *Thieme Dissector*.

S. D. Gangane, MBBS, MS, FAIMS

Thieme has taken a positive step by introducing this book for imparting anatomy education to medical students worldwide. The process of depicting videos and pictures of actual cadaver dissections in a textbook is indeed a monumental task. It starts with planning of the region to be dissected. This is followed by meticulous dissection of the region itself, which can take hours if not days. Then comes the process of accurate live narration of the dissection of the region on camera, while the video recording is in progress. The back-breaking task of editing and captioning the video frames and clips follows next, because many anatomical and medical terms used in the narration may otherwise be incomprehensible to the student. Since clinical students like content related to radiology, some videos have radiological images embedded within the frames. The relevant still shots from the dissections are then edited and labeled. Finally, of course, comes the task of publishing the finished product.

There are many digital anatomy tools available to the medical academia, ranging in size and versatility from usage in classrooms and digital labs to those used in individual laptops and tablets. Some have virtual reality–like, immersive three-dimensional, or augmented reality applications. They vary in accuracy, comprehensiveness, and versatility. They are good study tools, which are interactive and interesting to use in teaching and learning anatomy. They show body parts and spatial relationships. They are available offline, accessible anytime, anywhere, and can even show rare pathology. They present consolidated anatomy information to suit users' learning styles. They do not have the legal, ethical, religious, social, regional, and logistical constraints of human cadaver procurement. These factors are weaning away institutions from the hoary art of cadaver dissection.

However, cadaver dissection is still the gold standard for learning human anatomy and surgery. It is the benchmark for measuring the success of newer learning technologies. Cadavers are medical students' first "patients." Digital resources are to be considered as supplements to the armamentarium of learning methods in human anatomy. Digital technologies lack haptic qualities of human tissue, which are essential for a surgeon. Therefore, they can never completely replace cadaver dissection for anatomy students and surgical residents under training. Nobody would want to be treated by surgeons who acquired their entire quantum of expertise in operating on the human body through virtual reality alone, just like nobody would want to be flown by an airline pilot whose only flying experience was in the digital flight simulator.

The author is truly gratified knowing that students have learned the subject of anatomy and mastered the intricacies of the human body by watching *Thieme Dissector* videos and illustrations.

Sanjoy Sanyal, MBBS, MS, MSc, ADPHA

About the Authors

Vishram Singh
(Editor-in-Chief and Author, Volume II, Abdomen and Lower Limb)
Vishram Singh, MBBS, MS, PhD (hc), MICPS, FASI, FIMSA, is currently the Adjunct Professor, Department of Anatomy, KMC, Manipal Academy of Higher Education, Mangalore, Karnataka, India; Editor-in-Chief, *Journal of the Anatomical Society of India*; and Member, Federative International Committee for Scientific Publications (FICSP), International Federation of Association on Anatomists (IFAA), Geneva, Switzerland.

A renowned anatomist, Prof. Singh has taught undergraduate and postgraduate students at several colleges and institutes, such as GSVM Medical College, Kanpur; King George Medical College, Lucknow; All India Institute of Medical Sciences, New Delhi; and Al Arab Medical University, Benghazi, Libya. He has more than 50 years of experience in teaching, research, and clinical practice. He has various bestselling titles to his credit, such as *Textbook of Clinical Neuroanatomy, Textbook of Anatomy*—three volumes, and *Textbook of Clinical Embryology*. He has published more than 20 books and more than 100 research articles in reputed national and international journals.

Prof. Singh has received various recognitions and awards for his contributions in the field of gross anatomy, neuroanatomy, and embryology.

He has been elected Vice President of the Anatomical Society of India many times. He is currently Editor-in-Chief, *Journal of Anatomical Society of India* (JASI).

G. P. Pal
(Author, Volume III, Head, Neck, and Brain)
G. P. Pal, MBBS, MS, DSc, FASI, FAMS, FNASc, FASc, Bhatnagar Laureate, is currently the Director Professor of Anatomy at the Index Medical College; Emeritus Professor at MGM Medical College, Indore, Madhya Pradesh, India. Dr. Pal is an eminent teacher with almost five decades of teaching experience in various medical colleges of India and the United States. He has to his credit numerous publications in journals of international repute. He has received several national awards and honors for his research works, which includes Shakuntala Amir Chand Prize of Indian Council of Medical Research (ICMR), Shanti Swarup Bhatnagar Prize of Council of Scientific and Industrial Research (CSIR), and several gold medals, oration awards, and Lifetime Achievement Award by the Anatomical Society of India. He has been elected Fellow at various leading academies of sciences in India—Anatomical Society of India; National Academy of Medical Sciences (New Delhi), National Academy of Sciences (Allahabad), and Indian Academy of Sciences (Bengaluru). His research work is cited in more than 100 standard medical textbooks throughout the world. Recently, his name featured in the list of top 2% scientists of the world. As per a survey conducted by the Stanford University, USA, in 2020, he is ranked as no. 1 Anatomy Scientist in India and 102 in the world. Dr. Pal has authored many well-received books such as *Textbook of Histology, Illustrated Textbook of Neuroanatomy, Medical Genetics, Genetics in Dentistry, General Anatomy, Basics of Medical Genetics, Human Osteology, Genetics for Dental Student, Neuroanatomy for Medical Students*, and *Thieme Dissector*. He has edited 1st South Asian edition of *Grant's Atlas of Anatomy* (in press). He has also coauthored Prof. Inderbir Singh's *Human Embryology* from the 7th to 9th editions. For more information about the author and his works, Google "Indian Anatomists - Wikipedia" or "Gaya Prasad Pal - Wikipedia."

S. D. Gangane
(Author, Volume I, Upper Limb and Thorax)

S. D. Gangane, MBBS, MS, FAIMS, is currently serving as Professor and Head, Department of Anatomy at Terna Medical College, Navi Mumbai, Maharashtra, India. He has been Professor and Head, Department of Anatomy and Genetic Division at Grant Medical College, Mumbai and Sir J. J. Group of Hospitals, Mumbai. This is a unique Anatomy Department offering services to patients having genetic disorders. Prof. Gangane has authored a bestselling book titled *Human Genetics* which has been widely accepted by faculty and both undergraduate and postgraduate students.

Prof. Gangane has over four decades of teaching experience and has been guiding students for MD Anatomy, and MSc and PhD in Applied Biology courses at the Mumbai University. He has also been a guide for the MD Anatomy and PhD Genetics courses at Maharashtra University of Health Sciences (the State Health University). He has published several articles in national and international journals and is also a coauthor of the recently published *Textbook of Pathology and Genetics for Nurses*. In addition, he has been on the national advisory board and the executive editorial board for a few journals, including *Indian Journal of Anatomy* and *National Journal of Medical Sciences*.

Prof. Gangane has also worked as an Officer of Special Duty (OSD) for the Government of Maharashtra under the Directorate of Medical Education and Research. He is a member of the advisory panel for the South Asian region of the international publishing house, Lippincott Williams and Wilkins. He is the founder Trustee of "Sandnya Sanwardhan Sanstha", an organization that takes care of mentally challenged children by imparting vocational training and enabling them to lead better lives.

Sanjoy Sanyal
(Contributor of Videos, Volumes I, II, and III)

Sanjoy Sanyal, MBBS, MS, MSc, ADPHA, is the Provost and Dean of Richmond Gabriel University College of Medicine, St. Vincent and the Grenadines, Canada. He is also the Professor and Department Chair of Anatomical Sciences in the same university. With medical degrees from India and the United Kingdom, Dr. Sanyal has 39 years of clinical, surgical, and teaching experience as a surgeon, surgical anatomist, neuroscientist, and medical informatician.

A prolific medical and educational researcher, he has published 25 original research papers in peer-reviewed journals and presented 15 papers in many international conferences in 11 countries. He is the recipient of five Outstanding Professor Awards from several different universities and medical schools.

He is a surgical skills instructor to American Medical Students' Association (AMSA). He is a life-member of Indian Medical Association (IMA), and annual member of American Association for Anatomy (AAA) and American Association of Clinical Anatomists (AACA). He is a provisional patent holder (January 2014) of a computerized medical program from the United States Patent and Trademark Office (USPTO). He is peer reviewer of several medical journals.

Dr. Sanjoy Sanyal is honorary faculty of the Multimedia Educational Resource for Learning and Online Teaching (MERLOT), a program of the California State University (CSU), Long Beach, partnering with educational institutions, professional societies, and industry. He is Gold-level MERLOT contributor, having authored more than 350 learning materials. He is a member of Virtual Speaker's Bureau (VSB) of MERLOT. He is also the recipient of Innovative Use of MERLOT award.

With an underpinning philosophy of lifelong learning, his motto is to make each succeeding generation better than the previous.

Contributors to Volume II

Poonam Kharb, MSc, PhD
Ex-Professor
Department of Anatomy
Associate Dean
Sharda University
Greater Noida, Delhi NCR, India

D. Krishna Chaitanya Reddy, MSc, Ph.D., FHPE
Assistant Professor
Department of Anatomy
Kamineni Academy of Medical Sciences and Research Center
Hyderabad, Telangana, India

Introduction and an Overview of the Bones of the Lower Limb

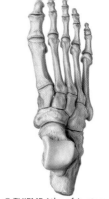

Introduction

The lower limbs are caudal extensions (appendages) from the trunk, specialized for the transmission of the body weight and locomotion. The lower limb extends from hip to the toes. It comprises four major parts or regions: the gluteal, thigh, leg, and foot (**Fig. 1.1**).

The Common people's reference of lower limb as the leg, is in fact the part of lower limb between knee and foot.

Gluteal region: The gluteal region overlies the side and back of the pelvis. The gluteal region comprises a rounded prominent region, the buttock, and a less prominent region, the hip. It extends from the waist down to the gluteal fold, which limits the buttock inferiorly and to the hollow on the lateral side of the hip. Usually, the hip and buttock are not clearly distinguished from each other. The hip is the lateral aspect of region while buttock is rounded bulge behind. The groove between the buttocks is called the *natal cleft*. The lower part of the sacrum and coccyx can be felt in this groove. Anterior to the gluteal region lies the perineum, in the depth of the cleft, and continues forward between the thighs.

This region contains the hip bone. It comprises three parts, the ilium, ischium, and pubis, which are fused together at the acetabulum where the head of the femur articulates with it. The *ilium* is the expanded upper part with a crest, the *iliac crest*, which can be felt in the lower margin of the waist at the level between the L3 and L4 vertebrae. The ischium is the posteroinferior part. It consists of the ischial tuberosity and ramus on which the body rests during the sitting position. The *pubis* is the anterior part and comprises a body and superior and inferior pubic rami. The body of the pubis articulates with its fellow of the opposite side through a median fibrocartilaginous pad, the pubic *symphysis*. It may be felt at the lower end of the abdominal wall in the median plane. Draw your finger laterally from the symphysis on the anterosuperior surface of the body of the pubis. The bone felt is the *pubic crest* which ends in a small, blunt prominence, the pubic tubercle 2.5 cm laterally. In males, it is not easily palpable as it is covered by the spermatic cord.

Thigh region: The thigh region lies between the gluteal, abdominal, and perineal regions proximally and the knee region distally. It contains the femur, which connects the hip and the knee. The femur articulates at the upper end with the hip bone to form the hip joint and at the lower end with the tibia and patella to form the knee joint.

The junction between the trunk and lower limb is abrupt anteromedially. The boundary between abdomen and lower limb, the inguinal ligament extends between anterior superior iliac spine and pubic tubercle. This junction between the two regions is called the inguinal region or groin.

Leg (L. crus) or *leg region*: The leg region extends from the knee joint to the ankle joint. The leg contains two bones, the tibia and fibula which are united along the length by interosseous membrane. The soft fleshy prominence on the back of the leg is called the *calf* and is formed by the triceps surae muscle. The lower end of the tibia and fibula form prominences on the medial and lateral sides of the ankle to form the *medial and lateral malleoli*. The flattened upper surface of the expanded proximal end of the tibia articulates with the lower end of the femur at the knee joint. The proximal end of the fibula articulates with the inferolateral surfaces of the lateral condyle of the tibia and does not take part in the formation of the knee joint.

Foot (*L. Pes*) or *foot region*: The foot region is the distal part of the lower limb and extends from the heel to the tips of the toes. It contains the tarsus, metatarsals, and phalanges. Its superior surface is the *dorsum of the foot*, while its inferior surface is the *sole of the foot*, which comes in contact with the ground.

An Overview of the Bones of the Lower Limb

A brief account of the bones of the lower limb is necessary before beginning to dissect so that the student studies the surface anatomy and relates it to the appropriate dried bone. The bones of the lower limb include the hip bone, femur, patella, tibia, fibula, and foot bones (**Fig. 1.2**).

Hip bone (**Fig. 1.3**): Hip bone is a large, flat bone formed by the fusion of three primary bones, the ilium, ischium, and pubis. At birth, the components are joined with each other by a Y-shaped triradiate hyaline cartilage (**Fig. 1.3**). By adulthood, they are ossified.

The hip bone looks like a propeller with a large sinuous blade directed upward and a smaller blade directed downward. The upper blade is called the ilium and the lower blade consists of the ischium and pubis. It is perforated by a large aperture, the *obturator foramen*. The lateral aspect of the hip bone at the junction of the two blades presents a cup-shaped hollow called the *acetabulum*. Posteriorly, each hip bone articulates with the sacrum at the sacroiliac joint.

Ilium: Ilium's flattened upper border is called the iliac crest. It runs backward from the anterior superior iliac spine to the posterior superior iliac spine. It can be felt at the lower margin of the waist and below each of these spines are the corresponding inferior spines. The outer surface of the ilium is termed the "gluteal surface," which provides attachment to the gluteal muscles. The inferior, anterior, and posterior *gluteal* lines demarcate bony attachments of these muscles. The inner surface of the ilium is smooth and hollowed out to form the *iliac fossa*. It provides attachment to the iliacus muscle. The articular surface of the ilium articulates with the sacrum at the sacroiliac joints. The iliopectineal line runs anteriorly on the inner surface of the ilium, from the auricular surface to the pubis.

Ischium: Ischium forms the posteroinferior part of the hip bone. It comprises a spine on its posterior part which demarcates the greater sciatic notch (above) from the lesser sciatic notch (below). The ischial tuberosity is a thickening on the lower part of the body of the ischium which bears the body's weight in the sitting position. The *ischial ramus* projects forward from the tuberosity to meet with the *inferior pubic ramus* to form the *ischiopubic ramus*.

Pubis: Pubis forms the anteromedial part of the hip bone. It comprises a body and superior and inferior pubic rami. It articulates with the pubic bone of the contralateral side by a secondary cartilaginous joint (the symphysis pubis). The superior surface of the body bears the pubic crest and the pubic tubercle. The large obturator foramen is bounded by the pubis, ischium, and their rami.

Femur (**Fig. 1.4**): The femur is the longest and heaviest bone in the body. It transmits the body weight from the hip bone to the tibia. It presents the following characteristic features:

1. *Femoral head*: It articulates with the acetabulum of the hip bone at the hip joint. It extends from the femoral neck and is rounded and smooth. It forms two-thirds of the sphere and is covered with articular cartilage except for a medially placed depression or pit called the fovea to which the ligamentum teres is attached. This configuration permits a wide range of movement. The head faces medially, upward and forward into the acetabulum.

2. *Femoral neck*: It forms an angle of 125 degrees with the femoral shaft, the *neck shaft angle*. This angle is less in females because of the increased width of the pelvis.

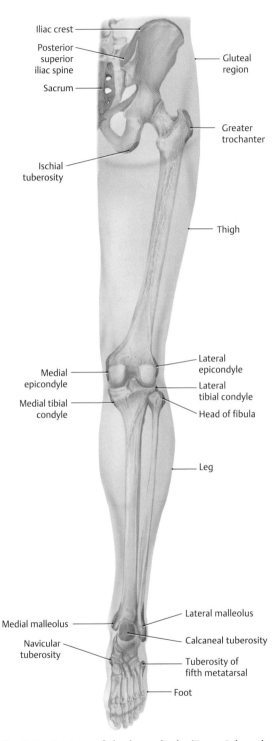

Fig. 1.1 Regions of the lower limb. (From Schuenke M, Schulte E, Schumacher U. THIEME Atlas of Anatomy. General Anatomy and Musculoskeletal System. Illustrations by Voll M and Wesker K. © Thieme 2020)

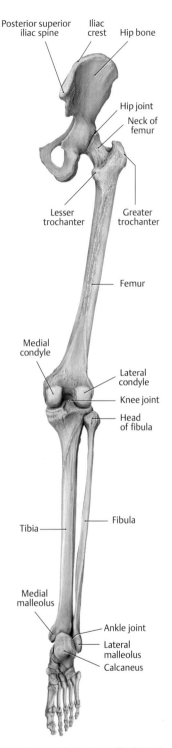

Fig. 1.2 Bones of the lower limb (posterior view). (From Schuenke M, Schulte E, Schumacher U. THIEME Atlas of Anatomy. General Anatomy and Musculoskeletal System. Illustrations by Voll M and Wesker K. © Thieme 2020)

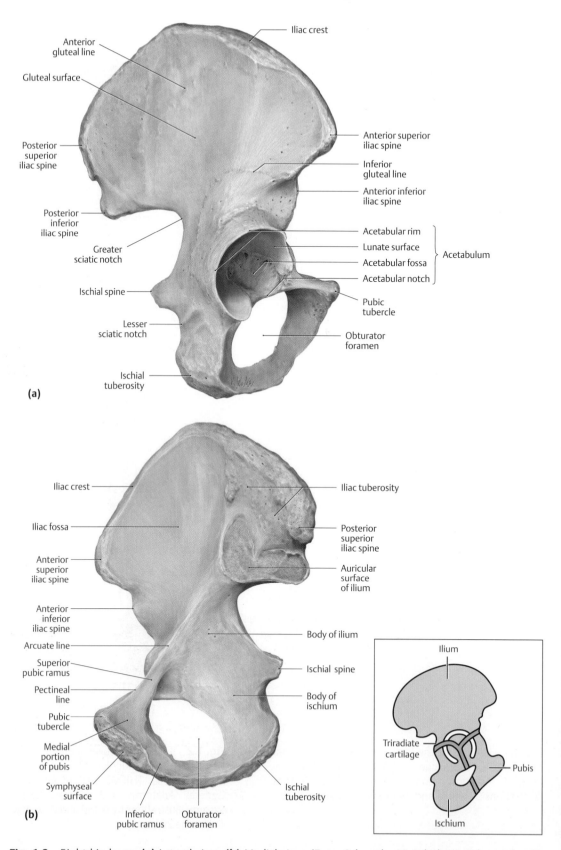

Fig. 1.3 Right hip bone. **(a)** Lateral view. **(b)** Medial view. (From Schuenke M, Schulte E, Schumacher U. THIEME Atlas of Anatomy. General Anatomy and Musculoskeletal System. Illustrations by Voll M and Wesker K. © Thieme 2020). Figure in the insert shows three primary components of hip bone.

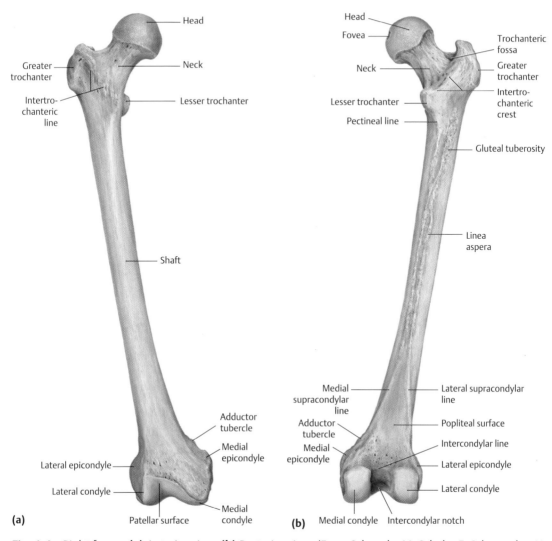

Fig. 1.4 Right femur. **(a)** Anterior view. **(b)** Posterior view. (From Schuenke M, Schulte E, Schumacher U. THIEME Atlas of Anatomy. General Anatomy and Musculoskeletal System. Illustrations by Voll M and Wesker K. © Thieme 2020)

3. *Femoral shaft*: It constitutes the length of the bone. At its upper end, it carries the greater trochanter placed superolaterally and the lesser trochanter placed posteromedially. Anteriorly the rough intertrochanteric line and posteriorly the smooth trochanteric crest demarcate the junction between the shaft and the neck. The linea aspera is the crest seen running longitudinally along the posterior surface of the femur. It splits in the lower portion into the medial and lateral supracondylar lines. The medial supracondylar line terminates at the adductor tubercle.

The lower end of the femur presents the medial and lateral condyles. These condyles bear the articular surfaces for articulation with the tibia at the knee joint. The two condyles are in the same horizontal plane when the femur is in its anatomical position. The lateral condyle is more prominent than the medial condyle, which prevents the lateral displacement of the patella. The condyles are separated posteriorly and inferiorly by a deep *intercondylar notch/fossa*. Anteriorly, the lower femoral aspect presents a saddle-shaped smooth surface for articulation with the posterior surface of the patella to form the patellofemoral joint.

Tibia (shin bone) (**Fig. 1.5**): The tibia is the medial bone of the leg. It is the second largest bone of the body and transfers the body weight from the femur to the talus. It presents the following characteristic features:

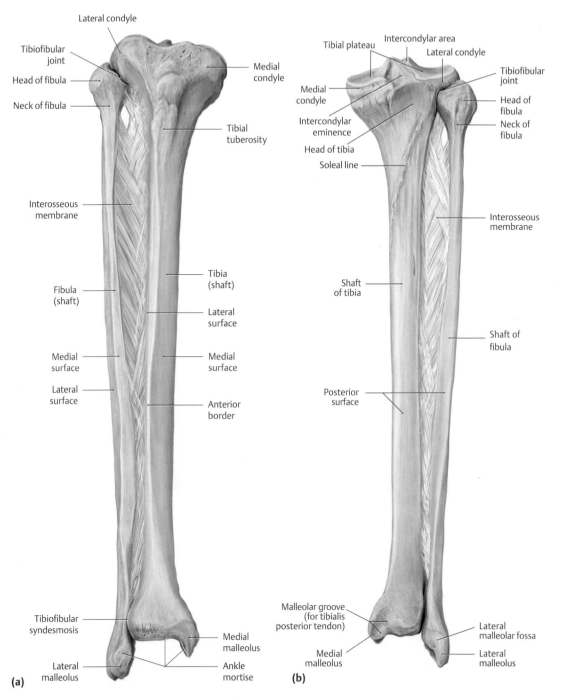

Fig. 1.5 Tibia and fibula (right side). **(a)** Anterior view. **(b)** Posterior view. (From Schuenke M, Schulte E, Schumacher U. THIEME Atlas of Anatomy. General Anatomy and Musculoskeletal System. Illustrations by Voll M and Wesker K. © Thieme 2020)

1. The proximal end of the tibia widens to form the medial and lateral condyles. The flattened upper end of the *tibia–tibial plateau*–comprises two smooth articular cartilages over the medial and lateral tibial condyles for articulation with the respective femoral condyles. In contrast to the femur, the medial tibial condyle is larger of the two.

2. The intercondylar area is the space between the two articular surfaces on the tibial condyles. It presents two projections, the *medial* and *lateral intercondylar tubercles*. Together, these tubercles constitute the *intercondylar eminence*.

3. The shaft of the tibia is triangular in cross-section. It has anterior, medial, and lateral borders and posterior, lateral, and medial surfaces.

4. The anterior border of the tibia is the most prominent border. At its upper end, there is a *tibial tuberosity* which is easily identifiable. It provides attachment to the ligamentum patellae.

5. The anterior border and medial surface of the shaft are subcutaneous throughout its length and are often termed as the *shin*.

6. On the posterior surface of the proximal part of the tibial shaft, there is an oblique line, the soleal line, which provides the tibial origin of soleus. The popliteus muscle is often inserted into the triangular area above the soleal line.

7. The fibula articulates with the tibia superiorly at an articular facet on the posteroinferior aspect of the lateral condyle to form the *superior tibiofibular joint*.

8. The fibular notch situated laterally on the lower end of the tibia articulates with the fibula to form the *inferior tibiofibular joint*.

9. The tibia projects inferiorly as the *medial malleolus*, which constitutes the medial part of the mortise that stabilizes the talus. The medial malleolus is grooved posteriorly for the passage of the tendon of the tibialis posterior muscle.

Fibula (**Fig. 1.5**): The fibula is the lateral bone of the leg. It is not a part of the knee joint and has no function in weight transmission. The main functions of the fibula are to provide attachment to the muscles and also to participate in the formation of the ankle joint. It presents the following characteristic features:

1. Its upper end is called the *head of the fibula*, which presents styloid process, a prominence on to which tendon of biceps femoris is inserted.

2. A constriction below the head is called the *fibular neck*. It separates the head from the fibular shaft. The common peroneal nerve is in close relation, as it winds around the lateral aspect of the neck before it divides into the superficial and deep peroneal nerves.

3. The fibula is triangular in cross-section. It has anterior, medial (interosseous), and posterior borders with anterior, lateral, and posterior surfaces. A vertical ridge, the medial crest, is on the posterior surface which divides into the medial and lateral parts.

4. The lower end of the fibula enlarges and is prolonged inferiorly to form the *lateral malleolus*. It is the lateral part of the mortise that stabilizes the talus. It bears a smooth triangular articular facet on the medial surface for articulation with the talus. The area above the articular facet is rough to provide attachment to the tibiofibular ligament. The posterior aspect of the malleolus bears a groove for the passage of the tendons of the peroneus longus and brevis muscles. The lateral malleolus projects more downward than the medial malleolus.

Patella (knee cap) (**Fig. 1.6**):

1. The patella is the largest sesamoid bone in the tendon of the quadriceps femoris. It is triangular in shape and lies in front of the knee joint.

2. The ligamentum patellae, which extends between the apex of the patella and the tibial tuberosity, is the true insertion of the quadriceps femoris.

3. The posterior surface of the patella bears a smooth articular surface, which is covered with the articular cartilage. It is divided into a large lateral facet and a smaller medial facet for articulation with the femoral condyles.

4. The anterior surface of the patella is subcutaneous.

Bones of the foot (**Fig. 1.7**): The foot bones comprise the following:

1. Tarsal bones.

2. Metatarsals.

3. Phalanges.

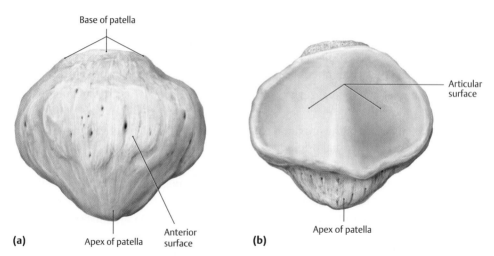

Base of patella

Articular surface

(a)   Apex of patella   Anterior surface   **(b)**   Apex of patella

Fig. 1.6   Patella. **(a)** Anterior view. **(b)** Posterior view (From Schuenke M, Schulte E, Schumacher U. THIEME Atlas of Anatomy. General Anatomy and Musculoskeletal System. Illustrations by Voll M and Wesker K. © Thieme 2020)

Tarsal bones: The tarsal bones are arranged in two rows. The proximal row consists of two large bones (calcaneus and talus) set one above the other.

Calcaneus (**Fig. 1.8a**): The calcaneus is the largest tarsal bone forming the skeleton of the foot. Its superior surface articulates with the talus to form the *subtalar joint*. The inferior surface presents the medial and lateral tubercles at the proximal end. The medial surface presents a distinctive shelf-like projection called the *sustentaculum tali*. The lateral surface presents a *peroneal tubercle*. The anterior surface presents a facet for articulation with the cuboid. The posterior surface presents a roughened middle part for attachment to the tendo calcaneus.

Talus (**Fig. 1.8b**): The talus forms a connecting link between the bones of the foot and leg. It presents the head, neck, and body. The body presents facets on its superior, medial, and lateral surfaces for articulation with the tibia, medial malleolus, and lateral malleolus, respectively. There is a groove on the posterior surface for the tendon of the flexor hallucis longus. The head projects distally and articulates with the navicular bone. The neck connecting the body and head presents a groove called the sinus tarsi.

Cuboid (**Fig. 1.7**): As the name implies, it is cuboid in shape. It articulates proximally with the calcaneus and distally with the fourth and fifth metatarsals. Its undersurface is grooved for the tendon of the peroneus longus.

Navicular (**Fig. 1.7**): Navicular is boat-shaped. It articulates proximally by the concave facet with the head of the talus and distally with the three cuneiforms. It presents a tuberosity on its medial aspect for attachment to the tibialis posterior.

Cuneiforms (**Fig. 1.7**): There are three cuneiforms: medial, intermediate, and lateral. They articulate anteriorly with the first, second, and third metatarsals, respectively.

Metatarsals (**Fig. 1.7**): The metatarsals are five miniature long bones and are numbered 1 to 5 from the medial side. Their proximal ends articulate with the tarsal bones. The distal end (bead) of each metatarsal articulates with the base of the proximal phalanx of the corresponding toe. The first metatarsal is the largest and the inferior surface of its head is grooved for two sesamoid bones.

Phalanges (**Fig. 1.7**): The phalanges are miniature long bones of the toes. In each toe, there are three phalanges: proximal, middle, and distal, except in the great toe which has only two phalanges (proximal and distal). The proximal end of each phalanx is its base and the distal end is its head. The phalanges articulate with each other at the interphalangeal joints.

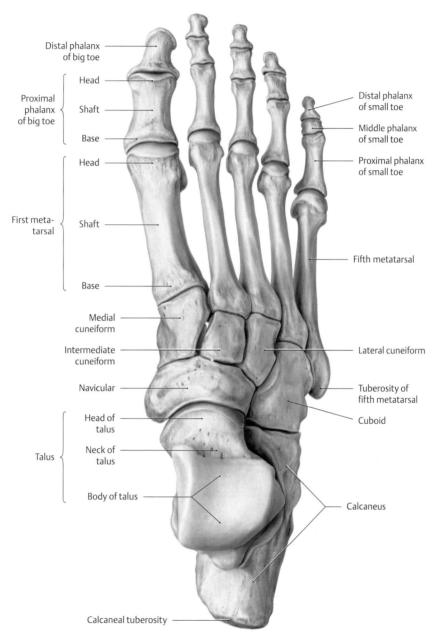

(a)

Fig. 1.7 (a) Bones of the right foot (dorsal view). (From Schuenke M, Schulte E, Schumacher U. THIEME Atlas of Anatomy. General Anatomy and Musculoskeletal System. Illustrations by Voll M and Wesker K. © Thieme 2020) *(Continued)*

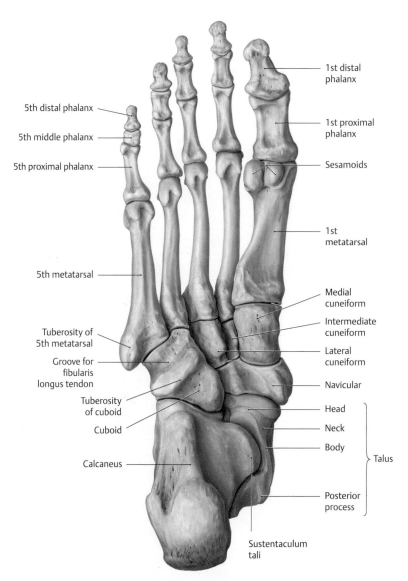

5th distal phalanx

5th middle phalanx

5th proximal phalanx

5th metatarsal

Tuberosity of
5th metatarsal

Groove for
fibularis
longus tendon

Tuberosity
of cuboid

Cuboid

Calcaneus

1st distal
phalanx

1st proximal
phalanx

Sesamoids

1st
metatarsal

Medial
cuneiform

Intermediate
cuneiform

Lateral
cuneiform

Navicular

Head

Neck

Body

Posterior
process

Talus

Sustentaculum
tali

(b)

Fig. 1.7   *(Continued)* **(b)** Bones of the right foot (ventral view). (From Schuenke M, Schulte E, Schumacher U. THIEME Atlas of Anatomy. General Anatomy and Musculoskeletal System. Illustrations by Voll M and Wesker K. © Thieme 2020)

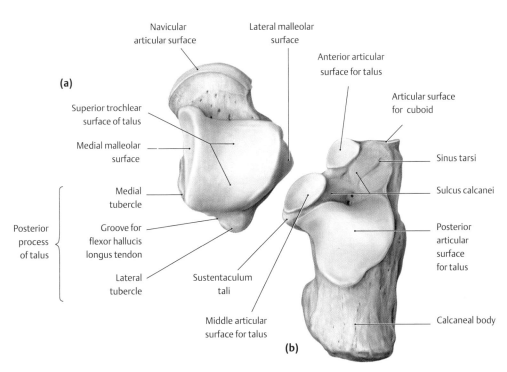

Fig. 1.8 **(a)** Right talus (dorsal view) and **(b)** Right calcaneus (dorsal view). (From Schuenke M, Schulte E, Schumacher U. THIEME Atlas of Anatomy. General Anatomy and Musculoskeletal System. Illustrations by Voll M and Wesker K. © Thieme 2020)

Anterior and Medial Compartments of the Thigh

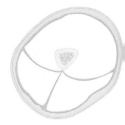

Introduction

The thigh extends from the hip joint to the knee joint. The deep fascia of the thigh (fascia lata) encloses the entire thigh like a sleeve/stocking. From the deep aspect of the fascia lata, three fibrous intermuscular septa—lateral, medial, and posterior—pass to the linea aspera of the femur and divide the thigh into three compartments—anterior, medial, and posterior (**Fig. 2.1**). The anterior (extensor) compartment of the thigh lies between the lateral and medial intermuscular septa, and the medial compartment lies between the medial and posterior septa.

The superficial fascia on the front of the thigh close to inguinal ligament consists of two layers similar to that in the lower part of abdomen. They fuse with each other 1cm interior to inguinal ligament. An oval opening in the deep fascia 3-4 cm inferolateral to public tubercle is called *saphenous opening*, through which long saphenous vein enters into femoral vein. The superficial fascia on the front of the thigh contains:

1. *Cutaneous nerves:* derived from lumbar plexus, viz., femoral branch of genito femoral nerve, lateral cutaneous nerve of thigh, intermediate, lateral cutaneous nerve of thigh, and medial cutaneous nerve of thigh.

2. *Cutaneous arteries:* from femoral artery.

3. *Termination of great saphenous vein:* longest superficial vein of lower limb.

4. *Superficial inguinal lymph nodes:* lies below the inguinal ligament.

5. Some along the ligament and some along the upper part of long saphenous vein.

Surface Landmarks

1. Before starting the dissection, study the surface anatomy of the region. Palpate the bony land-marks and relate them to the respective bones on the articulated skeleton (refer to **Fig. 1.1** and **1.2**).

2. Run your finger along the *fold of the groin* (*inguinal groove*), a shallow groove extending from the pubic tubercle to the anterior superior iliac spine. It corresponds to the underlying inguinal ligament that separates the anterior abdominal wall from the front of the thigh. Feel the resilient

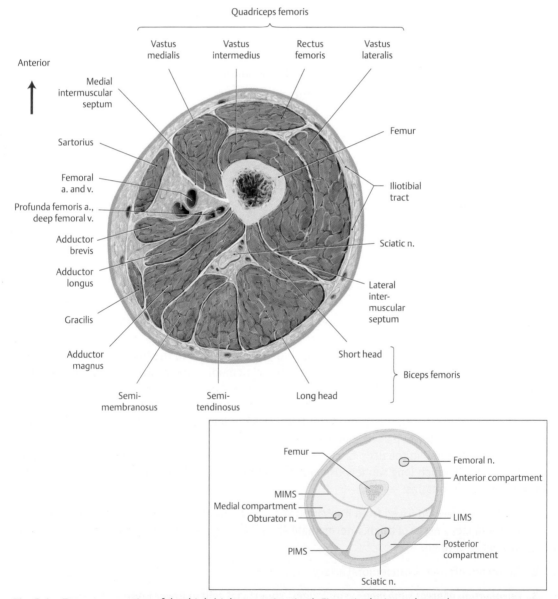

Fig. 2.1 Transverse section of the thigh (right, superior view). Figure in the inset shows three compartments of the right thigh. MIMS, medial intermuscular septum; LIMS, lateral intermuscular septum; PIMS, posterior intermuscular septum. (From Schuenke M, Schulte E, Schumacher U. THIEME Atlas of Anatomy. General Anatomy and Musculoskeletal System. Illustrations by Voll M and Wesker K. © Thieme 2020.)

band (inguinal ligament) in the groove extending between the anterior superior iliac spine and pubic tubercle.

3. Palpate the *anterior superior iliac spine* at the lateral end of the fold of the groin and observe that it forms the anterior end of the iliac crest of the hip bone.

4. Palpate the *pubic tubercle*, a small bony projection at the medial end of the fold of the groin. It lies approximately 2.5 cm lateral to the pubic symphysis. The tubercle is less easily felt in males as it is covered by the spermatic cord.

5. Use chalk to mark the *midinguinal point* and the *midpoint of the inguinal ligament* along the inguinal groove. The *midinguinal point* is a point midway between the anterior superior iliac spine and pubic symphysis, whereas the midpoint of the inguinal ligament is midway between the anterior superior iliac spine and pubic tubercle.

6. At the lower end of the thigh, identify the *medial* and *lateral condyles of the femur* and *tibia*. They form large bony masses on the medial and lateral sides of the knee, respectively.

7. *Feel the patella*, a triangular bone in front of the knee, and try to move it when the knee is extended.

8. Palpate the *tibial tuberosity*, a bony prominence in front of the upper part of the tibia.

9. *Ligamentum patellae* is a strong fibrous band that extends between the patella and tibial tuberosity.

Anterior Compartment of the Thigh

Dissection and Identification

1. Make a horizontal incision "A" through the skin from the anterior superior iliac spine to the midline and continue the incision downward lateral to the external genitalia. Make a vertical incision "B" from the lower end of the above incision till the medial condyle of the tibia. Make another horizontal incision "C" from the lower end of the vertical incision passing laterally till the lateral condyle of the tibia (**Fig. 2.2**).

2. Reflect the skin from the superficial fascia and turn it laterally, taking care not to damage the cutaneous nerves.

3. Strip the superficial fascia from the front and lateral aspects of the thigh by blunt dissection. Find the cutaneous nerves (lateral cutaneous nerve of the thigh, femoral branch of the genitofemoral nerve, intermediate cutaneous nerve of the thigh, and medial cutaneous nerve of the thigh) which pierce the deep fascia at different points (**Fig. 2.3**) and follow them distally.

4. Find the *great saphenous vein* in the superficial fascia of the medial part of the anterior surface of the thigh. Trace it downward till the knee and upward where it turns backward through the *saphenous opening* (hiatus) to enter the femoral vein. Note that this area is 3 to 4 cm inferolateral to the pubic tubercle and is about 3 cm long and 1.5 cm wide. In this area, the deep fascia is thin and perforated (*cribriform fascia*). Put your finger beside the upper end of the great saphenous vein to feel the sharp thick edge of the deep fascia (*falciform margin*) which limits the saphenous opening all around except medially (**Fig. 2.4**).

5. Identify the lower group of the superficial inguinal lymph nodes scattered along the upper part of the great saphenous vein.

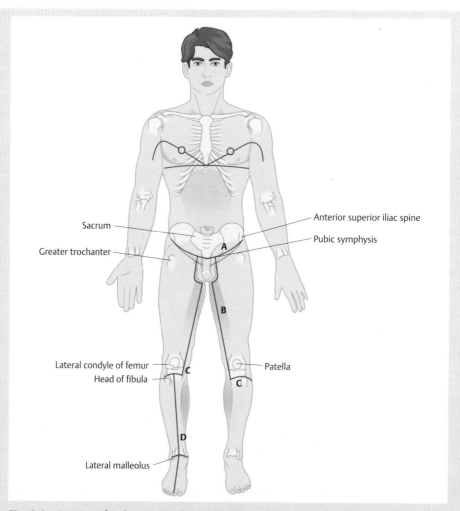

Fig. 2.2 Incisions for dissection of the front of the lower limb.

6. Observe that at least three small veins enter the great saphenous vein near its termination. Follow these veins along with the superficial branches of the femoral artery, which pierce the cribriform fascia, and accompany them. The superficial epigastric vessels course superiorly to the anterior abdominal wall, the superficial circumflex iliac artery courses laterally below the inguinal ligament, and the superficial external pudendal vessels pass medially to the external genitalia.

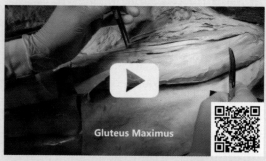

Video 2.1 Muscles of anterior compartment of thigh.

7. Use a pair of scissors to cut through the deep fascia to expose the muscles and deeper structures in the upper anterior compartment of the thigh. Expose the sartorius muscle extending from the anterior superior iliac spine to its insertion into the upper part of the medial surface of the tibia. Medially, expose the adductor longus muscle down to the point where it meets the sartorius muscle (**Video 2.1**).

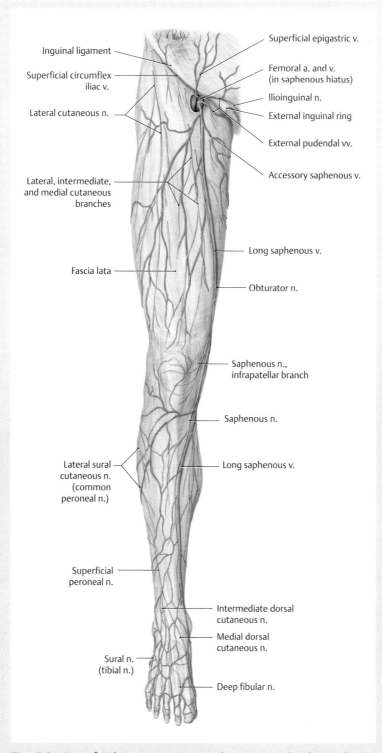

Fig. 2.3 Superficial cutaneous vein and nerves on the front of right lower limb. (From Schuenke M, Schulte E, Schumacher U. THIEME Atlas of Anatomy. General Anatomy and Musculoskeletal System. Illustrations by Voll M and Wesker K. © Thieme 2020)*

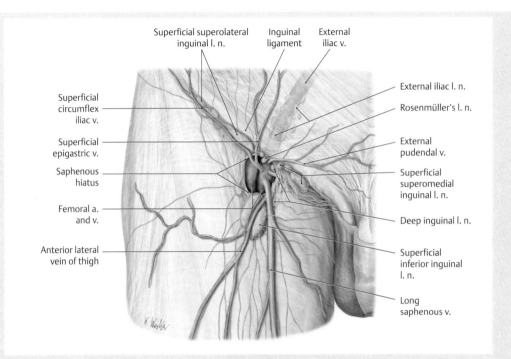

Fig. 2.4 Superficial dissection of proximal part of the front of thigh. The saphenous opening and the superficial lymph nodes of the groin. (From Schuenke M, Schulte E, Schumacher U. THIEME Atlas of Anatomy. General Anatomy and Musculoskeletal System. Illustrations by Voll M and Wesker K. © Thieme 2020)

8. Identify the boundaries of the femoral triangle: superiorly formed by the inguinal ligament, laterally by the sartorius and medially by the medial border of the adductor longus. Clean the structures, that is, the femoral nerve, femoral artery, and femoral vein within the triangle (**Fig. 2.5**).

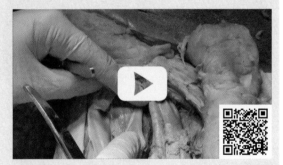

Video 2.2 Femoral nerve.

9. Follow the great saphenous vein to the femoral vein. Split the femoral sheath lateral and medial to the femoral vein to expose the femoral artery and femoral canal, respectively. Note the two septa of the femoral sheath that separate it into three compartments containing the femoral artery, femoral vein, and deep lymph node (from lateral to medial) (**Fig. 2.5**).

10. Put your little finger into the femoral canal and push it upward. Feel the peritoneum which covers the abdominal opening of the canal. Move the tip of your little finger to feel the structures bounding the abdominal opening of the femoral canal. Feel the inguinal ligament anteriorly, the edge of the lacunar ligament medially, and the pecten pubis posteriorly.

11. Find the femoral nerve lateral to the femoral artery in the groove between the muscles and observe that it immediately divides into anterior and posterior divisions from which arise a number of cutaneous and muscular branches. Trace the nerve to the pectineus passing medially posterior to the femoral artery. Follow the other cutaneous and muscular branches till they leave the femoral triangle (**Fig. 2.6**; **Video 2.2**).

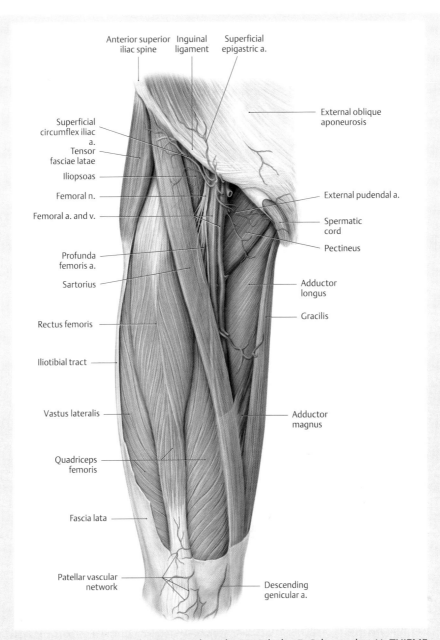

Fig. 2.5 Femoral triangle. (From Schuenke M, Schulte E, Schumacher U. THIEME Atlas of Anatomy. General Anatomy and Musculoskeletal System. Illustrations by Voll M and Wesker K. © Thieme 2020)

12. Remove the venae comitantes of the smaller arteries in this region to trace the deep branches of the femoral artery. Retract the femoral artery medially and identify the profunda femoris artery which arises from the posterolateral aspect of the femoral artery. Follow it downward along with the profunda femoris vein till the apex of the femoral triangle. Note that at the apex of the femoral triangle the femoral artery, femoral vein, profunda femoris vein, and profunda femoris artery lie in this order from before backward.

13. Find the lateral and medial circumflex arteries which usually arise from the profunda femoris near its origin. Trace the lateral circumflex artery as it passes laterally among the branches of the femoral nerve and deep to the upper part of the rectus femoris and gives three branches,

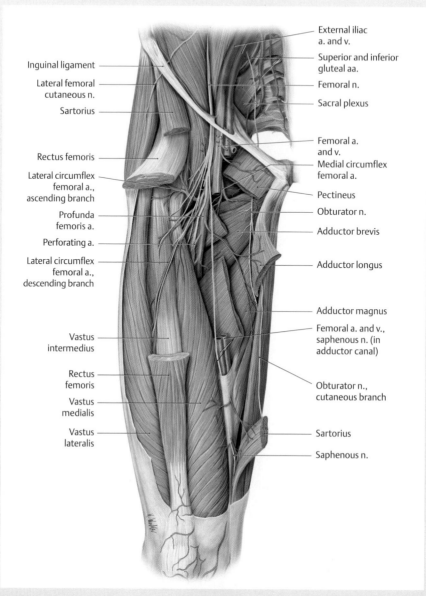

Fig. 2.6 Neurovascular structure of the anterior thigh. (From Schuenke M, Schulte E, Schumacher U. THIEME Atlas of Anatomy. General Anatomy and Musculoskeletal System. Illustrations by Voll M and Wesker K. © Thieme 2020)

that is, the ascending, transverse, and descending branches.

14. Strip the fascia from the iliacus and psoas major muscles in the floor of the femoral triangle. Place your finger on the tendon of the psoas major and push it downward and backward to reach its insertion to the lesser trochanter. Trace the medial circumflex artery as it passes backward between the psoas and pectineus

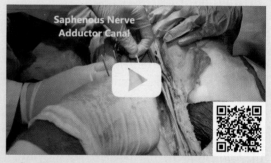

Video 2.3 Fascia lata.

muscles. Make a vertical incision in the fascia lata from the iliac crest to the lateral margin of the patella and remove the fascia between this incision and the sartorius. This would expose the underlying quadriceps femoris muscle and tensor fasciae lata (**Fig. 2.5**; **Video 2.3**).

15. Use your fingers to separate the sartorius muscle from the underlying fascia in the middle third of the thigh. Cut the sartorius muscle a little above the apex of the femoral triangle and turn the lower part downward to expose the narrow strip of the fascia extending between the vastus medialis and adductor muscles which forms the roof of the adductor canal. Using a pair of scissors, split the fascia to find the contents of the adductor canal, such as the femoral vessels, saphenous nerve, and nerve to the vastus medialis (**Fig. 2.6**).

16. Note the femoral vein lies posterior to the femoral artery and the femoral vessels leave the adductor canal to enter the popliteal fossa (at the back of the knee) by passing through the opening in the adductor magnus.

17. Observe the bipennate rectus femoris in the middle of the front of the thigh and obliquely running fibers of the vastus lateralis and medialis on either side of the rectus femoris. Retract the rectus femoris laterally or medially to expose the underlying vastus intermedius. Note that the four parts of the quadriceps femoris muscle mentioned above unite to form the quadriceps tendon which is attached to the patella, and the patellar ligament attaches the patella to the tibial tuberosity.

18. Femoral nerve.

Medial Compartment of the Thigh

1. Identify and clean the strap-like gracilis muscle extending from the pubic bone to its inferior attachment on the medial surface of the tibia posterior to the attachment of the sartorius muscle.

2. Use blunt dissection to remove the deep fascia to expose the other muscles of the adductor/medial compartment. Note the muscles are arranged in three layers.

3. Observe that the pectineus (in the floor of the femoral triangle) and adductor longus (forming the medial boundary of the femoral triangle) lie side by side and form the superficial layer.

4. Cut the adductor longus muscle about 4 to 5 cm inferior to its upper attachment to the pubic bone and reflect the lower part downward and laterally. This will expose the adductor brevis muscle which forms the middle layer and the anterior division of the obturator nerve overlying it. Follow the anterior division of the obturator nerve superiorly where it lies between the pectineus and adductor brevis. Note the branches of the anterior division of the obturator nerve supplying the adductor longus, adductor brevis, gracilis, and sometimes pectineus muscles (**Video 2.4**).

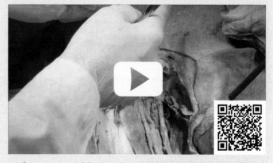

Video 2.4 Adductor brevis.

5. Cut the adductor brevis muscle close to its origin from the pubic bone taking care to preserve the posterior division of the obturator nerve which lies deep to it on the adductor magnus muscle (forms the deep layer).

6. Trace the posterior division of the obturator nerve superiorly and note that it reaches the adductor compartment by piercing the obturator muscle.

7. Find the muscular branches of the posterior division of the obturator nerve supplying the obturator externus, adductor brevis, and adductor magnus.

Muscles

Muscles of the anterior and medial compartments of the thigh are listed in **Table 2.1**.

Table 2.1   Muscles of the anterior and medial compartments of the thigh

Compartment	Muscles		Action	Nerve supply
Anterior	Quadriceps femoris	Rectus femoris	Flexion at the hip joint Extension at the knee joint	Femoral n.
		Vastus medialis	Extension at the knee joint	
		Vastus intermedius		
		Vastus lateralis		
	Sartorius		Flexion and lateral rotation at the hip joint Flexion at the knee joint	Femoral n.
Medial/adductor	Adductor longus		Adduction of the thigh	Obturator n.
	Adductor brevis		Adduction of the thigh	Obturator n.
	Adductor magnus		Adduction of the thigh Extension at the hip joint (ischial part)	Obturator and tibial division of the sciatic n.
	Pectineus		Flexion and adduction at the hip joint	Obturator and femoral n.
	Gracilis		Adduction of the thigh Flexion at the knee joint Medial rotation of the leg	Obturator n.

Abbreviation: n., nerve.

Arteries of the Anterior and Medial Compartments of the Thigh

Branches of the femoral artery:

1. Superficial branches:
   - Superficial epigastric.
   - Superficial circumflex iliac.
   - Superficial external pudendal.

2. Deep branches:
   - Deep external pudendal.
   - Profunda femoris:
     a. Medial circumflex femoral.
     b. Lateral circumflex femoral.
   - Muscular branches.
   - Descending genicular.

Branches of the profunda femoris artery:

1. Medial circumflex femoral artery.

2. Lateral circumflex femoral artery.

3. Muscular branches.

4. Three perforating arteries.

The profunda femoris artery ends by piercing the adductor magnus as the fourth perforating artery.

Nerves of the Anterior and Medial Compartments of the Thigh

Femoral Nerve–Root Value: L2, L3, and L4 (Dorsal Divisions)

The femoral nerve is the largest branch of lumbar plexus. It arises in the lumbar region within psoas major, runs in the groove between iliacus and psoas major and enter femoral triangle by passing deep to inguinal ligament, where it lies lateral to femoral artery.

Femoral nerve divides into anterior and posterior divisions:

1. Branches of the anterior division are:
   - Muscular branches to:
     a. Pectineus.
     b. Sartorius.
   - Cutaneous branches to:
     a. Medial cutaneous.
     b. Intermediate cutaneous.

2. Branches of the posterior division are:
   - Muscular branches to:
     a. Quadriceps femoris.
   - Cutaneous branches to:
     a. Saphenous nerve (longest cutaneous nerve of the body).
   - Articular branches to:
     a. Hip joint via nerve to the rectus femoris.
     b. Knee joint via branches to the vasti.

The effects of injury to the femoral nerve are as follows:

Motor loss: Paralysis of the quadriceps femoris and sartorius.

Sensory loss: Loss of sensations on the anterior and medial aspects of the thigh, medial aspect of the leg, and medial aspect of the foot till the head of the first metatarsal.

Obturator Nerve–Root Value: L2, L3, and L4 (Ventral Divisions)

The obturator nerve is the nerve of the adductor compartment of the thigh. It divides into the anterior and posterior divisions.

1. Muscles supplied by the anterior division:
   - Adductor longus.
   - Adductor brevis.
   - Gracilis.
   - Pectineus.
2. Muscles supplied by the posterior division:
   - Adductor brevis.
   - Adductor magnus.
   - Obturator externus.

Femoral Triangle

It is a triangular intermuscular space on the front of the upper one-third of the thigh. Its boundaries are as follows (**Fig. 2.7**):

1. *Lateral*: Medial border of the sartorius.

2. *Medial*: Medial border of the adductor longus.

3. *Apex*: It is where the sartorius overlaps the adductor longus.

4. *Base*: Inguinal ligament.

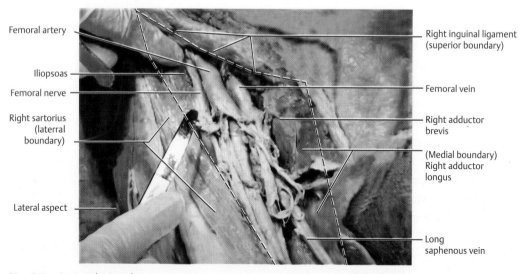

Fig. 2.7 Femoral triangle.

5. *Roof*: It is formed by the following:
   - Skin.
   - Superficial fascia with superficial blood vessels and superficial inguinal lymph nodes.
   - Deep fascia (fascia lata).

6. *Floor* is formed by the following muscles (lateral to medial):
   - Iliacus.
   - Psoas major.
   - Pectineus.
   - Adductor longus.

7. *Contents*:
   - *Arteries*: Femoral artery and its branches.
     a. *Superficial branches*: Superficial epigastric, superficial circumflex iliac, superficial external pudendal.
     b. Deep external pudendal.
     c. Profunda femoris and its branches: Lateral and medial circumflex femoral.
   - *Veins*: Femoral vein and its tributaries.
   - *Nerves*:
     a. Femoral nerve and its branches.
     b. Lateral cutaneous nerve of the thigh.
     c. Femoral branch of the genitofemoral nerve.
   - Deep inguinal lymph nodes.
   - Fibrofatty tissue.

Femoral Sheath

1. It is a funnel-shaped fascial sheath that surrounds the upper part of the femoral vessels and it also encloses the femoral canal.

2. It is formed:
   - Anteriorly by the fascia transversalis.
   - Posteriorly by the fascia iliaca.

3. It is divided into three compartments:
   - *Medial compartment*: It is called the femoral canal and is filled with areolar tissue and contains a lymph node (Gland of Cloquet) which drains the glans penis/clitoris.
   - *Intermediate compartment*: The femoral vein passes through it.
   - *Lateral compartment*: It allows the passage of the femoral artery and the femoral branch of the genitofemoral nerve.

The femoral nerve lies outside the femoral sheath, lateral to the femoral artery.

Femoral Canal

1. It is the funnel-shaped medial compartment of the femoral sheath.

2. It is 1.2 cm long.

3. It contains some areolar tissue and a lymph node of the deep inguinal group.

4. Its upper end opens toward the abdominal cavity and is bounded by the femoral ring.

5. Boundaries of the femoral ring are:
   - *Lateral*: The femoral vein.
   - *Medial*: The lacunar ligament.
   - *Anterior*: The inguinal ligament.
   - *Posterior*: The pectineal line of the pubic bone.

6. The femoral ring is closed by a plug of fat called the femoral septum.

The femoral canal is wider in females because:

1. The bony pelvis is wider.

2. The femoral vessels are smaller in diameter.

Therefore, *femoral hernia is more common in females*.

Adductor Canal/Subsartorial Canal/Hunter's Canal (Video 2.5)

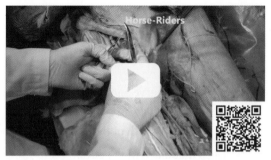

Video 2.5   Femoral triangle and adductor canal.

1. It is a narrow intermuscular canal located in the middle one-third of the medial aspect of the thigh.

2. It extends from the apex of the femoral triangle to the osseoaponeurotic opening in the adductor magnus.

3. It allows the passage of the femoral vessels from the femoral triangle to the popliteal fossa.

4. Its boundaries are:
   - *Anterolateral*: Vastus medialis.
   - *Anteromedial* (*roof*): Fibrous membrane sheath covered by the sartorius.
   - *Posterior*:
     a. Adductor longus (in the upper part).
     b. Adductor magnus (in the lower part).

5. Contents:
   - Femoral artery.
   - Femoral vein.
   - Saphenous nerve.
   - Nerve to the vastus medialis.
   - Branches of the obturator nerve.

- Descending genicular branch of the femoral artery.

All the contents enter the canal through the apex of the femoral triangle but femoral vessels leave it through the opening in the adductor hiatus (lower end), saphenous nerve by piercing the roof, and nerve to the vastus medialis by entering the vastus medialis (anterolateral wall).

▋ Clinical Notes

1. *Femoral pulse*: The pulsations of the femoral artery can be felt in the femoral triangle just below the midinguinal point against the head of the femur.

2. *Femoral hernia*:
   - It is an abnormal protrusion of the abdominal contents (e.g., small intestine) through the femoral canal.
   - Lies inferior and lateral to the pubic tubercle.
   - The herniated structure enters the canal through the femoral ring, then bulges anteriorly through the saphenous opening and bends superolaterally toward the inguinal ligament.
   - Strangulation of a femoral hernia may occur due to the sharp, stiff boundaries of the femoral ring.
   - Femoral hernia lies inferior and lateral to the pubic tubercle whereas the inguinal hernia lies above and medial to the pubic tubercle.
   - Surgical reduction of the femoral hernia: Lacunar ligament has to be divided to relieve strangulation. Care has to be taken to ligate the abnormal obturator artery which may run along the lateral margin of the lacunar ligament.
   - Abnormal obturator artery (enlargement of the anastomosis between the pubic branches of the inferior epigastric and pubic branch of the obturator artery) is in danger of being cut during surgery (femoral hernia reduction) as it lies close to the medial border of the femoral ring (along the lacunar ligament). This may cause severe bleeding.

3. Ligation of femoral artery in popliteal aneurysm. The femoral artery can be ligated in the adductor canal to treat popliteal aneurysm. Following ligation of the femoral artery, blood can reach the popliteal artery through the anastomotic channels around the knee. This was first described in the eighteenth century by John Hunter.

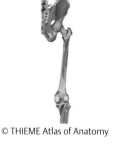

Learning Objectives

At the end of the dissection, you should be able to identify the following:

- Iliac crest, posterior and anterior superior iliac spines, greater and lesser sciatic notches, greater trochanter, and ischial tuberosity on the skeleton as well as on the cadaver.
- Attachments of the gluteal muscles, trace their nerve supply, and demonstrate their actions.
- Piriformis and quadratus femoris, obturator internus, gemelli, and the obturator externus, trace their nerve supply, and demonstrate their action on the hip joint.
- Sacrotuberous and sacrospinous ligaments.
- Structures entering the gluteal region through the greater sciatic foramen and the structures passing through the lesser sciatic foramen.
- Course of the sciatic nerve and its relations.
- Anatomical basis for the site selected for giving the intramuscular injection.

Introduction

The gluteal region overlies the back and the side of the lateral half of the pelvis. It extends from the iliac crest superiorly to the gluteal fold inferiorly. Medially, it extends up to the middorsal line and natal cleft and laterally up to an imaginary line joining the anterior superior iliac spine to the anterior edge of the greater trochanter.

Surface Landmarks

1. Note the gluteal fold, a transverse skin crease which forms the lower limit of the gluteal region (**Fig. 3.1**).

2. Note the natal cleft which is a midline cleft between the buttocks and has lower sacral spines and coccyx lying in its floor. Palpate the posterior superior iliac spine which lies deep to a skin dimple at the level of the second sacral spine.

3. Feel the iliac crest, a curved bony ridge at the lower limit of the waist extending between the anterior and posterior superior iliac spine. Note that the highest point of the iliac crest corresponds to the interval between the spines of L3 and L4 vertebrae.

4. Feel the ischial tuberosity by pressing your fingers upward into the medial part of the gluteal fold. It is 5 cm above the gluteal fold and about the same distance from the midline.

5. Palpate the tip of the greater trochanter as it lies just in front of the hollow on the side of the hip, about one hand's breadth below the tubercle of the iliac crest.

Dissection and Identification

1. Place the cadaver in a prone position (**Fig. 3.1**).

2. Make a curved incision "A" from the anterior superior iliac spine to the midline. Make a vertical incision "B" from this point down to the tip of the coccyx. Extend the incision from the tip of the coccyx curving laterally a little below the gluteal fold "C" (**Fig. 3.1**).

3. Reflect the flap of the skin laterally. Remove the superficial fascia from the region which may be heavily laden with fat and try to identify the cutaneous nerves (**Fig. 3.2**).

4. Remove the deep fascia from the underlying gluteus maximus muscle. Use the back of the forceps or your finger to define the superior border of the muscle extending from the iliac crest to its lateral attachment to the iliotibial tract. Clean the lower border of the muscle that runs obliquely deep to the gluteal fold (**Fig. 3.3**; **Video 3.1**).

5. Pass a blunt forceps deep to the inferior border of the muscle 3 to 4 cm medial to the gluteal tuberosity and cut upward across the gluteus maximus muscle to its superior border along the gap between the two limbs of the forceps to avoid damaging the nerve and blood vessels lying deep to it (**Fig. 3.4**).

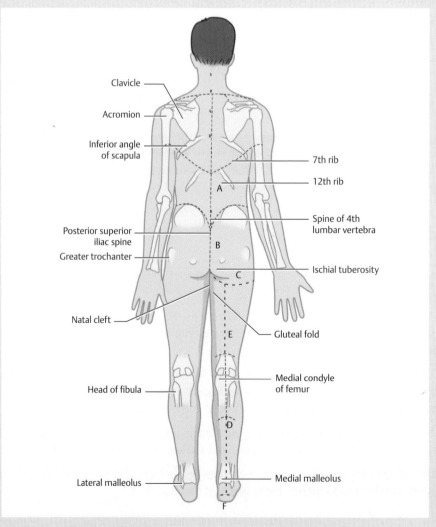

Fig. 3.1   Landmarks and incisions.

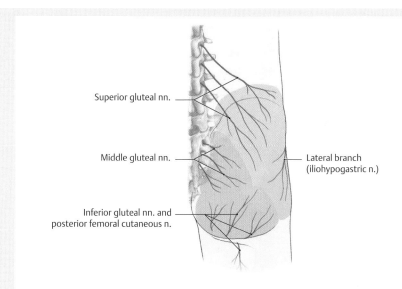

Fig. 3.2 Cutaneous nerves of the gluteal region. (From Schuenke M, Schulte E, Schumacher U. THIEME Atlas of Anatomy. General Anatomy and Musculoskeletal System. Illustrations by Voll M and Wesker K. © Thieme 2020)

6. Reflect the lateral part of the muscle and identify the bursa which separates it from the greater trochanter.

7. While reflecting the medial part of the gluteus maximus muscle, identify the inferior gluteal nerve and vessels entering the deep surface of its lower part and the superficial division of the superior gluteal vessels entering its upper part. Cut the inferior gluteal nerve and vessels and reflect the muscle further medially to uncover the ischial tuberosity and note the presence of the bursa superficial to it (**Fig. 3.5**).

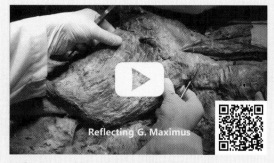

Video 3.1   Gluteal region—Part 1.

8. Trace the branch of the superior gluteal artery to the greater sciatic foramen where it emerges between the gluteus medius (superiorly) and piriformis (inferiorly). Identify the conical piriformis muscle that reaches the gluteal region by passing through the greater sciatic notch and taper toward its insertion to the greater trochanter (**Fig. 3.6**).

9. Identify and trace the large sciatic nerve from the inferior border of the piriformis down to the midpoint between the ischial tuberosity and the greater trochanter.

10. Remove the fascia from the muscles anterior to the sciatic nerve. From above downward they are the superior gemellus, tendon of the obturator internus, inferior gemellus, quadrates femoris, and adductor magnus.

11. Return to the inferior border of the piriformis and note the other structures besides the piriformis and sciatic nerve entering the gluteal region through the greater sciatic foramen. Lift the sciatic nerve laterally and observe the slender nerve to the quadratus femoris on the posterior surface of the acetabulum and then it disappears deep to the tendon of the obturator internus and the gemelli.

12. Medial to the upper part of the sciatic nerve, identify the ischial spine and tough fibrous structure, that is, the sacrospinous ligament medial to the ischial spine. Superficial to them, find

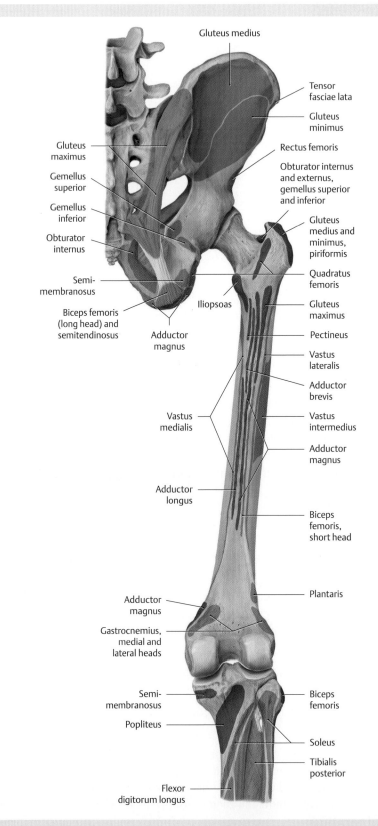

Fig. 3.3 Bony attachments to muscles of the gluteal region and back of thigh. (From Schuenke M, Schulte E, Schumacher U. THIEME Atlas of Anatomy. General Anatomy and Musculoskeletal System. Illustrations by Voll M and Wesker K. © Thieme 2020)

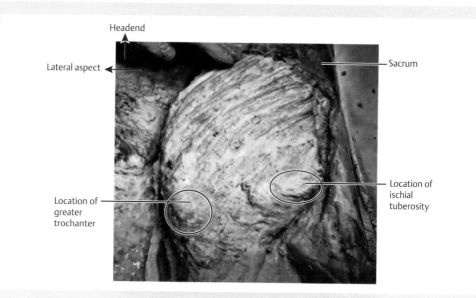

Fig. 3.4   Gluteus maximus muscle.

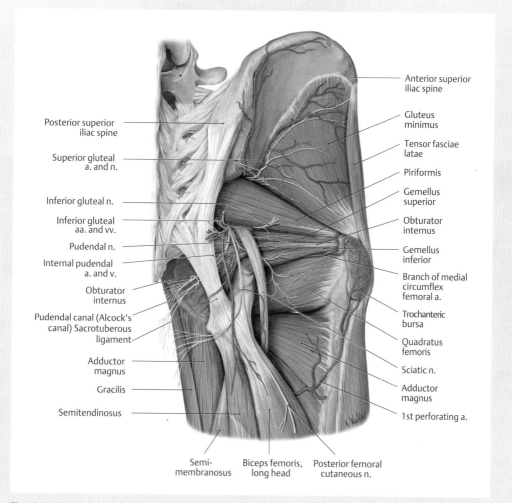

Fig. 3.5   Dissection of the gluteal region. (From Schuenke M, Schulte E, Schumacher U. THIEME Atlas of Anatomy. General Anatomy and Musculoskeletal System. Illustrations by Voll M and Wesker K. © Thieme 2020)

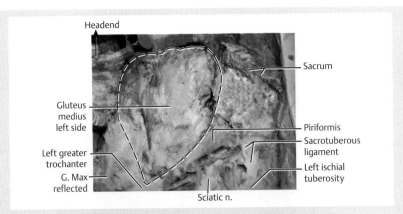

Fig. 3.6   Gluteus medius muscle.

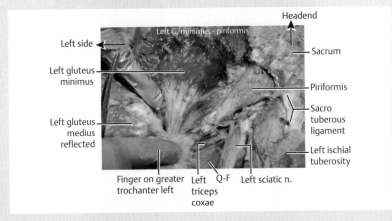

Fig. 3.7   Piriformis muscle.

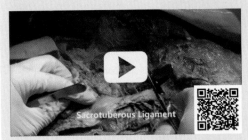

Video 3.2   Gluteal region—Part 2.

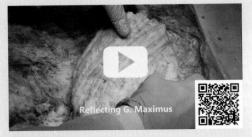

Video 3.3   Gluteal muscles.

the nerve to the obturator internus, internal pudendal vessels, and pudendal nerve from the lateral to the medial (**Video 3.2**).

13. Remove the fascia from the surface of the gluteus medius and separate its posterior border from the piriformis using the back of the forceps. Locate the branches of the superior gluteal vessels above the piriformis muscle. Push your fingers deep to the posterior border of the gluteus medius in the plane of the superior gluteal vessels and nerve to separate it from the underlying gluteus minimus (**Fig. 3.7**).

14. Cut across the gluteus medius about 4 to 5 cm above the greater trochanter and trace the branches of the superior gluteal nerve and vessels running between the gluteus medius and minimus muscles (**Video 3.3**).

15. Identify the tensor fasciae lata muscle enclosed in the fascia lata extending from the anterior part of the iliac crest to the iliotibial tract.

Muscles

Muscles of the gluteal region and their nerve supply along with attachment and action are described in **Tables 3.1** and **3.2**, respectively.

Table 3.1   Muscles of the gluteal region and their nerve supply

	Name	Nerve supply
Gluteal muscles	Gluteus maximus	Inferior gluteal nerve (L5, S1, S2)
	Gluteus medius	Superior gluteal nerve (L4, L5, S1)
	Gluteus minimus	Superior gluteal nerve (L4, L5, S1)
Lateral rotators of the thigh	Piriformis	Ventral rami of S1, S2
	Obturator internus	Nerve to the obturator internus (L5, S1, S2)
	Superior gemellus	Nerve to the obturator internus (L5, S1, S2)
	Inferior gemellus	Nerve to the quadratus femoris (L4, L5, S1)
	Quadratus femoris	Nerve to the quadratus femoris (L4, L5, S1)
	Obturator externus	Obturator nerve (L2, L3, L4)
	Tensor fasciae latae	Superior gluteal nerve (L4, L5, S1)

Table 3.2   Gluteal muscles: attachments and actions

Muscle	Origin	Insertion	Action/s
Gluteus maximus	Gluteal surface of the ilium behind the posterior gluteal line Dorsal surface of the sacrum and ileum Sacrotuberous ligament	Superficial three-fourth into the iliotibial tract Deep one-fourth into the gluteal tuberosity	Powerful extensor of the hip joint (in getting up from the sitting position, running, jumping, etc.)
Gluteus medius	Gluteal surface of the ilium between the anterior and posterior gluteal lines	Lateral surface of the greater trochanter	Abductors of the hip joint Medial rotators of the hip joint
Gluteus minimus	Gluteal surface of the ilium between the anterior and inferior gluteal lines	Anterior surface of the greater trochanter	Prevents sagging of the pelvis on the unsupported side

Structures Passing through the Greater Sciatic Foramen (Fig. 3.5)

1. Piriformis muscle.

2. Structures passing above the piriformis:
   - Superior gluteal nerve.
   - Superior gluteal vessels.

3. Structures passing below the piriformis:
   - Inferior gluteal nerve.
   - Inferior gluteal vessels.
   - Sciatic nerve.
   - Posterior cutaneous nerve of the thigh.
   - Nerve to the obturator internus.
   - Nerve to the quadratus femoris.
   - Internal pudendal vessels.
   - Pudendal nerve.

Structures Passing through the Lesser Sciatic Foramen (Fig. 3.5)

1. Tendon of the obturator internus.
2. Nerve to the obturator internus.
3. Internal pudendal vessels.
4. Pudendal nerve.

Arteries Participating in the Trochanteric Anastomosis (in the Trochanteric Fossa)

1. Descending branch of the superior gluteal artery.
2. Ascending branch of the lateral circumflex femoral artery.
3. Ascending branch of the medial circumflex femoral artery.
4. A branch from the inferior gluteal artery.

Arteries Participating in the Cruciate Anastomosis (at the Root of the Greater Trochanter)

1. Transverse branch of the medial circumflex femoral artery.
2. Transverse branch of the lateral circumflex femoral artery.
3. Descending branch of the inferior gluteal artery.
4. Ascending branch of the first perforating artery.

Course and Branches of the Sciatic Nerve

1. The sciatic nerve arises from the ventral rami of the L4 to S3 spinal nerves.
2. It leaves the pelvis through the greater sciatic foramen inferior to the piriformis.
3. It lies successively on the ischium, obturator internus, quadrates femoris, and adductor magnus.
4. It lies midway between the greater trochanter and ischial tuberosity.
5. It is crossed by the long head of the biceps femoris in the posterior compartment of the thigh.
6. It usually divides into the tibial and common peroneal nerves at the superior angle of the popliteal fossa.
7. It has no branches in the gluteal region.
8. It supplies all the hamstring muscles (semitendinosus, semimembranosus, biceps femoris, and ischial part of the adductor magnus) in the posterior compartment of the thigh.
9. The sciatic nerve injury leads to foot drop.
10. Compression of the sciatic nerve results in "sleeping foot."

▌Clinical Notes

1. *Trendelenburg sign:* If the gluteus medius and minimus of one side are paralyzed (due to injury to the superior gluteal nerve), then if the patient is asked to stand on the paralyzed side of the foot, the pelvis sinks on the unsupported side (opposite side, foot is off the ground). The affected person walks with a lurching gait.

2. *Intramuscular injections* in the gluteal region are given in its upper and outer quadrants into gluteus medius muscle to avoid injury to the sciatic nerve.

4 Posterior Compartment of the Thigh and Popliteal Fossa

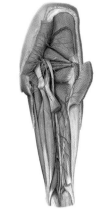

Learning Objectives

At the end of the dissection, you should be able to identify the following:

- Hamstring muscles, their attachments, and their actions.
- Branches of the sciatic nerve in the back of the thigh and popliteal fossa.
- Boundaries of the popliteal fossa and the contents.

Introduction

The back of the thigh extends from the gluteal fold above to the back of the knee below. The popliteal fossa is a diamond-shaped hollow on the back of the knee joint. It becomes prominent when the knee is flexed. The fossa is an important anatomical region as it provides passage to the main vessels from the thigh to the leg.

Surface Landmarks

Before starting the dissection, study the surface anatomy of the region. Palpate the bony landmarks and relate them to the respective bones on the articulated skeleton (refer to **Fig. 1.1**).

The surface landmarks are as follows:

1. Ischial tuberosity (refer to page 29, Chapter 3).
2. Tip of greater trochanter (refer to page 29, Chapter 3).
3. Medial and lateral condyles of tibia (refer to page 45, Chapter 5).
4. Medial and lateral malleoli (refer to page 45, Chapter 5).

Posterior Compartment of Thigh

Dissection and Identification

1. Make a horizontal incision "D" across the back of the leg about 8 to 10 cm below the knee.
2. Make a vertical incision "E" (refer to **Fig. 3.1**) along the midline of the back of the thigh extending till the horizontal incision on the back of the leg.
3. Reflect the skin flaps and strip the superficial fascia from the deep fascia by blunt dissection. Divide the deep fascia vertically and find the posterior cutaneous nerve running down the middle of the back of the thigh, superficial to the long head of the biceps femoris. Retract the long head of the biceps femoris laterally to expose the sciatic nerve which lies deep to it.

Find its muscular branches to the hamstring muscles. Follow the sciatic nerve inferiorly till the knee, where it divides into the tibial nerve which descends vertically down in line with the sciatic nerve and the common peroneal nerve which courses laterally (**Fig. 4.1**).

4. Find the short head of the biceps femoris deep to the long head as it takes origin from the posterior aspect of the femur. Find the upper end of the long head of the biceps femoris which

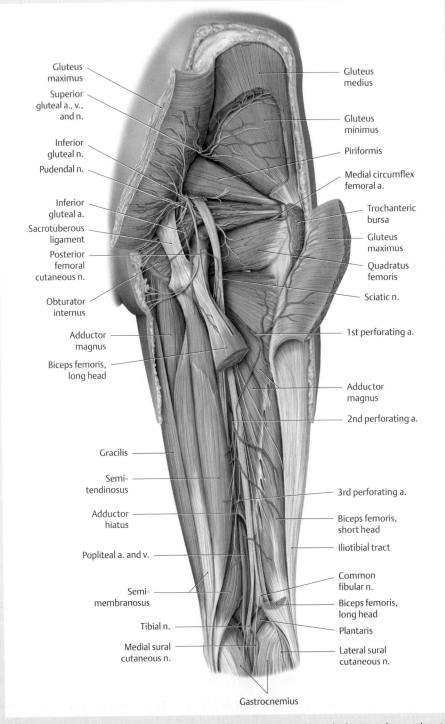

Fig. 4.1   Dissection of the back of thigh. (From Schuenke M, Schulte E, Schumacher U. THIEME Atlas of Anatomy. General Anatomy and Musculoskeletal System. Illustrations by Voll M and Wesker K. © Thieme 2020)

is attached to the ischial tuberosity. Observe that the semitendinosus muscle arises in common with the long head of the biceps femoris from the medial part of the ischial tuberosity, and semimembranosus arises from the lateral part of the ischial tuberosity (**Video 4.1**).

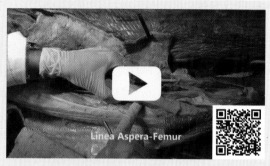

Video 4.1 Hamstring muscles.

5. Note that the lower part of the semitendinosus is a long cord-like tendon which is attached to the upper part of the medial surface of the tibia, posterior to the attachment of the sartorius and gracilis. The upper half of the semimembranosus is a broad flat tendon. Both the semitendinosus and semimembranosus pass downward along the medial aspect of the back of the thigh.

6. Cut the hamstring muscles near their origin from the ischial tuberosity and turn them downward to expose the ischial part of the adductor magnus. Expose the insertion of the adductor magnus to the femur and find the perforating arteries which pass between the femur and the adductor magnus.

Muscles

The muscles of the back of the thigh are called hamstring muscles.

Hamstring Muscles

1. Hamstring muscles are four in number (**Video 4.2; Fig. 4.2**) and cross both hip and knee joints.

2. They include the following:

   • Semimembranosus.
   • Semitendinosus.
   • Long head of the biceps femoris.
   • Ischial part of the adductor magnus.

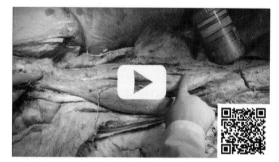

Video 4.2 Hamstring muscles and sciatic nerve.

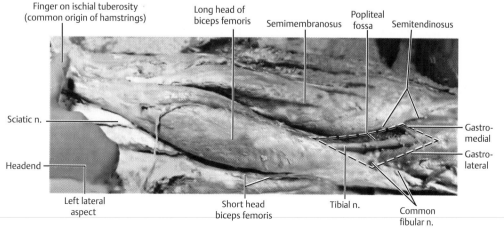

Fig. 4.2 Hamstring muscles.

3. They take origin from the ischial tuberosity.

4. They are inserted on one of the bones of the leg.

5. They are supplied by the tibial division of the sciatic nerve (all the branches arise from the medial side of the sciatic nerve).

6. They act as extensors of the hip joint and flexors of the knee joint.

7. The short head of biceps femoris takes origin from the lateral lip of the linea aspera and is supplied by the common peroneal part of the sciatic nerve.

Iliotibial Tract

1. It is a thickened fascia lata along the lateral surface of the thigh.

2. It is about 2.5 cm wide.

3. It receives insertion of two muscles, that is, the tensor fasciae latae and superficial three-fourth of the gluteus maximus.

4. Above, it splits to enclose the tensor fasciae latae; the superficial layer is attached to the iliac crest and the deep layer is attached to the capsule of the hip joint.

5. Inferiorly, it is attached to the flattened triangular area on the anterior surface of the lateral condyle of the tibia.

6. It maintains the knee in an extended position.

Popliteal Fossa

Dissection and Identification

1. Remove any traces of the superficial fascia left on the back of the knee. Find the branches of the posterior cutaneous nerve in the upper part of the region and the small saphenous vein in the lower part (**Fig. 4.3**).

2. Cut through the deep fascia and remove the deep fascia from the surface of the muscles forming boundaries of the popliteal fossa.

3. Superomedially, follow the semitendinosus to the medial surface of the tibia and the semimembranosus to the posterior aspect of the medial condyle of the tibia. Superolaterally, follow the tendon formed by the fusion of the long and short heads of the biceps femoris to the head of the tibia. Inferomedially and inferolaterally, observe the medial and lateral heads of the gastrocnemius forming the boundaries of the popliteal fossa. Find the short belly of the plantaris just medial to the lateral head of the gastrocnemius.

4. Follow the tibial nerve and find its branches: the sural nerve (the cutaneous branch) lies between the two heads of the gastrocnemius. Using your fingers, separate the heads of the gastrocnemius and find the muscular branches to the gastrocnemius, plantaris, soleus, and popliteus arising in the middle of the popliteal fossa. Find the superior, middle, and inferior genicular branches to the knee joint. Trace the common peroneal nerve medial to the tendon of the biceps femoris to the back of the head of the fibula.

5. Lift the tibial nerve to expose the popliteal vessels enclosed in a connective tissue sheath. Use a pair of scissors to cut through the sheath and note that the popliteal vein lies posterolateral to the artery. Observe the arrangement of the popliteal artery, vein, and tibial nerve in the upper, middle, and lower parts of the popliteal fossa (**Fig. 4.3**).

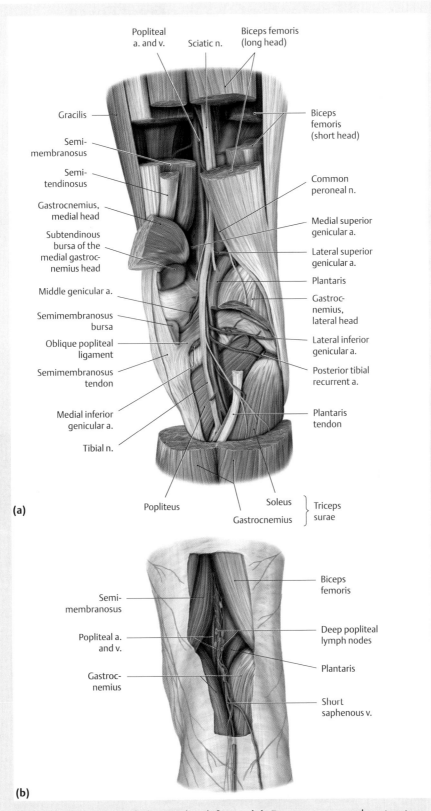

Fig. 4.3 Dissection of the popliteal fossa. **(a)** Deep neurovascular structures. **(b)** Deep lymph nodes of the popliteal region. (From Schuenke M, Schulte E, Schumacher U. THIEME Atlas of Anatomy. General Anatomy and Musculoskeletal System. Illustrations by Voll M and Wesker K. © Thieme 2020)

Boundaries and Contents of the Popliteal Fossa

Boundaries (Videos 4.3 and 4.4; Fig. 4.4):

1. Roof:
   - The roof is formed by the skin, superficial fascia, and deep fascia (popliteal fascia).
   - It is pierced by the posterior cutaneous nerve of the thigh and the small saphenous vein.
2. Floor:
   - The floor is formed by the popliteal surface of the femur, capsule of the knee joint, and fascia over the popliteus muscle (from above downward).
3. Side boundaries:
   - *Superolateral*: Biceps femoris.
   - *Superomedial*: Semitendinosus and semimembranosus.
   - *Inferolateral*: Lateral head of the gastrocnemius and plantaris.
   - *Inferomedial*: Medial head of the gastrocnemius.

Contents:

1. Popliteal artery and its branches.
2. Popliteal vein and its tributaries.
3. Tibial nerve and its branches.
4. Common peroneal nerve and its branches.
5. Popliteal group of lymph nodes.

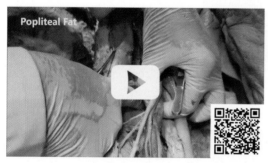

Video 4.3   Popliteal fossa—Part 1.

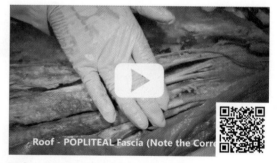

Video 4.4   Popliteal fossa—Part 2.

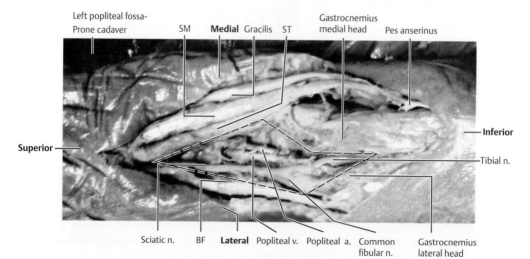

Fig. 4.4   Popliteal fossa. Abbreviations: SM, Semimembranosus; BF, Biceps femoris.

Neurovascular Structures and Lymph Nodes in the Popliteal Fossa

The popliteal artery lies deep along the floor of the fossa. The popliteal vein runs posterior to the artery. The tibial nerve descends through middle of fossa superficial to popliteal vessels. The common peroneal nerve runs posterolaterally along the tendon of biceps femoris. The lymph nodes lie along blood vessels.

Tibial Nerve

It is larger nerve and gives following branches.

1. *Muscular branches to the*:
   - Gastrocnemius.
   - Soleus.
   - Plantaris.
   - Popliteus.
2. *Cutaneous branch*: Sural nerve (supplies the skin of the lower part of the calf).

Common Peroneal Nerve

It is smaller nerve and gives following branches:
- Peroneal communicating nerve.
- Lateral cutaneous nerve of calf.

Popliteal Artery

It is the continuation of femoral artery at the adductor hiatus and runs on the anterior wall of fossa upto lower border of popliteus.

1. Terminal branches:
   - Anterior and posterior tibial arteries.
2. Other branches:
   - Superior, medial, and lateral genicular arteries.
   - Middle genicular artery.
   - Muscular branches.

The genicular arteries form anastomosis around the knee joint.

Popliteal Vein

It is formed at the lower border of popliteus muscle by the union of anterior and posterior tibial veins. It runs superficial to popliteal artery.

Tributaries of Popliteal Vein

1. Small saphenous vein.
2. Other small vein.

Popliteal Lymph Nodes

There are 4-6 lymph nodes lying deep in the popliteal fossa in relation to blood vessels. They drain the following areas.

Cutaneous lymphatics from the:
- Little toe.
- Lateral margin of the foot.
- Lateral side of the back of the leg.

Efferents from the popliteal lymph nodes drain into the deep inguinal lymph nodes.

▌Clinical Notes

1. *Popliteal aneurysm*: The popliteal artery is more prone to aneurysm than any other artery in the body. The popliteal aneurysm presents as a midline pulsatile swelling in the popliteal fossa.

2. *Moren Baker cyst*: It is the herniation of the synovial cavity of knee joint in the region of popliteal fossa.

5 Anterior and Lateral Compartments of the Leg and Dorsum of the Foot

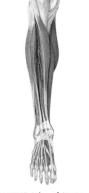

© THIEME Atlas of Anatomy

Introduction

The leg is that part of the lower limb that lies between the knee and ankle. The bones of the leg are the tibia medially and the fibula laterally. The larger bone tibia is weight bearing, whereas the thinner fibula provides attachment to most of the muscles of the leg. The tibia and fibula are joined by an interosseous membrane. The deep fascia of the leg is attached to the fibula by the anterior and posterior intramuscular septa. The tibia, fibula, interosseous membrane, and the two intermuscular septa divide the leg into three compartments, such as anterior, lateral, and posterior compartments (**Fig. 5.1**).

Surface Landmarks

1. Flex the knee and palpate the medial and lateral condyles of the tibia on either side of the ligamentum patellae.

2. Observe the bony prominence called the tibial tuberosity on the front of the upper part of the tibia, 2.5 cm distal to the knee joint.

3. Feel the sharp sinuously curved anterior border (shin) of the tibia extending downward from the tibial tuberosity to the anterior margin of the medial malleolus.

4. Locate the medial and lateral malleoli, the bony prominences on the medial and lateral sides of the ankles, respectively.

5. Feel the sustentaculum tali, a thumb breadth below the medial malleolus, and the peroneal trochlea, a small bony prominence about a fingerbreadth below the lateral malleolus.

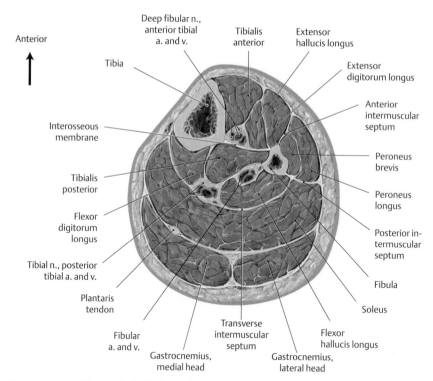

Fig. 5.1 Transverse section of right leg showing compartments. (From Schuenke M, Schulte E, Schumacher U. THIEME Atlas of Anatomy. General Anatomy and Musculoskeletal System. Illustrations by Voll M and Wesker K. © Thieme 2020)

Anterior Compartment of Leg

Dissection and Identification

1. Place the cadaver in a supine position. Make a midline incision on the front of the leg extending from incision 'C' down to the ankle upto incision 'D'. Extend the incision along the middle of the dorsum of the foot till the nail bed of the middle toe. Make a transverse incision 'D' across the front of the ankle connecting the two malleoli. Make another transverse incision at the root of the toes (refer to **Fig. 2.2**).

2. Reflect the skin flaps on the front of the leg as well as on the dorsum of the foot. Note the dorsal venous arch on the dorsum of the foot located transversely opposite the anterior parts of the metatarsals. Medially, the arch is continuous with the great saphenous vein. Follow the vein as it passes in front of the medial malleolus and then along the medial aspect of the leg to reach behind the knee. Find the saphenous nerve just anterior to the great saphenous vein.

3. Observe that laterally the dorsal venous arch is continuous with the small saphenous vein. Trace the vein till a point below the lateral malleolus and find the sural nerve beside it (**Fig. 5.2**).

4. Find the superficial peroneal nerve as it pierces the deep fascia at the junction of the middle third and lower third of the lateral side of the leg. Trace the nerve and its branches into the dorsum of the foot and toes. Find the digital nerves to the adjacent sides of the big and second toes and follow them proximally as they arise from the deep peroneal nerve.

5. Remove the superficial fascia and expose the deep fascia. Note that it is firmly attached to the anterior border of the tibia. Identify the thickenings of the deep fascia in front of the ankle, the thickenings of the fascia, and superior and inferior extensor retinacula (**Fig. 5.3**).

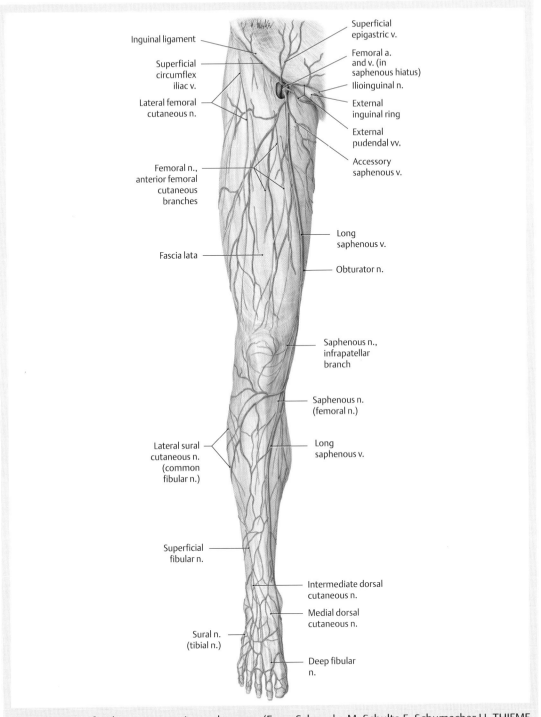

Fig. 5.2 Superficial cutaneous veins and nerves. (From Schuenke M, Schulte E, Schumacher U. THIEME Atlas of Anatomy. General Anatomy and Musculoskeletal System. Illustrations by Voll M and Wesker K. © Thieme 2020)

Divide the deep fascia on the front of the leg longitudinally but leave the retinacula intact. Pass a blunt seeker deep to the retinacula and define its margins. Superior extensor retinaculum extends across the tendons of the muscles of the anterior compartment between the lower ends of the tibia and fibula just above the ankle joint. Inferior extensor retinaculum is Y-shaped and lies across the ankle joint. Note that the stem of the Y is attached laterally to the calcaneus.

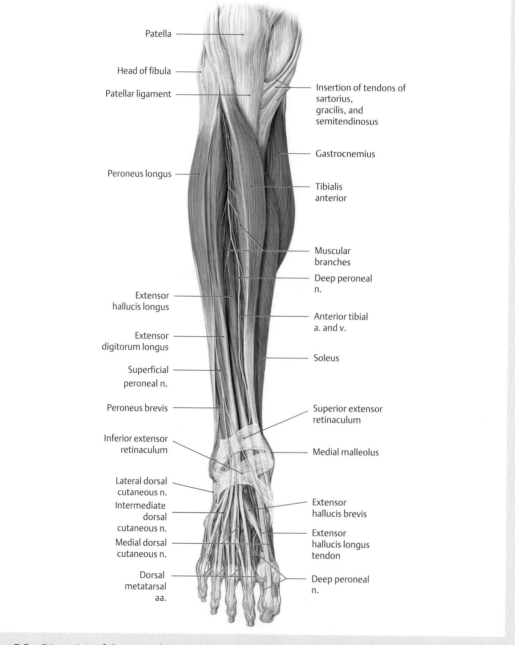

Fig. 5.3 Dissection of the anterolateral aspect of the leg. (From Schuenke M, Schulte E, Schumacher U. THIEME Atlas of Anatomy. General Anatomy and Musculoskeletal System. Illustrations by Voll M and Wesker K. © Thieme 2020)

6. Observe the tendons of the muscles of the extensor compartment which are enclosed in the synovial sheath and pass deep to the extensor retinaculum. From medial to lateral, these tendons are the tibialis anterior, extensor hallucis longus, extensor digitorum longus, and peroneus tertius. Follow the tendons upward (**Video 5.1**).

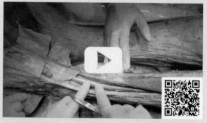

Video 5.1 Tendons on dorsum of foot.

7. Separate the tibialis anterior from the other muscles deep to the interosseous membrane. Find the anterior tibial vessels and the deep peroneal nerve on the membrane. Trace them upward and downward. Divide the superior extensor retinaculum and identify the anterior tibial vessels and deep peroneal nerve lying between the tendons of the extensor hallucis longus and extensor digitorum longus. Trace the artery on the dorsum of the foot where it continues as the dorsalis pedis artery toward the first intermetatarsal space. Identify the arcuate artery, a branch of the dorsalis pedis artery that crosses the proximal ends of the metatarsal bones. Note the lateral three dorsal metatarsal branches of the arcuate artery (**Figs. 5.4** and **5.5**).

8. On the dorsum of the foot, find the extensor digitorum brevis muscle arising from the calcaneus and dividing into four tendons for medial four toes.

9. On the second or third toe, clean the extensor expansion formed by the extensor tendons.

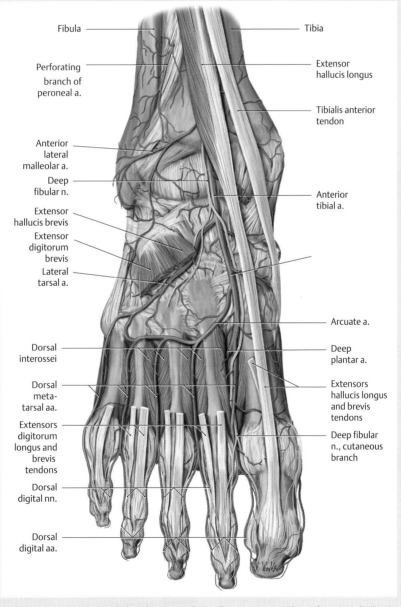

Fig. 5.4   Dissection of the dorsum of the foot. (From Schuenke M, Schulte E, Schumacher U. THIEME Atlas of Anatomy. General Anatomy and Musculoskeletal System. Illustrations by Voll M and Wesker K. © Thieme 2020)

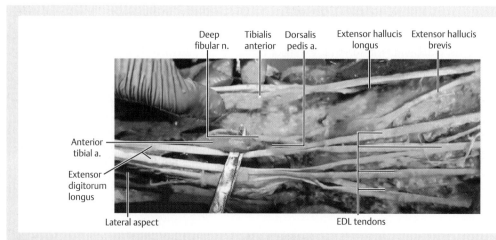

Fig. 5.5   Anterior tibial and dorsalis pedis arteries.

Muscles of the Anterior Compartment of the Leg

Muscles of the anterior compartment of the leg are described in **Table 5.1** and **Fig. 5.6** (**Video 5.2**).

Table 5.1   Muscles of the anterior compartment of the leg

Muscle	Origin	Insertion	Nerve supply	Action
Tibialis anterior	Lateral surface of the shaft of the tibia and interosseous membrane	Medial cuneiform and base of the first metatarsal	Deep peroneal nerve	Dorsiflexes the foot, inverts the foot, and supports the medial longitudinal arch
Extensor digitorum	Medial surface of the shaft of the fibula and interosseous membrane	Extensor expansion of the lateral four toes	Deep peroneal nerve	Extends the toes, dorsiflexes (extends) the foot
Peroneus tertius	Medial surface of the shaft of the fibula and interosseous membrane	Base of the fifth metatarsal bone	Deep peroneal nerve	Dorsiflexes the foot and everts the foot
Extensor hallucis longus	Medial surface of the shaft of the fibula and interosseous membrane	Base of the distal phalanx of the big toe	Deep peroneal nerve	Extends the big toe, dorsiflexes the foot, and inverts the foot

Structures Passing Deep to the Superior Extensor Retinaculum from the Medial to the Lateral Side

1. Tibialis anterior.

2. Extensor hallucis longus.

3. Anterior tibial vessels.

4. Deep peroneal nerve.

5. Extensor digitorum longus.

6. Peroneus tertius.

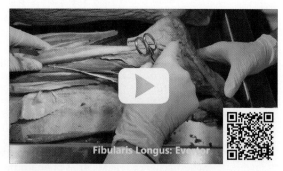

Video 5.2   Anterior compartment of leg.

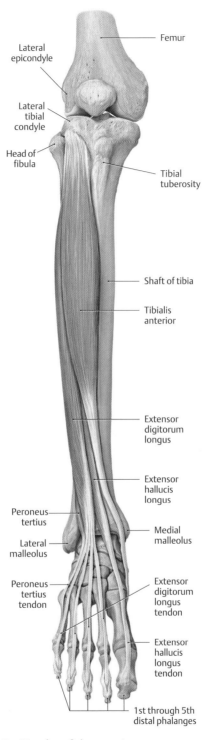

Fig. 5.6 Muscles of the anterior compartment of the leg. (Reproduced with permission from Schuenke M, (From Schuenke M, Schulte E, Schumacher U. THIEME Atlas of Anatomy. General Anatomy and Musculoskeletal System. Illustrations by Voll M and Wesker K. © Thieme 2020)

Branches of the Dorsalis Pedis Artery:

1. Medial tarsal artery.

2. Lateral tarsal artery.

3. Arcuate artery (gives second to fourth dorsal metatarsal arteries).

4. First dorsal metatarsal artery.

Pulsations of the dorsalis pedis artery can be felt between the tendon of the extensor hallucis and tendon of the extensor digitorum longus.

Lateral Compartment of the Leg

Dissection and Identification

1. Observe the deep fascia on the lateral aspect of the leg and identify the superior peroneal retinaculum on the lateral side of the ankle posterior to the lateral malleolus (**Figs. 5.7** and **5.8**).

2. Make a longitudinal incision to divide the deep fascia over the peroneal muscles and turn the flaps aside. Using your fingers, separate the superficial peroneus longus from the underlying peroneus brevis. Follow the tendons of the peroneus longus and brevis inferiorly as their tendons pass behind the lateral malleolus deep to the superior and inferior peroneal retinacula. Follow the insertion of the peroneus brevis to the tuberosity of the fifth metatarsal.

3. Trace the common peroneal nerve as it winds around the neck of the fibula to enter the peroneus longus. Cut through the upper part of the peroneus longus muscle to expose its terminal branches, deep and superficial peroneal nerves. Follow the superficial peroneal nerve distally as it gives branches to the peroneus longus and brevis.

4. Trace the deep peroneal nerve into the anterior compartment of the leg.

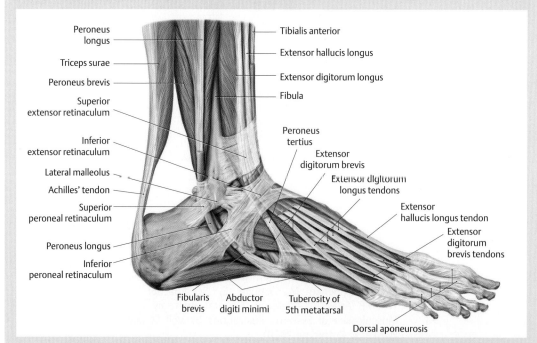

Fig. 5.7   Dissection of lateral aspect of ankle to show peroneal retinacula. (From Schuenke M, Schulte E, Schumacher U. THIEME Atlas of Anatomy. General Anatomy and Musculoskeletal System. Illustrations by Voll M and Wesker K. © Thieme 2020)

Muscles of the Lateral Compartment of the Leg

Muscles of the lateral compartment of the leg are described in **Table 5.2** and **Fig. 5.8** (**Video 5.3**).

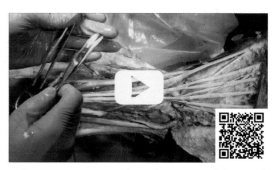

Video 5.3 Anterior lateral aspect of leg and dorsum of foot.

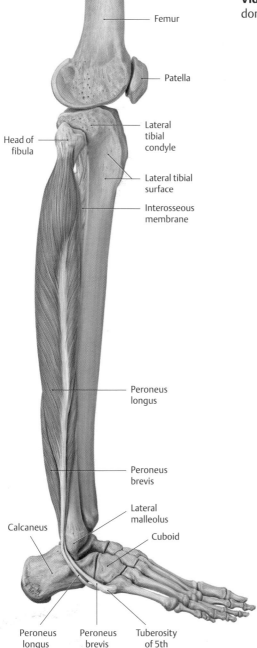

Femur

Patella

Head of fibula

Lateral tibial condyle

Lateral tibial surface

Interosseous membrane

Peroneus longus

Peroneus brevis

Lateral malleolus

Calcaneus

Cuboid

Peroneus longus tendon

Peroneus brevis tendon

Tuberosity of 5th metatarsal

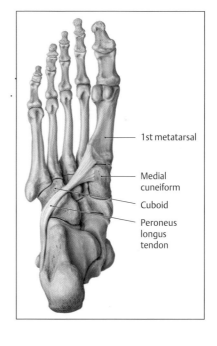

1st metatarsal

Medial cuneiform

Cuboid

Peroneus longus tendon

Fig. 5.8   Muscles of the lateral compartment of leg. Figure on the right in the insert shows the insertion of peroneus longus tendon. (From Schuenke M, Schulte E, Schumacher U. THIEME Atlas of Anatomy. General Anatomy and Musculoskeletal System. Illustrations by Voll M and Wesker K. © Thieme 2020)

Table 5.2   Muscles of the lateral compartment of the leg

Muscle	Origin	Insertion	Nerve supply	Action
Peroneus longus	Lateral surface of the shaft of the fibula	Base of the first metatarsal and medial cuneiform	Superficial peroneal nerve	Plantar flexes the foot, everts the foot, and supports the lateral longitudinal and transverse arches of the foot
Peroneus brevis	Lateral surface of the shaft of the fibula	Base of the fifth metatarsal bone	Superficial peroneal nerve	Plantar flexes the foot, everts the foot, and supports the lateral longitudinal arch

▌Clinical Notes

1. *Foot drop*: The foot is plantar flexed and dorsiflexors of the foot are paralyzed. It is caused due to injury to the sciatic or common peroneal or deep peroneal nerves.

2. *Anterior tibial compartment syndrome*: Anterior tibial compartment syndrome occurs following excessive exertion of the muscles of the anterior compartment of the leg. Muscles within the tight compartment swell resulting in compression of the anterior tibial artery and its branches, leading to ischemia and pain. The boundaries of the anterior compartment of the leg are:

   a. *Anterior*: Deep fascia.

   b. *Posterior*: Interosseous membrane.

   c. *Lateral*: Anterior intermuscular septum and fibula.

   d. *Medial*: Lateral surface of the tibia.

3. *Intermittent claudication* (derived from the word claudicare [Latin] which means "to limp"): Intermittent claudication occurs due to ischemia of the muscles of the lower limb, chiefly the calf muscles. It is seen in occlusive peripheral arterial diseases, particularly involving the popliteal artery and its branches. The pain usually causes the person to limp. Pain is typically felt while walking and it subsides with rest.

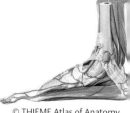
Posterior Compartment of the Leg

Introduction

The back of the leg, also known as the calf, is the bulkiest of the three compartments of the leg as it contains large powerful muscles (gastrocnemius and soleus). The posterior compartment of the leg is continuous superiorly with the popliteal fossa and inferiorly with the sole of the foot. The posterior compartment of the leg is subdivided by two transverse fascial septae (superficial and deep) into three parts: superficial, middle, and deep (**Fig. 6.1**). The superficial part contains the gastrocnemius, soleus, and plantaris muscles; the middle part contains the flexor digitorum longus, flexor hallucis longus, tibial nerve, and posterior tibial vessels; and the deep part contains the popliteus and tibialis posterior muscles. The deep fascia on the posterior aspect of the leg is thickened near the ankle to form the flexor retinaculum on the medial side of the ankle.

Dissection and Identification

1. Place the cadaver in a prone position (**Fig. 3.1**). Make a transverse incision 'F' on the distal part of heal and carry it along the borders of the foot. Now give a vertical incision to join the incision 'D' and 'F' . Strip off the skin from the posterior surface of the leg till the heel. Find the sural nerve and small saphenous vein behind the lateral malleolus. Trace the small saphenous vein in the middle of the posterior aspect of the leg till it joins the popliteal vein at the back of the knee (**Fig. 6.2a**).

2. Identify the thickening of the deep fascia, flexor retinaculum extending from the medial malleolus to the calcaneus.

3. Use a pair of scissors to make a vertical incision through the deep fascia and turn the flaps to expose the superficial muscles. Follow the two heads of the gastrocnemius muscle inferiorly to the thick tendon, tendo calcaneus, which is attached to the calcaneal tuberosity.

4. Use your fingers to separate the two heads of the gastrocnemius and find the plantaris, a small muscle posteromedial to the lateral head of the gastrocnemius. Follow its tendon between the

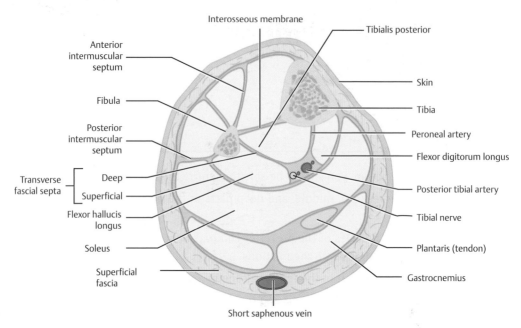

Fig. 6.1 A transverse section of middle third of the left leg showing subdivisions of posterior compartment.

gastrocnemius and underlying soleus to the medial side of the gastrocnemius (**Fig. 6.3**).

5. Cut across the two heads of the gastrocnemius just above the point where they meet. Turn the inferior part of the gastrocnemius inferiorly. This will uncover the slipper-shaped soleus muscle. Follow the fibers of the soleus muscle to the deep surface of the tendo calcaneus.

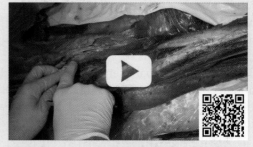

Video 6.1 Posterior aspect of leg—Part 1.

6. Note the tibial nerve and the popliteal vessels passing deep to the tendinous arch of the soleus muscle.

7. Divide the tendo calcaneus tendon about 5 cm above the tuberosity of the calcaneus and use your fingers to separate it from the deep muscles (**Video 6.1**).

8. Using a scalpel, detach the soleus muscle from its attachment on the tibia but leave the muscle attached to the fibula. Retract the soleus along with the distal part of the gastrocnemius laterally to expose the middle layer of the muscles and the neurovascular bundle (**Fig. 6.2b**).

9. Retract the contents of the popliteal fossa laterally to see the triangular popliteus muscle. Observe that the popliteal artery divides into the anterior and posterior tibial artery at the lower border of the popliteus muscle. Follow the posterior tibial vessels inferiorly to the ankle. Note that the anterior tibial vessels enter the anterior compartment of the leg through the gap above the interosseous membrane.

10. Find the thin nerve to the popliteus, a branch of the tibial nerve that arises in the popliteal fossa and descends over popliteus to it lower border. It then turns around the inferior border to enter the deep surface of the muscle.

11. Identify the long flexors of the toes. The larger flexor hallucis muscle is located laterally and the flexor digitorum longus, which takes origin from the tibia, is present medially.

12. Retract the flexor hallucis longus laterally to uncover the deep layer of the muscle formed by the tibialis posterior.

13. Observe that beneath the flexor retinaculum, posteroinferior to the medial malleolus, lie the tendons of the tibialis posterior, flexor digitorum longus, and flexor hallucis longus. The posterior tibial vessels and tibial nerve lie between the flexor digitorum longus and flexor hallucis longus (**Videos 6.2** and **6.3**).

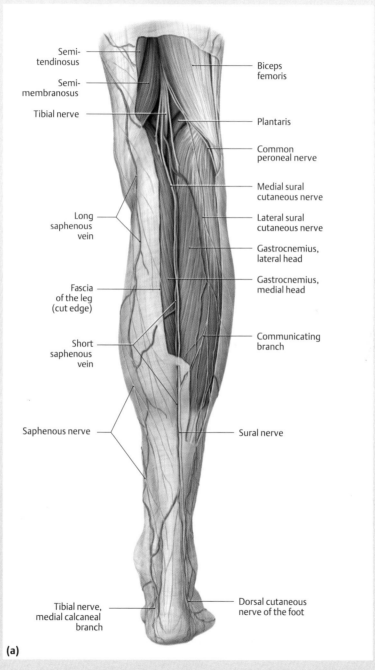

(a)

Fig. 6.2 **(a)** Superficial neurovascular structures on the back of the leg. (From Schuenke M, Schulte E, Schumacher U. THIEME Atlas of Anatomy. General Anatomy and Musculoskeletal System. Illustrations by Voll M and Wesker K. © Thieme 2020) *(Continued)*

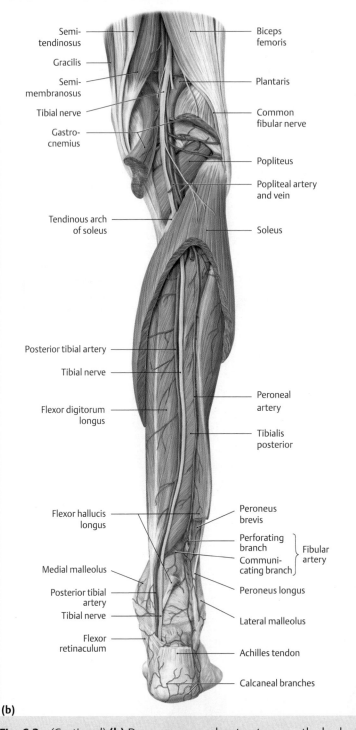

Fig. 6.2 *(Continued)* **(b)** Deep neurovascular structures on the back of the leg. (From Schuenke M, Schulte E, Schumacher U. THIEME Atlas of Anatomy. General Anatomy and Musculoskeletal System. Illustrations by Voll M and Wesker K. © Thieme 2020)

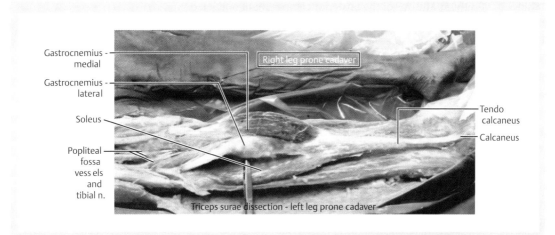

Fig. 6.3 Triceps surae.

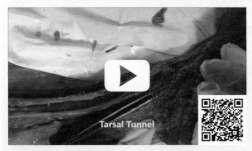

Video 6.2 Posterior aspect of leg—Part 2.

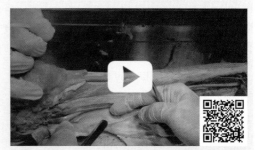

Video 6.3 Posterior aspect of leg—Part 3.

Muscles of the Posterior Compartment of the Leg

These are given in **Table 6.1** and shown in **Figs. 6.4–6.6**.

Table 6.1 Muscles of the posterior compartment of the leg

Muscle	Origin	Insertion	Nerve supply	Action
Gastrocnemius	Medial and lateral condyles of the femur	Via tendo calcaneus to the calcaneus	Tibial nerve	Plantar flexes the foot and the leg
Plantaris	Lateral supracondylar ridge of the femur	Calcaneus	Tibial nerve	Plantar flexes the foot and the leg
Soleus	Shafts of the tibia and fibula	Via tendo calcaneus to the calcaneus	Tibial nerve	Powerful plantar flexor of the foot, provides main propulsive force in walking and running
Popliteus	Lateral condyle of the femur	Triangular area above the soleal line on the posterior sur face of the tibia	Tibial nerve	Flexes the leg, unlocks the knee joint by laterally rotating the femur on the tibia

(Continued)

Table 6.1 *(Continued)* Muscles of the posterior compartment of the leg

Muscle	Origin	Insertion	Nerve supply	Action
Flexor digitorum longus	Posterior surface of the shaft of the tibia	Distal phalanges of the lateral four toes	Tibial nerve	Flexes the distal phalanges of the lateral four toes, plantar flexes the foot, supports the medial and lateral longitudinal arches of the foot
Flexor hallucis longus	Posterior surface of the shaft of the fibula	Base of the distal phalanx of the big toe	Tibial nerve	Flexes the distal phalanx of the big toe, plantar flexes the foot, supports the medial longitudinal arch of the foot
Tibialis posterior	Posterior surface of the shafts of the tibia and fibula and interosseous membrane	Tuberosity of the navicular bone	Tibial nerve	Plantar flexes the foot, inverts the foot, supports the medial longitudinal arch of the foot

Muscles Inserted on the Upper Part of the Medial Surface of the Tibia and Their Nerve Supply

1. Sartorius: Supplied by the femoral nerve.

2. Gracilis: Supplied by the obturator nerve.

3. Semitendinosus: Supplied by the tibial part of the sciatic nerve.

Muscles Responsible for Dorsiflexion of the Toes

1. Tibialis anterior.

2. Extensor hallucis longus.

3. Extensor digitorum longus.

4. Peroneus tertius.

Muscles Responsible for Flexion of the Toes

1. Flexor digitorum longus: flexes 2–5 toes.

2. Flexor hallucis longus: flexes great toe.

Muscles Responsible for Inversion of the Foot

1. Tibialis anterior.

2. Tibialis posterior.

Muscles Responsible for Eversion of the Foot

1. Peroneus longus.

2. Peroneus brevis.

3. Peroneus tertius.

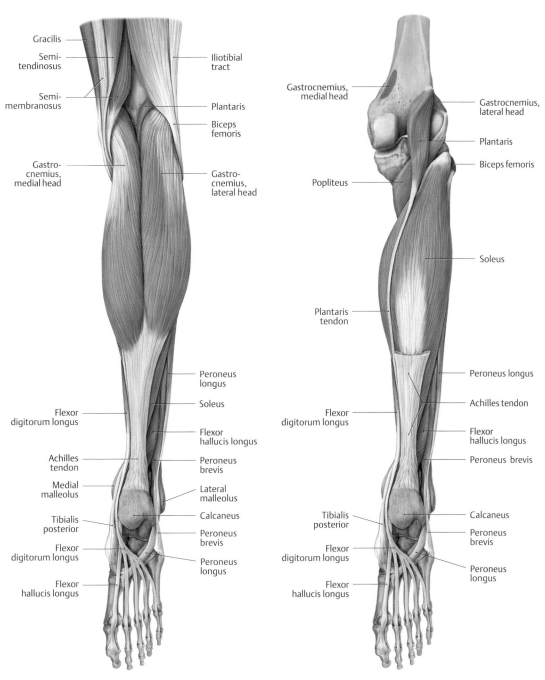

Fig. 6.4 Dissection to expose the muscles of posterior compartment of right leg. (From Schuenke M, Schulte E, Schumacher U. THIEME Atlas of Anatomy. General Anatomy and Musculoskeletal System. Illustrations by Voll M and Wesker K. © Thieme 2020)

Fig. 6.5 Dissection to expose the plantaris and soleus muscles. (From Schuenke M, Schulte E, Schumacher U. THIEME Atlas of Anatomy. General Anatomy and Musculoskeletal System. Illustrations by Voll M and Wesker K. © Thieme 2020)

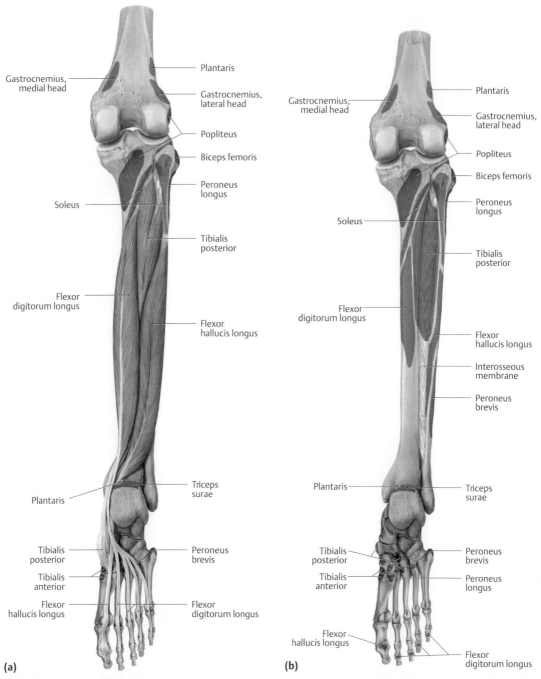

Fig. 6.6 **(a)** Deep muscles on the back of the leg. **(b)** Deep muscles on the back of the leg (attachments). (From Schuenke M, Schulte E, Schumacher U. THIEME Atlas of Anatomy. General Anatomy and Musculoskeletal System. Illustrations by Voll M and Wesker K. © Thieme 2020)

▌Clinical Note

Peripheral heart: It is the name given to the soleus muscle. This muscle contains venous sinuses/ soleal sinuses which communicate both with superficial and deep veins. The contraction of soleus helps return the venous blood from leg toward the heart; hence the name *peripheral heart*.

7 Sole of the Foot

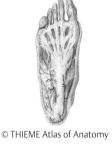

Learning Objectives

At the end of the dissection, you should be able to identify the following:

- Plantar aponeurosis and discuss its functions.
- Four muscular layers of the sole of the foot and the muscles of each layer.
- Attachment of the muscles present in each layer and locate their nerve supply and discuss their actions.
- Plantar nerves, trace their muscular branches, and demonstrate their areas of cutaneous distribution.
- Course and distribution of the plantar arteries and note the formation of the plantar arch and trace its branches.

Introduction

The undersurface of the foot that meets the ground is termed as the *sole of the foot*. The skin of the sole is thick and hairless and is firmly bound by the underlying deep fascia (plantar aponeurosis). In the region of the toes, the deep fascia forms the fibrous flexor sheaths. The flexor sheaths along with the inferior surfaces of the phalanges and interphalangeal joints form a blind tunnel through which pass the long flexor tendons of the toes. The muscles of the sole, 18 intrinsic muscles and four tendons of the extrinsic muscles, are arranged in four layers from the superficial to the deep surface. There are two neurovascular planes between the muscle layers of the sole. In the superficial neuromuscular plane, between the first and second layers lie the trunks of the medial and lateral plantar nerves and arteries. In the deep neurovascular plane, between the third and fourth layers of the muscles lie the deep branches of the lateral plantar nerve and plantar arch.

Dissection and Identification

1. Make a midline incision 'X' in the skin of the sole from the heel to the tip of the middle toe. Make a transverse incision 'Y' across the roots of the toes (**Fig. 7.1**). Reflect the skin flaps.

2. Using a scalpel, strip the superficial fascia from the deep fascia to which it is firmly attached. Take care not to cut into the plantar aponeurosis (deep fascia). It is difficult to preserve the cutaneous vessels and nerves; however, try to find the digital nerves to the medial side of the big toe and the lateral side of the little toe. These become superficial further proximally than the other plantar digital nerves (**Fig. 7.1**).

3. Make a longitudinal incision through the skin of the plantar surface of each toe and reflect the skin. Find the plantar digital vessels and nerves. Remove the superficial fascia to expose the deep fascia which is thickened here to form the fibrous flexor sheaths enclosing the flexor tendons of the digits.

4. Define the plantar aponeurosis, the thick layer of the plantar fascia in the middle of the sole. Note that the plantar aponeurosis is attached to the calcaneus posteriorly and splits into five

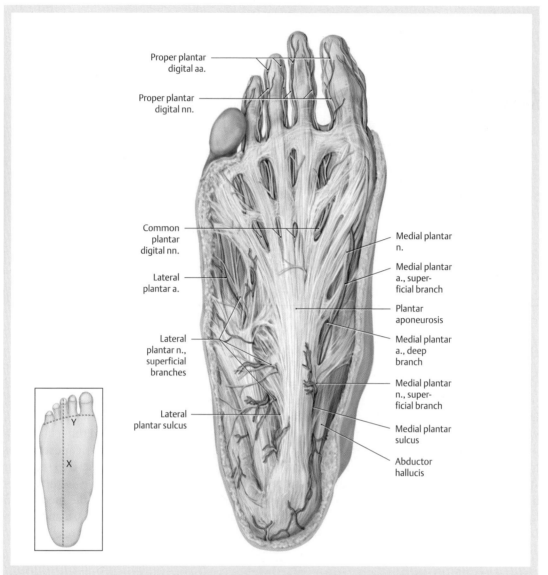

Fig. 7.1 Superficial dissection of the sole of the foot to show plantar aponeurosis. The skin, subcutaneous tissue, and fascia have been removed. (From Schuenke M, Schulte E, Schumacher U. THIEME Atlas of Anatomy. General Anatomy and Musculoskeletal System. Illustrations by Voll M and Wesker K. © Thieme 2020). Figure in the insert shows incisions to be made in the sole.

slips anteriorly, which curve dorsally over the flexor tendons to get attached to the plantar ligaments of the metatarsophalangeal joints.

5. Find the branches of the lateral and medial plantar vessels and nerves in the furrows along the edges of the plantar aponeurosis.

6. Cut across the plantar aponeurosis 3 to 4 cm in front of the heel. Divide the

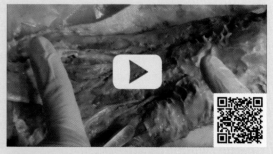

Video 7.1 Sole of foot aponeurosis muscle layers and plantar nerves.

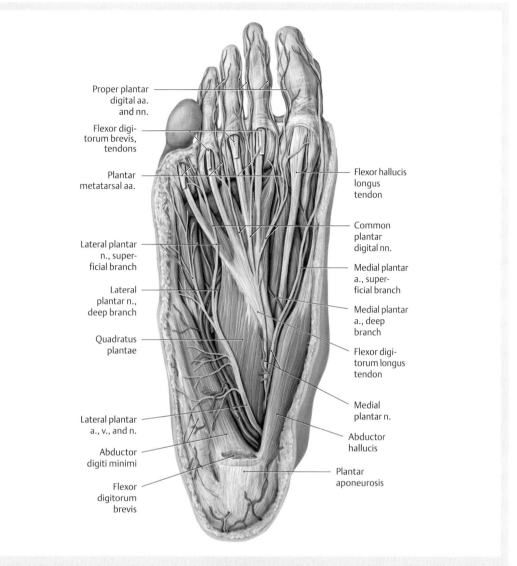

Proper plantar
digital aa.
and nn.

Flexor digi-
torum brevis,
tendons

Plantar
metatarsal aa.

Lateral plantar
n., super-
ficial branch

Lateral
plantar n.,
deep branch

Quadratus
plantae

Lateral plantar
a., v., and n.

Abductor
digiti minimi

Flexor
digitorum
brevis

Flexor hallucis
longus
tendon

Common
plantar
digital nn.

Medial plantar
a., super-
ficial branch

Medial plantar
a., deep
branch

Flexor digi-
torum longus
tendon

Medial
plantar n.

Abductor
hallucis

Plantar
aponeurosis

Fig. 7.2 Superficial dissection of the sole of the foot. The plantar aponeurosis and flexor digitorum brevis have been removed. (From Schuenke M, Schulte E, Schumacher U. THIEME Atlas of Anatomy. General Anatomy and Musculoskeletal System. Illustrations by Voll M and Wesker K. © Thieme 2020)

medial and lateral intermuscular septa passing deeply from the aponeurosis. Lift its part away to expose the flexor digitorum brevis. Remove the deep fascia from the medial and lateral sides of the foot to uncover the other muscles of the first layer of muscles, that is, the abductor hallucis and abductor digiti minimi, respectively (**Fig. 7.2**).

7. Find the medial plantar nerve and vessels between the abductor hallucis and flexor digitorum brevis. Trace the cutaneous branches of the nerve to the medial three-and-a-half toes.

8. Push a probe deep to the abductor hallucis muscle near its attachment to the calcaneus and cut across the muscle over the probe. Turn the muscle medially and this will uncover the greater parts of the medial and lateral plantar arteries and nerves. Find the nerve to the abductor hallucis, a branch of the medial plantar nerve. Remove the connective tissue surrounding the nerve and vessels and trace their branches in continuity with the digital branches already exposed.

9. Detach the abductor hallucis from the flexor retinaculum and cut across the flexor retinaculum and follow the plantar nerves and arteries to their origin from the tibial nerve and posterior tibial artery.

10. Detach the flexor digitorum brevis from its origin from the calcaneus and reflect it forward to trace the lateral plantar nerve and artery toward the lateral aspect of the foot.

11. Identify the tendon of the tibialis posterior, placed most medially deep to the flexor retinaculum and follow it to its insertion on the navicular tuberosity. Follow the tendons of the flexor digitorum longus and flexor hallucis longus into the sole of the foot where they cross each other. Reflect the abductor digitorum minimi from its origin which exposes the flexor accessorius muscle. Note the insertion of the flexor accessorius into the lateral aspect of the tendon of the flexor digitorum longus.

12. Using blunt dissection, remove the connective tissue from the long flexor tendons and identify the four lumbricals taking origin from them and trace the lumbricals to the proximal phalanx and to the extensor expansion. Trace one of the four tendons of the flexor digitorum longus through the fibrous flexor sheath to its insertion on the distal phalanx. Observe that the tendon of the flexor digitorum longus passes through the gap between the two slips of the tendon of the flexor digitorum brevis.

13. Cut across the flexor digitorum longus tendon where it is joined by the flexor accessories and reflect the tendons distally along with the lumbricals. This exposes the three muscles, that is, the flexor hallucis brevis, adductor hallucis, and flexor digiti minimi, forming the third layer of the muscles (**Figs. 7.3** and **7.4**).

14. Note that the flexor hallucis brevis divides into two slips: the medial slip joins the abductor hallucis tendon, while the lateral one joins the adductor hallucis to be inserted to the respective sides of the proximal phalanx. Note the sesamoid bones at their insertion. Observe the transverse and oblique heads of the adductor hallucis muscle.

15. Trace the deep branch of the lateral plantar nerve which arises at the base of the fifth metatarsal bone and crosses the foot on the proximal parts of the metatarsal bones deep to the oblique head of the adductor hallucis.

16. Observe that the lateral plantar artery turns medially and forms the plantar arch. Follow it until it passes deep to the oblique head of the adductor hallucis. Note the metatarsal and digital arteries arising from the plantar arch.

17. Clean the intrinsic muscles that lie deep to the plantar arch and between the metatarsal ligaments. Expose the deep transverse metatarsal ligament by detaching the transverse head of the adductor hallucis from the deep transverse metatarsal ligaments and turn it medially.

18. Insert a probe deep to the flexor digiti minimi and abductor digiti minimi and cut across them above the probe and reflect them to expose the tendon of the peroneus longus.

19. Locate the tendon of the peroneus longus tendon curving around the cuboid bone and pull it. The tendon passes through a groove on the inferior surface of the cuboid which is converted into a tunnel by the long plantar ligament that extends from the calcaneus to the cuboid.

20. Pass a probe along the superficial surface of the peroneus longus through the tunnel and cut the long plantar ligament above the probe. Follow the tendon of the peroneus longus to its insertion on the medial cuneiform bone.

21. Locate the tendon of the tibialis posterior and pull it. Note its main attachment to the navicular bone and its extensions to the other tarsals (except talus) and metatarsal bones.

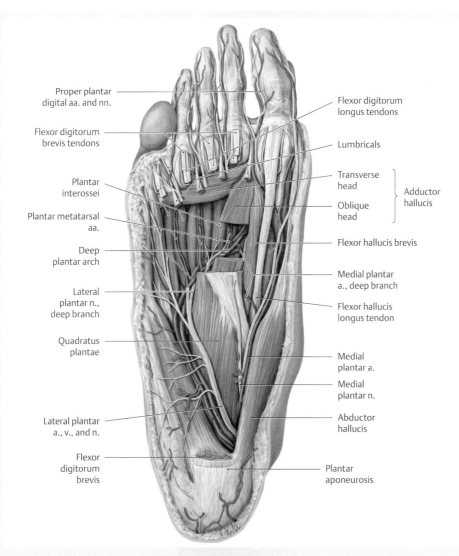

Proper plantar digital aa. and nn.

Flexor digitorum brevis tendons

Plantar interossei

Plantar metatarsal aa.

Deep plantar arch

Lateral plantar n., deep branch

Quadratus plantae

Lateral plantar a., v., and n.

Flexor digitorum brevis

Flexor digitorum longus tendons

Lumbricals

Transverse head ⎫
Oblique head ⎬ Adductor hallucis

Flexor hallucis brevis

Medial plantar a., deep branch

Flexor hallucis longus tendon

Medial plantar a.

Medial plantar n.

Abductor hallucis

Plantar aponeurosis

Fig. 7.3 Deep dissection of the sole of the foot. The flexor digitorum longus is removed. (From Schuenke M, Schulte E, Schumacher U. THIEME Atlas of Anatomy. General Anatomy and Musculoskeletal System. Illustrations by Voll M and Wesker K. © Thieme 2020)

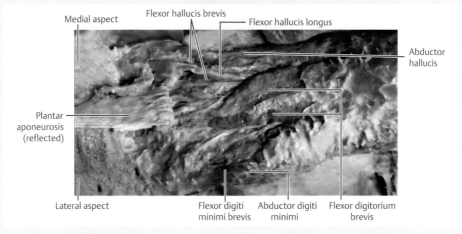

Medial aspect

Flexor hallucis brevis

Flexor hallucis longus

Abductor hallucis

Plantar aponeurosis (reflected)

Lateral aspect

Flexor digiti minimi brevis

Abductor digiti minimi

Flexor digitorium brevis

Fig. 7.4 Layers of the sole.

Muscles of the Sole of the Foot

1. *First muscular layer* of the sole (two abductors and a flexor) (**Fig. 7.5**):
   - Abductor hallucis.
   - Flexor digitorum brevis.
   - Abductor digiti minimi.

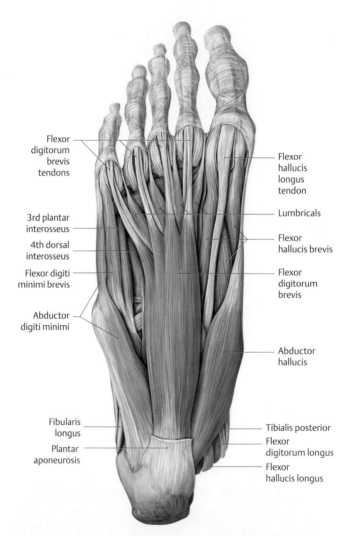

Fig. 7.5   First muscular layer of the sole of the foot. (From Schuenke M, Schulte E, Schumacher U. THIEME Atlas of Anatomy. General Anatomy and Musculoskeletal System. Illustrations by Voll M and Wesker K. © Thieme 2020)

2. *Second muscular layer* of the sole (two tendons of the longus muscles of the toes and two associated muscles) (**Fig. 7.6**):

- Tendon of the flexor digitorum longus.
- Tendon of the flexor hallucis longus.
- Flexor digitorum accessorius (quadratus plantae).
- Four lumbricals.

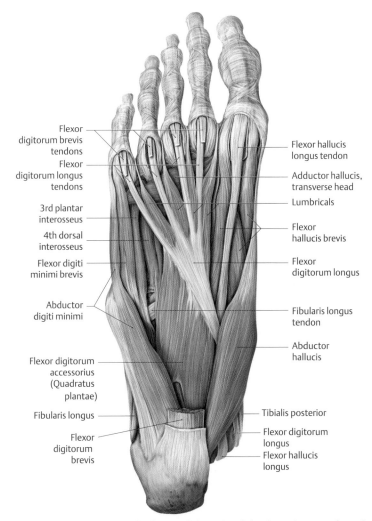

Fig. 7.6 Second muscular layer of the sole of the foot. (From Schuenke M, Schulte E, Schumacher U. THIEME Atlas of Anatomy. General Anatomy and Musculoskeletal System. Illustrations by Voll M and Wesker K. © Thieme 2020)

3. *Third muscular layer* of the sole (two flexors and one adductor) (**Fig. 7.7**):

- Flexor hallucis brevis.
- Flexor digiti minimi brevis.
- Adductor hallucis.

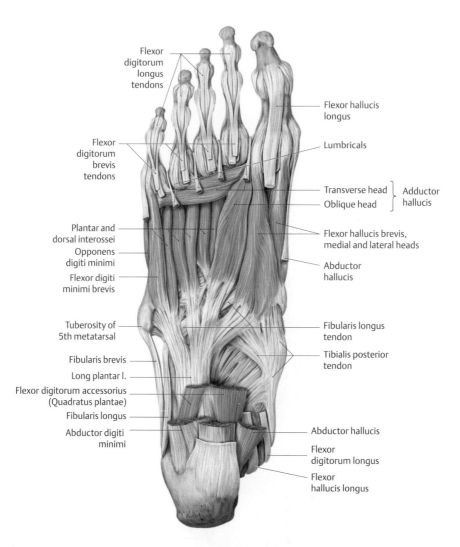

Fig. 7.7   Third muscular layer of the sole of the foot. (From Schuenke M, Schulte E, Schumacher U. THIEME Atlas of Anatomy. General Anatomy and Musculoskeletal System. Illustrations by Voll M and Wesker K. © Thieme 2020)

4. *Fourth muscular layer* of the sole (all interossei) (**Fig. 7.8**):

- Three plantar interossei.
- Four dorsal interossei.

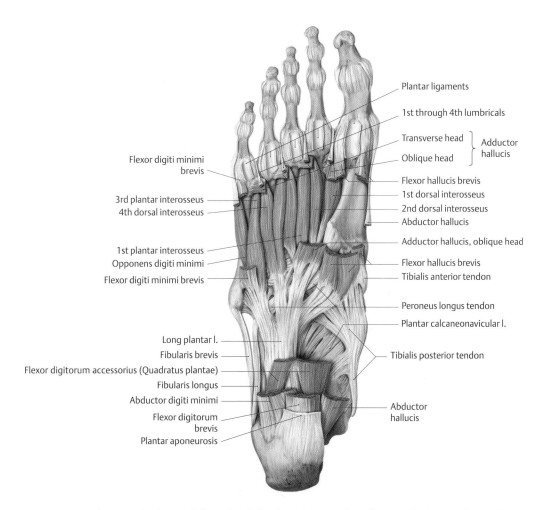

Fig. 7.8   Fourth muscular layer of the sole of the foot. (From Schuenke M, Schulte E, Schumacher U. THIEME Atlas of Anatomy. General Anatomy and Musculoskeletal System. Illustrations by Voll M and Wesker K. © Thieme 2020)

5. Branches of the dorsalis pedis artery:
   - Medial tarsal artery.
   - Lateral tarsal artery.
   - Arcuate artery (gives second to fourth dorsal metatarsal arteries).
   - First dorsal metatarsal artery.

The bony attachments of muscles on the plantar aspect of skeleton of foot are shown in **Fig. 7.9**. Pulsations of the dorsalis pedis artery can be felt between the tendon of the extensor hallucis and tendon of the extensor digitorum longus.

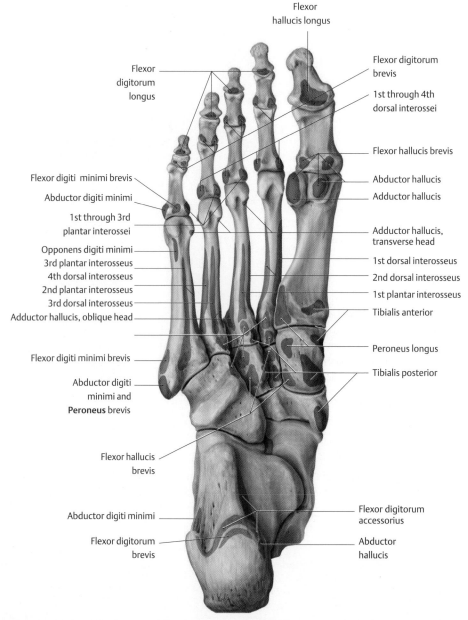

Fig. 7.9   Bony attachments of muscles on the plantar aspect of the skeleton of the foot. (From Schuenke M, Schulte E, Schumacher U. THIEME Atlas of Anatomy. General Anatomy and Musculoskeletal System. Illustrations by Voll M and Wesker K. © Thieme 2020)

Nerves of the Sole of the Foot (Fig. 7.10)

Branches of the Medial Plantar Nerve (Similar to the Median Nerve in the Palm)

Muscular Branches

The muscular branches of medial plantar nerve supply the following four muscles:

1. Abductor hallucis.

2. Flexor hallucis brevis.

3. Flexor digitorum brevis.

4. First lumbrical.

Cutaneous Branches

The cutaneous branches of medial plantar nerve innervate the following regions:

1. Skin of the medial part of the sole.

2. Skin of the plantar surface of the medial three-and-a-half toes.

3. Dorsum of the terminal phalanx including the nail bed of the medial three-and-a-half toes.

4. One proper digital and three common digital branches.

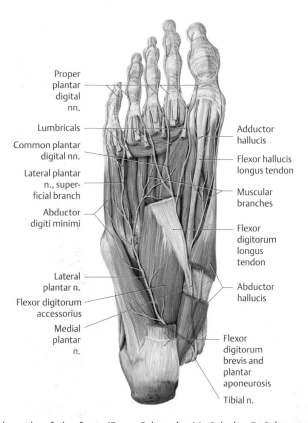

Fig. 7.10   Nerves of the sole of the foot. (From Schuenke M, Schulte E, Schumacher U. THIEME Atlas of Anatomy. General Anatomy and Musculoskeletal System. Illustrations by Voll M and Wesker K. © Thieme 2020)

Branches of the Lateral Plantar Nerve (Similar to the Ulnar Nerve in the Palm)

Muscular branches (supply all the intrinsic muscles of the sole, except the four muscles supplied by the medial plantar nerve, see pg 69):

1. Abductor digiti minimi.
2. Flexor digiti minimi brevis.
3. Flexor digitorum accessorius.
4. Adductor hallucis.
5. All plantar interossei.
6. All dorsal interossei.
7. 2nd, 3rd, and 4th lumbricals.

Cutaneous branches supply lateral 1/3rd of sole and lateral one and half digits including their nail beds.

Arches of the Foot

The skeleton of the foot is arched, both longitudinally and transversely with the concavity directed toward the plantar surface. The arches of the foot are present right from birth, but due to the presence of excessive subcutaneous fat in the sole they are not apparent during infancy and childhood. The presence of arches makes the foot a pliable platform to support the body weight during the standing position.

Functions of the Arches

1. Distribution of body weight to the weight-bearing points.
2. They act as shock absorbers (e.g., during jumping).
3. The concavity of the arches protects underlying vessels and nerves.
4. They help in walking on uneven surfaces.

Classification (Fig. 7.11)

1. Two longitudinal arches:
   - Medial longitudinal arch.
   - Lateral longitudinal arch.
2. Two transverse arches:
   - Posterior (incomplete) transverse arch.
   - Anterior (complete) transverse arch.

Bony Components of the Arches (Fig. 7.11)

Longitudinal arches

1. *Medial longitudinal arch* (medial half of the calcaneus, talus, navicular, three cuneiforms, and three metatarsals).
   - Posterior pillar: Medial tubercle of the calcaneus.

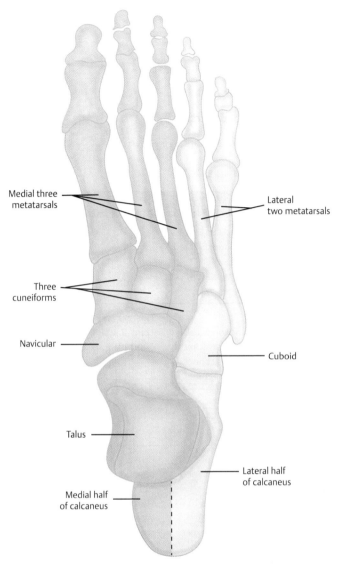

Fig. 7.11 Bones forming longitudinal arches of foot. Medial longitudinal arch (dark color); Lateral longitudinal arch (light color).

- Anterior pillar: Heads of the medial three metatarsals.
- Keystone: Talus.

2. *Lateral longitudinal arch* (lateral half of the calcaneus, cuboid, and lateral two metatarsals).
   - Posterior pillar: Lateral tubercle of the calcaneus.
   - Anterior pillar: Heads of the lateral two metatarsals.
   - Summit: At calcaneocuboid joint.

Transverse Arches

1. *Posterior transverse arch* (is incomplete as its medial end does not touch the ground during standing position). It consists of the following:

   - Bases of the metatarsals, cuboid, and cuneiforms.

2. *Anterior transverse arch* (is complete as its medial and lateral ends touch the ground during standing position). It consists of the following:
   - Heads of the metatarsals.

Factors Maintaining Arches of the Foot

1. Shapes of the bones.

2. Intersegmental ties (connecting adjacent bones).

3. Slings (suspending arch from above).

4. Tie beams (connecting the ends of the arches).

Further details are given in **Table 7.1**.

Table 7.1   Factors maintaining arches of foot

Factors maintaining arches	Medial longitudinal arch	Lateral longitudinal arch	Transverse arches
Shape of the bones	Wedge-shaped cuneiforms with narrow edge directed to the plantar surface Sustentaculum tali supports the head of the talus	–	Wedge-shaped cuneiforms and bases of the middle three metacarpals with narrow edge directed to the plantar surface
Intersegmental ties	Ligaments: Plantar calcaneonavicular Interosseous talocalcaneal Dorsal ligaments connecting the bony components	Ligaments: Long plantar ligament Short plantar ligament	Deep transverse ligaments Transverse and oblique heads of the adductor hallucis
Slings	Tibialis anterior Tibialis posterior Deltoid ligament	Peroneus longus Peroneus brevis	Medially: Tibialis anterior Laterally: Peroneus tertius Peroneus brevis
Tie beams	Medial part of the plantar aponeurosis Abductor hallucis Flexor hallucis brevis Flexor hallucis longus Medial half of the flexor digitorum brevis	Lateral part of the plantar aponeurosis Abductor digiti minimi Flexor digiti minimi Lateral half of the flexor digitorum brevis	Tendons of: Peroneus longus Tibialis posterior

▌Clinical Notes

1. *Pes planus (flat foot)*: Collapse of arches (especially the medial longitudinal) of the foot. It leads to compression of the nerves and vessels in the sole of the foot.

2. *Pes cavus*: Arches (mainly the medial longitudinal) of the foot are exaggerated.

3. *Talipes equinovarus (club foot)*:

   a. It is a congenital deformity.

   b. The foot is plantar flexed, inverted and adducted.

   c. The four primary types are:

   • *Talipes equinus*: The foot is plantar flexed and toes touch the ground.
   • *Talipes calcaneus*: The foot is dorsiflexed and heel touches the ground.
   • *Talipes varus*: The foot is inverted and adducted.
   • *Talipes valgus*: The foot is everted and abducted.

Joints of the Lower Limb

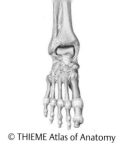

© THIEME Atlas of Anatomy

Introduction

The joints of the lower limb comprise the hip joint, the knee joint, the ankle joint, and the joints of the foot. The classification of the joints of the lower limb is given in **Table 8.1**.

Table 8.1   Classification of the joints of the lower limb

Joint	Type
Hip joint	Ball-and-socket type of synovial joint
Knee joint	Modified hinge type of synovial joint
Superior tibiofibular	Plane type of synovial joint
Intermediate tibiofibular	Syndesmosis
Ankle joint	Hinge type of synovial joint
Inferior tibiofibular	Syndesmosis

Intertarsal joints:
   Subtalar
   Talocalcaneonavicular
   Calcaneocuboid
	
	Plane type of synovial joint
	Ball-and-socket type of synovial joint
	Saddle type of synovial joint

Tarsometatarsal joints	Plane type of synovial joint
Metatarsophalangeal joints	Ellipsoid type of synovial joint
Interphalangeal joints	Hinge type of synovial joint

Hip Joint

Learning Objectives

At the end of the dissection of hip, the student should be able to identify the following:

- Articular surfaces of the hip joint and name their special features which have a bearing on the stability of the joint.
- Attachment of the capsule on the femur and hip bone.
- Iliofemoral, pubofemoral, and ischiofemoral ligaments and note their attachments and describe their functions.
- Movements possible at the hip joint and list the muscles responsible for these movements.

Dissection and Identification

1. Place the cadaver in supine position. Cut the femoral nerve and vessels immediately below the inguinal ligament.

2. Cut the sartorius and rectus femoris approximately 5 cm below their origin and reflect the parts superiorly and inferiorly, respectively.

3. Trace the insertion of the iliopsoas to the lesser trochanter and cut them close to the lesser trochanter. The psoas bursa and the capsule of the hip joint would be exposed.

4. Identify the iliofemoral ligament (**Fig. 8.1**) and note its two thickened bands (lateral and medial) attached to the upper and lower parts of the intertrochanteric line.

5. Cut transversely through the anterior part of the capsule, including the iliofemoral ligament, to open the joint. Abduct and laterally rotate the femur and note the ligament of the head of the femur (ligamentum teres) attached to the fovea on the head of the femur.

6. Cut the ligamentum teres and pull it from the acetabulum. Note the fibrocartilaginous labrum acetabulare attached to the margins of the acetabulum. Identify the acetabular notch along the inferior margin of the acetabulum and note that the notch is bridged across by the transverse ligament.

7. Identify the obturator externus and note that it passes inferior to the neck of the femur. Remove the muscle to expose the pubofemoral ligament.

8. Turn the cadaver to prone position.

9. Detach the piriformis, superior and inferior gemelli, tendon of the obturator internus, and quadratus femoris from the femur to expose the posterior surface of the joint capsule. Identify the ischiofemoral ligament below and behind the acetabulum and passing upward and laterally to fuse with the posterior part of the capsule.

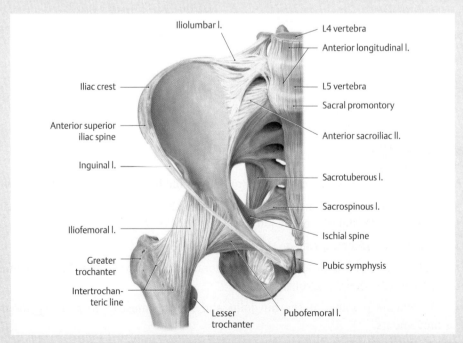

Fig. 8.1 Ligament of the hip joint (anterior view). (From Schuenke M, Schulte E, Schumacher U. THIEME Atlas of Anatomy. General Anatomy and Musculoskeletal System. Illustrations by Voll M and Wesker K. © Thieme 2020)

General Features

1. *Type*: It is a multiaxial ball-and-socket type of synovial joint.

2. *Bones and articular surfaces*: It is formed by the articulation of the head of the femur (ball) with the acetabulum (socket) of the hip bone (**Fig. 8.2**).

3. *Acetabulum labrum*: It is a fibrocartilaginous rim attached to the margin of acetabulum that deepens the articular socket.

Articular Capsule (Fig. 8.3)

1. Articular capsule is attached proximally to the margins of the acetabulum and to the transverse acetabular ligament.

2. It is attached distally to the neck of the femur as follows:
   - Anteriorly to the intertrochanteric line.
   - Posteriorly 1 cm medial to the intertrochanteric line.

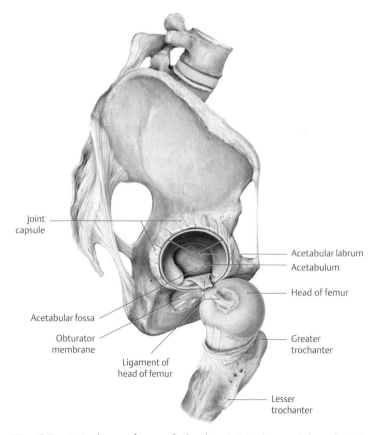

Fig. 8.2 Articular surfaces of the hip joint. (From Schuenke M, Schulte E, Schumacher U. THIEME Atlas of Anatomy. General Anatomy and Musculoskeletal System. Illustrations by Voll M and Wesker K. © Thieme 2020)

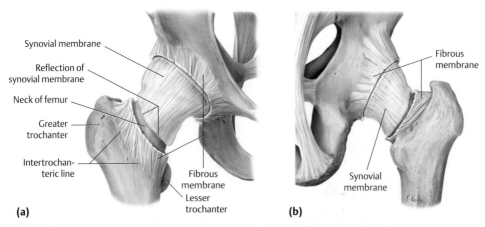

Fig. 8.3 Joint capsule. **(a)** Anterior view. **(b)** Posterior view. (From Schuenke M, Schulte E, Schumacher U. THIEME Atlas of Anatomy. General Anatomy and Musculoskeletal System. Illustrations by Voll M and Wesker K. © Thieme 2020)

Ligaments (Fig. 8.1)

1. *Iliofemoral ligament*: Iliofemoral ligament is an inverted V-shaped ligament that extends from the anterior inferior iliac spine to the intertrochanteric line. It reinforces the capsule anteriorly and resists/prevents hyperextension.

2. *Pubofemoral ligament*: Pubofemoral ligament is a triangular ligament with the base above and the apex below. It reinforces the capsule inferiorly and extends from the iliopubic eminence and obturator crest to the lower part of the neck of the femur. It prevents hyperabduction.

3. *Ischiofemoral ligament*: Ischiofemoral ligament reinforces the capsule posteriorly and extends from the ischium posteroinferior to the acetabulum to the intertrochanteric crest near the base of the greater trochanter.

4. *Ligament of the head of the femur (ligamentum teres or round ligament)*: It is a triangular ligament with its apex attached to the fovea of the head of the femur and the base is attached to the transverse acetabular ligament.

5. *Transverse acetabular ligament*: It bridges the acetabular notch.

Relations (Fig. 8.4)

1. *Anteriorly*: The iliopsoas and pectineus separate the femoral nerve and vessels from the hip joint.

2. *Posteriorly*: Lateral rotators of the hip joint and sciatic nerve.

3. *Superiorly*: Gluteus medius, minimus, and piriformis.

4. *Inferiorly*: Obturator externus.

Movements

1. *Flexion*: Iliopsoas, rectus femoris, and sartorius.

2. *Extension*: Gluteus maximus and hamstring muscles.

3. *Abduction*: Gluteus medius and gluteus minimus.

4. *Adduction*: Adductor longus, adductor fibers of the adductor magnus and adductor brevis.

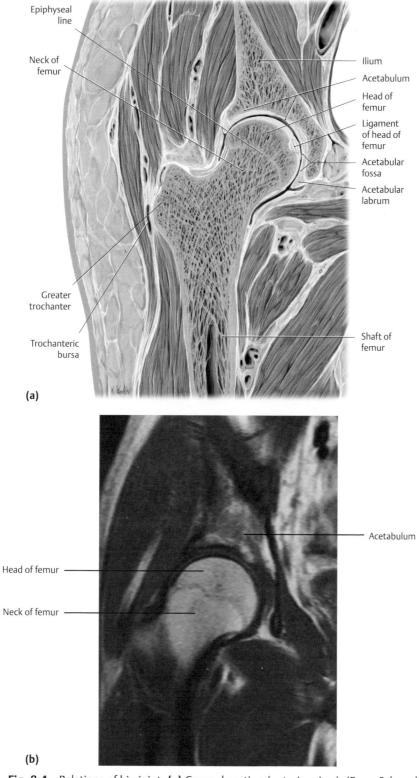

Epiphyseal line

Neck of femur

Ilium

Acetabulum

Head of femur

Ligament of head of femur

Acetabular fossa

Acetabular labrum

Greater trochanter

Trochanteric bursa

Shaft of femur

(a)

Acetabulum

Head of femur

Neck of femur

(b)

Fig. 8.4   Relations of hip joint. **(a)** Coronal section (anterior view). (From Schuenke M, Schulte E, Schumacher U. THIEME Atlas of Anatomy. General Anatomy and Musculoskeletal System. Illustrations by Voll M and Wesker K. © Thieme 2020) **(b)** T1-weighted magnetic resonance imaging (MRI). (From Vahlensieck M, Reiser M. MRI of the musculoskeletal system. 3rd edition Stuttgart: Thieme; 2006)

5. *Lateral rotation*: Piriformis, obturator internus and externus, quadratus femoris, superior and inferior gemelli.

6. *Medial rotation*: Anterior fibers of the gluteus medius, gluteus minimus, and tensor fasciae latae.

Nerve supply: Femoral, obturator, sciatic, and nerve to the obturator externus.

Blood supply: Medial and lateral circumflex femoral, superior, and inferior gluteal and obturator arteries.

Dislocation of the Hip Joint

1. *Congenital dislocation*: The upper margin of the acetabulum is developmentally deficient. Therefore, the head of the femur slips into the gluteal region. The affected limb is shorter in length, and the patient has a lurching gait with a positive Trendelenburg sign.

2. *Acquired posterior dislocation*: This may occur during an automobile accident and is also called the dashboard dislocation. It results in shortening and medial rotation of the lower limb. The sciatic nerve may get injured.

3. *Fracture of the neck of the femur*: This can damage the blood vessels supplying the femoral head resulting in nonunion and avascular necrosis of the head of the femur. Generally, the more proximal the fracture, the greater are its chances of interrupting the vascular supply. It is usually seen in elderly women, especially those who suffer from osteoporosis.

Knee Joint

Learning Objectives

At the end of the dissection of the knee joint, the student should be able to identify the following:

- Articular surfaces of the knee joint.
- Attachment of the capsule on the femur and tibia.
- Medial and lateral collateral ligaments, cruciate ligaments and menisci, their attachments, and describe their functions.
- Movements possible at the knee joint and list the muscles responsible for these movements.
- Mechanism of locking and unlocking of the knee joint.

Dissection and Identification

1. Place the cadaver in supine position. Review the muscles that are closely related to the knee joint.

2. Using a scalpel, detach the tendons of the sartorius, gracilis, and semitendinosus muscles from their attachment on the upper part of the medial surface of the tibia. Reflect the muscles upward and identify the broad flat band of the tibial collateral ligament extending from the medial epicondyle of the femur to the medial surface of the tibia. Note that the deep part of the ligament is attached to the medial meniscus via the capsule.

3. On the lateral side of the knee, cut the tendon of the biceps femoris close to the head of the fibula to expose the cord-like fibular collateral ligament extending from the lateral epicondyle of the femur to the head of the fibula. Note that it is separated from the capsule by the fatty tissue in which the inferior lateral genicular vessels run.

4. Cut transversely the tendon of the quadriceps femoris just above the patella and extend the incisions inferiorly around the patella to the tibia passing 2 to 3 cm on either side of the ligamentum patellae. Turn the patella along with the ligamentum patellae downward to expose the cavity of the knee joint. Lift the tendon of the quadriceps femoris upward and note that the cavity of the joint is continuous with the suprapatellar bursa present deep to the quadriceps femoris. Note that at the upper end of the bursa, the fibers of the vastus intermedius (articularis genu) are inserted into it (**Fig. 8.5; Video 8.1**).

5. Examine the infrapatellar and alar folds of the synovial membrane and the infrapatellar pad of fat (**Fig. 8.6**). Remove the infrapatellar fold and pad of fat. Flex and extend the knee joint and examine the anterior and posterior cruciate ligaments crossing each other like the letter X. Observe the medial and lateral menisci which are C-shaped fibrocartilaginous plates on the articular surface of the tibial condyles (**Video 8.2**).

6. Place the cadaver in a prone position. Remove the popliteal vessels, tibial, and common peroneal nerves from the posterior surface of the knee. Cut the semimembranosus muscle close to its attachment to the posterior surface of the medial condyle of the tibia. Observe the oblique popliteal ligament passing upward and laterally from the attachment of the semimembranosus. Using blunt forceps separate the two heads of the gastrocnemius and plantaris from the capsule and detach them from their attachment on the femur.

7. Follow the tendon of the popliteus muscle and note that it lies between the lateral meniscus and the fibrous capsule. Note the arcuate ligament, the fibers which arch over the aperture for the popliteus muscle in the fibrous capsule. Cut the tendon of the popliteus and turn the muscle downward and medially. As you do this, the posterior wall of the joint capsule will be opened. Remove the remnants of the posterior wall of the joint capsule to expose the joint cavity and identify the posterior cruciate ligament.

8. Again, place the cadaver in the supine position. To obtain a clear view of the articulate surfaces of the femur and tibia and the menisci, cut the cruciate ligaments close to their attachment on the intercondylar area of the femur, incise the fibular collateral ligaments, and flex the joint to observe the details.

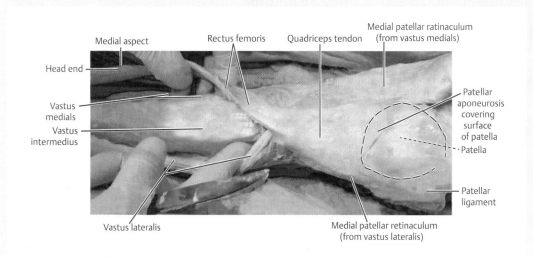

Fig. 8.5   Quadriceps tendon right knee.

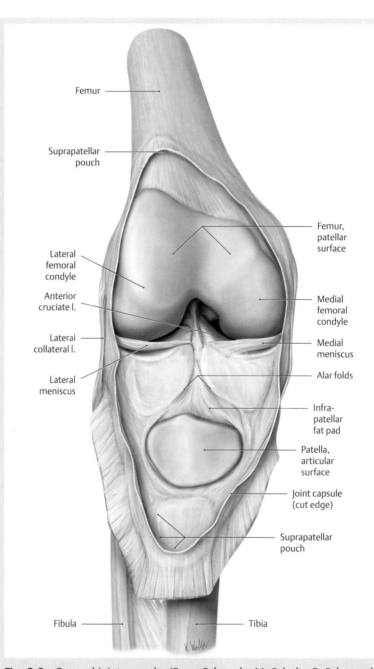

Femur

Suprapatellar pouch

Femur, patellar surface

Lateral femoral condyle

Medial femoral condyle

Anterior cruciate l.

Medial meniscus

Lateral collateral l.

Alar folds

Lateral meniscus

Infra-patellar fat pad

Patella, articular surface

Joint capsule (cut edge)

Suprapatellar pouch

Fibula

Tibia

Fig. 8.6 Opened joint capsule. (From Schuenke M, Schulte E, Schumacher U. THIEME Atlas of Anatomy. General Anatomy and Musculoskeletal System. Illustrations by Voll M and Wesker K. © Thieme 2020)

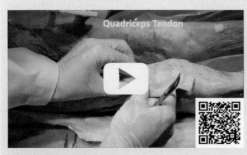

Video 8.1 Knee—Part 1.

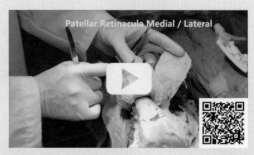

Video 8.2 Knee—Part 2.

General Features

The knee joint is the largest joint of the body. It is a compound (more than two bones articulate) and complex (joint cavity is divided into two compartments, meniscofemoral and meniscotibial) joint.

Type: It is a condylar (modified hinge) type of synovial joint.

Articular surfaces: Femoral and tibial condyles and patella.

Articular capsule: It is thin and incomplete anteriorly. It is attached to the femoral and tibial condyles and the patella and patellar ligament.

Ligaments (Figs. 8.7 and 8.8)

Extracapsular ligaments:

1. *Ligamentum patellae*: Extends from the apex of the patella to the tibial tuberosity.
2. *Tibial collateral ligament*: Has superficial and deep parts. Both the parts are attached to the medial epicondyle of the femur above. The superficial part is attached to the medial condyle and the upper part of the medial border to the tibia. Deep part blends with the fibrous capsule and is attached to the medial meniscus.
3. *Fibular collateral ligament*: Extends as a fibrous cord from the lateral epicondyle of the femur to the head of the fibula.
4. *Oblique popliteal ligament*: Extends from the medial condyle of the tibia to the lateral part of the intercondylar line of the femur.

Intracapsular ligaments: They are intracapsular but extrasynovial (**Fig. 8.9**).

1. *Anterior cruciate ligament*:
   - It is attached below to the anterior part of the intercondylar area of the tibia.
   - It passes upward, backward, and laterally.
   - It is attached above to the medial surface of the lateral condyle of the femur.
   - It is taut during extension and prevents hyperextension of the knee joint.
2. *Posterior cruciate ligament*:
   - It is attached below to the posterior part of the intercondylar area of the tibia.
   - It passes upward, forward, and medially.
   - It is attached above to the lateral surface of the medial condyle of the femur.
   - It is taut during flexion and prevents hyperflexion of the knee joint.
3. *Medial and lateral menisci*:
   - They act as shock absorbers and lubricate the articular surfaces by distributing the synovial fluid.
   - They are semilunar plates of rubbery fibrocartilage. The medial meniscus is "C" shaped and the lateral is "O" shaped.
   - The medial meniscus is attached to the tibial collateral ligament and the lateral meniscus is attached to the popliteus, which separates it from the fibular collateral ligament.

The medial meniscus is more prone to injury than the lateral meniscus as its movement is restricted because of its attachment to the tibial collateral ligament, whereas the medial fibers of the popliteus attached to the lateral meniscus pull it backward and prevent it from being trapped between the articular surfaces.

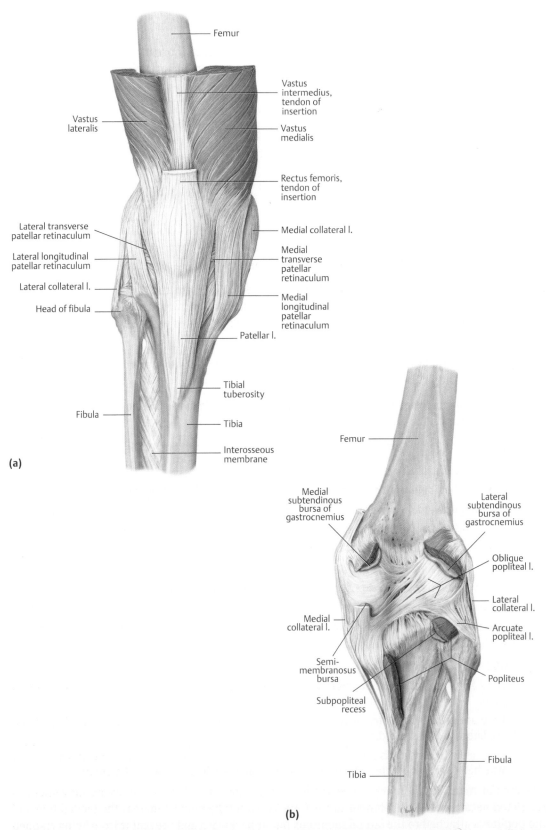

Fig. 8.7 Ligaments of the knee joint. **(a)** Anterior view. **(b)** Posterior view. (From Schuenke M, Schulte E, Schumacher U. THIEME Atlas of Anatomy. General Anatomy and Musculoskeletal System. Illustrations by Voll M and Wesker K. © Thieme 2020)

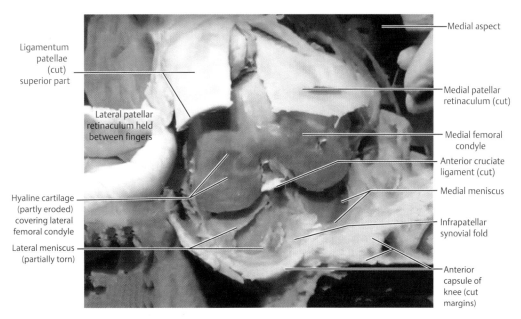

Fig. 8.8 Interior of right knee joint.

Movements

1. *Extension*: Quadriceps femoris and tensor fasciae latae.

2. *Flexion*: Semimembranosus, semitendinosus, biceps femoris, sartorius, gracilis, and popliteus.

3. *Medial rotation*: Semitendinosus, semimembranosus, sartorius, gracilis, and popliteus.

4. *Lateral rotation*: Biceps femoris.

Locking of the knee joint: The lateral femoral condyle is smaller than the medial femoral condyle. As the knee is extended, the smaller condyle moves through its arc before the medial condyle which continues to move further posteriorly. This movement results in a medial rotation of the femur. Therefore, at the end of extension, there is a slight medial rotation, which makes all the ligaments tightened and the joint move in a close-packed position called the *locking of the knee joint*.

Unlocking of the knee joint: In the beginning of flexion of the knee joint, there is either lateral rotation of the femur (foot on the ground) or medial rotation of the tibia (foot off the ground) to unlock the knee joint from its tight-packed position. This is done by the popliteus muscle which is, therefore, also known as the key muscle of the knee joint.

Bursae around the knee joint:

1. *Suprapatellar bursa*: It lies deep to the quadriceps femoris and communicates with the knee joint cavity.

2. *Subcutaneous prepatellar bursa*: It lies superficial to the lower part of the patella and upper half of the ligamentum patellae. Housemaid's knee: It is an inflammation of the subcutaneous prepatellar bursa.

3. *Subcutaneous infrapatellar bursa*: It lies between the skin and lower half of the ligamentum patellae. Clergyman's knee: It is an inflammation of the subcutaneous infrapatellar bursa.

4. *Deep infrapatellar bursa*: It lies deep to the ligamentum patellae.

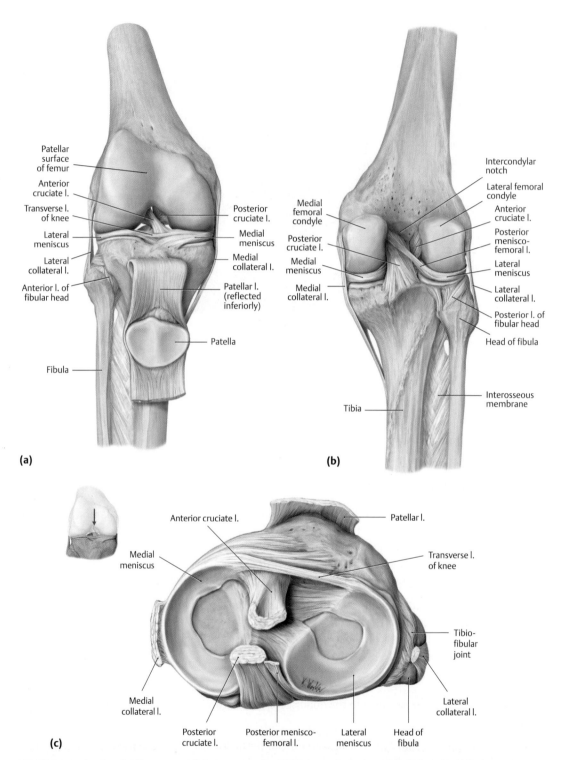

Fig. 8.9   Intracapsular ligaments. **(a)** Anterior view. **(b)** Posterior view. **(c)** Right tibial plateau (proximal view). (From Schuenke M, Schulte E, Schumacher U. THIEME Atlas of Anatomy. General Anatomy and Musculoskeletal System. Illustrations by Voll M and Wesker K. © Thieme 2020)

Blood and nerve supply:

Blood supply: By anastomosis around the knee joint which is formed by the following:

1. Five genicular branches of the popliteal artery.

2. Descending genicular branch of the femoral artery.

3. Descending branch of the lateral circumflex femoral artery.

4. Anterior and posterior recurrent branches of the anterior tibial artery.

5. Circumflex fibular branch of the posterior tibial artery.

Nerve supply: By the femoral, obturator, tibial, and common peroneal nerves. The femoral and obturator nerves supply both the hip and knee joints; therefore, pain in one joint is referred to the other.

▌Clinical Note

Meniscal Tear: The medial meniscus is more prone to injury (tear) than the lateral meniscus as its movement is restricted because of its attachment to the tibial collateral ligament, whereas the medial fibers of the popliteus attached to the lateral meniscus pull it backward and prevent it from being trapped between the articular surfaces. This injury commonly occurs in football players.

Ankle Joint

Learning Objectives

At the end of the dissection of ankle joint, the student should be able to:

- Describe the articular surfaces of the ankle joint and mark the attachment of the capsule on the tibia, fibula, and talus.

- Identify the deltoid, lateral collateral, plantar calcaneonavicular ligaments, and note their attachments and describe their functions.

- Discuss the movements possible at the ankle joint and list the muscles responsible for these movements.

Dissection and Identification

1. Remove the remains of the extensor retinacula. Cut vessels and nerves that cross the anterior aspect of the ankle and reflect the tendons. Observe the anterior part of the fibrous capsule, which is thin and can be easily damaged.

2. On the medial side of the ankle, retract the tendon of the tibialis muscle anteriorly and cut and reflect the tendons of the flexor digitorum longus and flexor hallucis longus. Clean and define the triangular deltoid ligament (medial ligament) with its blunt apex attached to the margins of the medial malleolus and base attached to the sustentaculum tali of the calcaneus, medial surface and neck of the talus, plantar calcaneonavicular (spring) ligament, and navicular bone.

3. On the lateral side, cut open the peroneal retinacula. Retract the tendons of the peroneus longus and brevis anteriorly and clean and define the lateral ligament of the ankle. Observe the three bands of the ligament, that is, the anterior talofibular, calcaneofibular, and posterior talofibular.

General Features (Fig. 8.10)

Type: Hinge type of synovial joint.

Articular surfaces: The distal ends of the tibia and fibula superiorly and the trochlea of the talus inferiorly.

The Inferior aspect of distal end of tibia with medial and lateral malleolus form *tibio-fibular mortise*.

Articular capsule: It is thin anteriorly and posteriorly to allow movements. It is reinforced medially by the deltoid ligament and laterally by the lateral ligament.

Ligaments (Fig. 8.10; Video 8.3)

1. Medial (deltoid) ligament (**Fig. 8.10a–c**):
   - It is a strong triangular ligament on the medial side of the ankle.
   - It extends from the medial malleolus to the navicular, talus, and calcaneus.
   - It is divided into superficial and deep parts.
   - The superficial part is further subdivided into three parts: tibionavicular, tibiocalcanean, and posterior tibiotalar.
   - The deep part comprises the anterior tibiotalar.
   - It prevents overeversion of the foot and helps maintain the medial longitudinal arch.
2. Lateral ligament (**Fig. 8.10d**):
   - It extends from the lateral malleolus to the calcaneus and talus.
   - It is divided into three parts: anterior talofibular, posterior talofibular, and calcaneofibular.

Movements

1. Dorsiflexion:
   - The angle between the leg and the foot decreases.
   - It is the close-packed position (stable position) of the ankle joint.

Muscles responsible: The tibialis anterior, extensor hallucis longus, extensor digitorum longus, and peroneus tertius.

2. Plantar flexion:
   - The angle between the leg and the foot increases.
   - It is the loose-packed position (unstable position) of the ankle joint.

Muscles responsible: The gastrocnemius, soleus, tibialis posterior, flexor hallucis longus, and flexor digitorum longus.

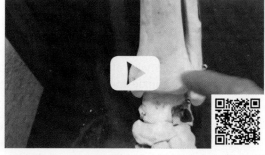

Video 8.3 Ankle joint/Talocrural joint (movements and axis).

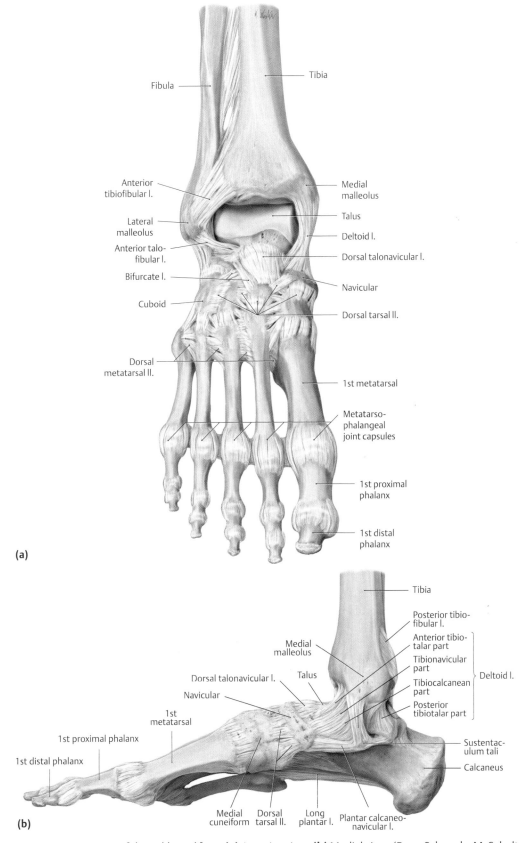

Fig. 8.10   Ligaments of the ankle and foot. **(a)** Anterior view. **(b)** Medial view. (From Schuenke M, Schulte E, Schumacher U. THIEME Atlas of Anatomy. General Anatomy and Musculoskeletal System. Illustrations by Voll M and Wesker K. © Thieme 2020) *(Continued)*

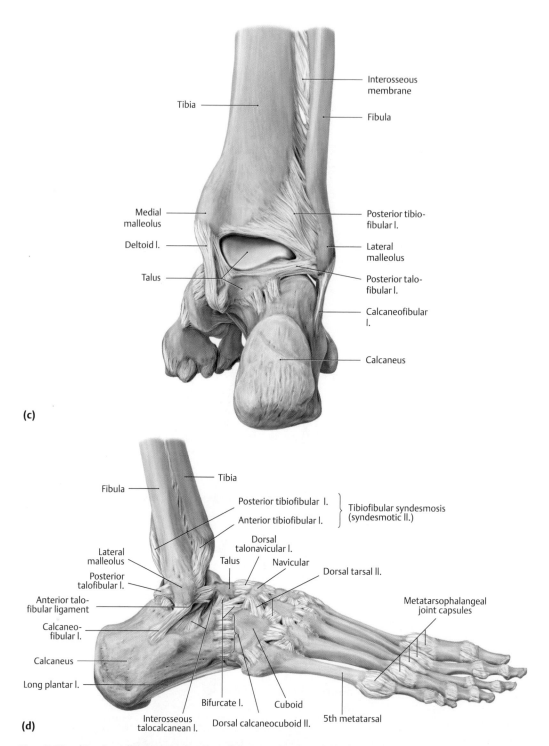

Fig. 8.10 *(Continued)* **(c)** Posterior view. **(d)** Lateral view. (From Schuenke M, Schulte E, Schumacher U. THIEME Atlas of Anatomy. General Anatomy and Musculoskeletal System. Illustrations by Voll M and Wesker K. © Thieme 2020)

■ Clinical Notes

1. *Ankle sprains*: They occur due to injury to the medial/lateral ligaments because of excessive eversion/inversion, respectively. Inversion type of lateral ligament injuries are about 85%.

2. *Pott fracture*: It occurs when the foot is everted forcibly when caught in a hole. It may result in:

   a. Torn deltoid ligament.

   b. Oblique fracture of the lower end of the fibula.

   c. Fracture of the medial malleolus.

   d. Fracture of the posterior margin of the lower end of the tibia.

Joints of the Foot

The joints of the foot involve tarsals, metatarsals, and phalanges (see **Table 8.1**).

Learning Objectives

At the end of the dissection, students should be able to:

- Describe the articular surfaces of the subtalar and calcaneocuboid joints.
- Identify the bifurcate, cervical, long and short plantar ligaments, and note their attachments.
- Discuss the inversion and eversion movements and name the muscles responsible for these movements.
- Describe the medial and lateral longitudinal arches and the transverse arches of the foot and list the factors which maintain these arches.

Dissection and Identification

1. Remove the muscles and tendons from the tarsal and metatarsal bones and note the important ligaments on the dorsal and plantar surfaces.

2. On the dorsal surface, clean and identify the calcaneonavicular and calcaneocuboid parts of the bifurcate ligament extending from the superior surface of the calcaneus to the navicular and cuboid bone, respectively.

3. Place the cadaver in the prone position. Inferomedially, examine the thick plantar calcaneonavicular (spring) ligament extending from the sustentaculum tali to the plantar surface of the navicular bone. Cut the spring ligament and open the subtalar joint to examine the interosseous ligament that extends between the talus and calcaneus.

4. Clean and define the margins of the long plantar ligament extending from the plantar surface of the calcaneus in front of the tuberosity to the lips of the groove on the cuboid for the tendon of the peroneus longus. Separate it from the underlying short plantar (calcaneocuboid) ligament by placing a probe between them. Detach the long plantar ligament from its attachment on the calcaneus to expose the short plantar ligament, which spans the calcaneocuboid joint and is attached close to it.

General Features

Following text deals with the general features of the joints of the foot (**Video 8.4**).

Subtalar joint (**Fig. 8.11**):

1. *Type*: Plane synovial joint.

2. *Articular surfaces*: The inferior surface of the talus and superior surface of the calcaneus.

3. *Ligaments*: The lateral and medial talocalcaneal, interosseous talocalcaneal, and cervical.

Talocalcaneonavicular joint:

1. *Type*: Ball-and-socket type of synovial joint.

2. *Articular surfaces*: The head of the talus fits into the socket formed by the calcaneus, navicular, and spring ligaments.

3. *Ligaments*: The plantar calcaneonavicular ligament (spring ligament) and the calcaneonavicular part of the bifurcate ligament.

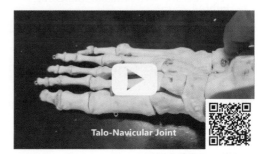

Video 8.4   Joints of foot.

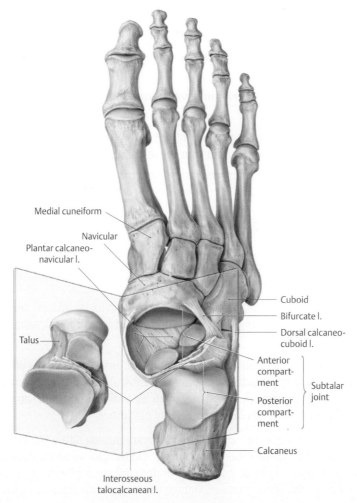

Fig. 8.11   Joints of the foot: subtalar joint and ligaments. (From Schuenke M, Schulte E, Schumacher U. THIEME Atlas of Anatomy. General Anatomy and Musculoskeletal System. Illustrations by Voll M and Wesker K. © Thieme 2020)

Calcaneocuboid joint (**Fig. 8.12**):

1. *Type*: Saddle type of synovial joint.

2. *Articular surfaces*: Reciprocally concavoconvex surfaces of the calcaneus and cuboid.

3. *Ligaments*: The calcaneocuboid part of the bifurcate ligament and long and short plantar ligaments.

Transverse talar joint (**Fig. 8.12**):

1. Collective term used for the talonavicular part of the talocalcaneonavicular joint and calcaneocuboid joint.

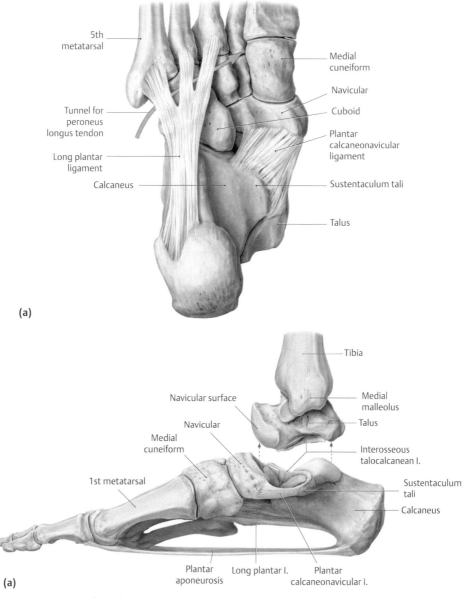

(a)

(a)

Fig. 8.12 Joints of the foot. **(a)** Plantar view. **(b)** Medial view. (From Schuenke M, Schulte E, Schumacher U. THIEME Atlas of Anatomy. General Anatomy and Musculoskeletal System. Illustrations by Voll M and Wesker K. © Thieme 2020)

Movements occurring at the subtalar and intertarsal joints:

1. Inversion.
   - The medial border of the foot is raised so that the sole faces medially.
   - *Muscles responsible*: The tibialis anterior, tibialis posterior, flexor hallucis longus, and flexor digitorum longus.
2. Eversion.
   - The lateral border of the foot is raised so that the sole faces laterally.
   - *Muscles responsible*: The peroneus longus, peroneus brevis, and peroneus tertius.
3. *Axis of movement*: Passes obliquely from the back of the calcaneus through the sinus tarsi to the neck of the talus.

▊ Clinical Notes

1. *Claw toes*: It is a clinical condition characterized by hyperextension of metatarsophalangeal joints and flexion of distal interphalangeal joints.

2. *Loss of inversion and eversion*: The important tarsal joints are subtalar and transverse tarsal joint (calcaneocuboid and talonavicular). These joints play an important role in inversion and eversion of the foot. Any derangement of these movements leads to difficulty on the sloping surface.

Introduction and Overview of the Bones of the Abdomen

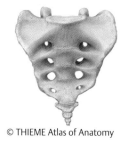

© THIEME Atlas of Anatomy

Introduction

Before students begin dissection, it is important for them to know the position of the abdomen in relation to other parts of the body. The abdomen is the lower part of the trunk which lies below the thorax. Its cavity is called the abdominal cavity. It is much more extensive than what it appears from the outside. It extends upward deep to the costal margin up to the diaphragm, and thus, it lies deep to lower parts of thoracic cage, pleura, and lungs but separated from them by a dome-shaped muscular diaphragm. The abdominal contents reach up to the T8 vertebra in the median plane and fifth rib in midclavicular line downward within the bony pelvis. The plane of the pelvic inlet/pelvic brim is used as a landmark to divide the abdominal cavity into a larger upper part, that is the abdominal cavity proper, and a smaller lower part, that is pelvic cavity. It is important to note that these two parts functionally and developmentally form a single unit.

The part of serous membrane lining the inner aspect of the abdominal wall is called parietal peritoneum, while the part which covers the viscera is called visceral peritoneum. The two parts are continuous with each other. The space between these two layers is called the peritoneal cavity, which is a potential space and contains a thin film of fluid for lubrication of serous membrane. This permits varying degrees of freedom for movement of the abdominal and pelvic viscera. Due to the overlapping of the abdominal cavity above by thoracic cage and below by gluteal regions, the penetrating wounds of these regions frequently inflict wounds to the abdominopelvic viscera.

Since the mobile muscular diaphragm forms the upper limit of the abdominal cavity, the abdominal viscera descend with it during inspiration. This is used by the clinicians during physical examinations of the abdominal organs.

Bones

The bones of the abdomen and pelvis comprise lower ribs and costal cartilages, lumbar vertebrae, sacrum, coccyx, and hip bones.

Lower Ribs and Costal Cartilages

They are 12 pairs of ribs. The anterior ends of ribs are attached with bar of hyaline cartilage called costal cartilages. They are described in Chapter 12, Vol. I. The costal cartilages of 7th to 10th ribs articulate with each other to form *costal margin*. The 11th and 12th ribs differ from the remainder, in that they are shorter and do not articulate anteriorly with adjacent cartilages. Thus, their anterior ends remain free and for this reason, they are able to move independently of other ribs and, hence, are termed as *floating ribs*.

Lumbar Vertebrae

The five lumbar vertebrae are the largest vertebrae and do not possess facets for articulation with the ribs. They are more massive in keeping with the greater load which they have to transmit. They are easily identified by their heavy bodies and blunt hatchet-shaped spinous processes (seen in profile view) for the attachment of powerful back muscles. The body of L5 is much deeper anteriorly than posteriorly (**Fig. 9.1**). This helps produce a *lumbosacral angle* with the wedge-shaped *lumbosacral intervertebral disc.*

The pedicles are thick and project backward from the upper two-thirds of the posterolateral surfaces of the body, superior to a deep inferior vertebral notch; as a result, inferior vertebral notches are much deeper than the superior ones. The pedicles join relatively narrow, short, and broad plates of laminae which pass downward and backward to meet in a thick rectangular spine. The quadrilateral spine projects backward posterior to the lower two-thirds of the vertebral body. The laminae and pedicles surround a large, triangular vertebral foramina which is larger than that of the thoracic vertebrae and smaller than that of the cervical vertebrae.

The articular processes are distinctive in the sense that the superior articular processes are directed medially instead of superiorly and inferior articular processes are directed laterally instead of inferiorly. The inferior articular processes project inferiorly from the laminae with a V-shaped gap between them which is wider in the lower than the upper lumbar vertebrae. The interlocking of the articular processes effectively prevents rotation. When two adjacent lumbar vertebrae are articulated, the V-shaped gap exists between the laminae. This deficiency in the posterior wall of the vertebral canal is filled by the ligamentum flava through which a needle is introduced into the lumbar vertebral canal during lumbar puncture. This gap is further increased by the forward bending of the vertebral column.

The transverse processes are thin and tapering in the upper lumbar vertebrae, but thicker in the fourth and fifth. In the fifth, the bases of these processes extend forward on the vertebral body, further thickening the pedicles. In an articulated vertebral column, the lumbar transverse processes are seen to lie in series with the ribs. Embryologically they represent lumbar ribs fused to the vertebrae. The posterolateral aspect of true lumbar transverse process near its base presents a small rough elevation, the accessory process. The rounded mammillary process projects posteriorly from the superior articular process. The accessory and mammillary processes give attachment to the erector spinae muscle (**Fig. 9.1**).

Sacrum

It is a wedge-shaped bone consisting of five fused sacral vertebrae. The sacrum together with the two hip bones and the coccyx forms the skeleton of the pelvis. It is functionally adapted to provide a strong foundation to the pelvic girdle. The sacrum is concave anteriorly. The bodies of the sacral vertebrae are separated on the pelvic surface by the transverse ridges which have the remnants of intervertebral discs deep to them. The sacral canal is the continuation of vertebral canal in the sacrum. It communicates posteriorly with a dorsal/posterior sacral foramina and anteriorly with pelvic/anterior sacral intervertebral foramen which leads into the sacral canal. The tubular sacral canal is continuous with the vertebral canal posterior to the sacral foramina. It contains the caudal parts of the meninges (dura, arachnoid, and pia mater) of the central nervous system and transmits the sacral nerves; in addition, it also transmits the branches of the internal vertebral venous plexus to the sacral intervertebral foramina. Here the sacral nerves divide into ventral and dorsal rami, which emerge through the pelvic and dorsal foramina, respectively (**Fig. 9.2**).

The sacrum is wedge-shaped superoinferiorly and anteroposteriorly. Its broad base lies anterosuperiorly at the lumbosacral angle. Here the anterior margin of the superior surface of the first sacral vertebral body forms the promontory. It is an important obstetric landmark for pelvic measurements. The concave pelvic surface of the sacrum forms the posterior wall of the lesser pelvis and ends in a blunt apex which articulates with the coccyx.

The dorsal surface of the sacrum shows five longitudinal crests (e.g., median, intermediate, and lateral). The median sacral crest is formed by the fusion of the upper three or four sacral spines. The spine and corresponding laminae of the fifth vertebrae fail to fuse and produce the sacral hiatus—a dorsal opening into the lower part of the sacral canal. The hiatus is of variable length. The intermediate crests are formed by the fusion of articular processes on either side of median crest and medial to

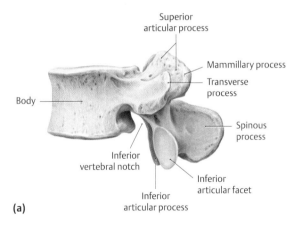

(a)

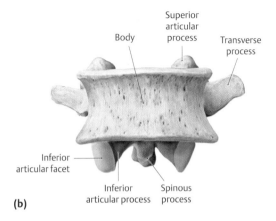

(b)

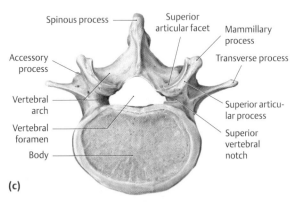

(c)

Fig. 9.1 Typical lumbar vertebra. **(a)** Left lateral view. **(b)** Anterior view. **(c)** Superior view. (From Schuenke M, Schulte E, Schumacher U. THIEME Atlas of Anatomy. General Anatomy and Musculoskeletal System. Illustrations by Voll M and Wesker K. © Thieme 2020)

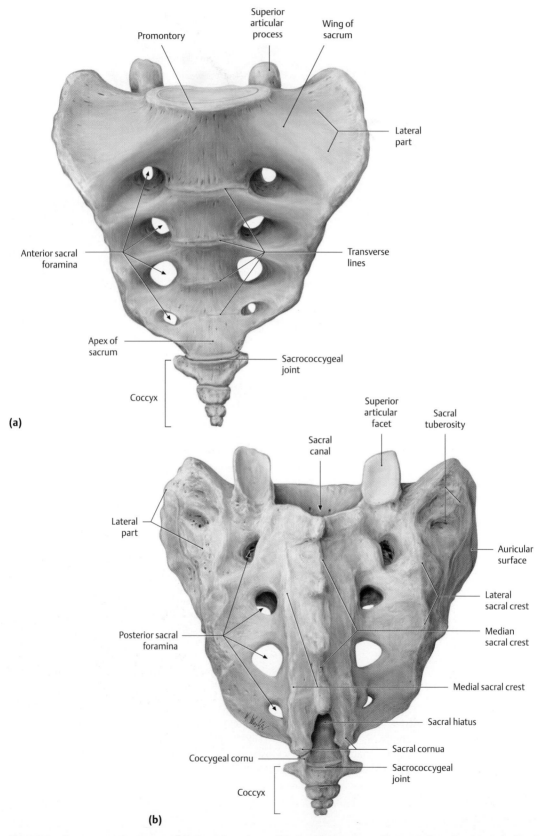

Fig. 9.2 Sacrum and coccyx. **(a)** Anterior view. **(b)** Posterior view. (From Schuenke M, Schulte E, Schumacher U. THIEME Atlas of Anatomy. General Anatomy and Musculoskeletal System. Illustrations by Voll M and Wesker K. © Thieme 2020)

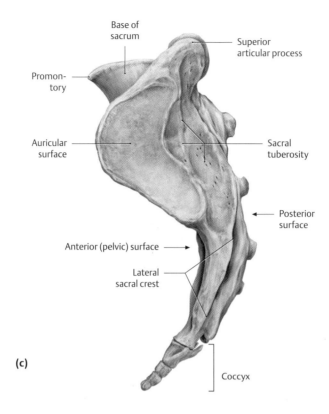

Base of
sacrum

Superior
articular process

Promon-
tory

Auricular
surface

Sacral
tuberosity

Posterior
surface

Anterior (pelvic) surface

Lateral
sacral crest

(c)

Coccyx

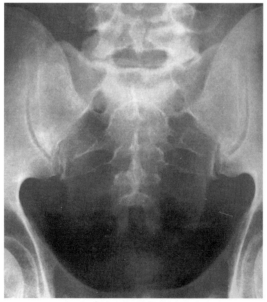

(d)

Fig. 9.2 Sacrum and coccyx. **(c)** Left lateral view. (From Schuenke M, Schulte E, Schumacher U. THIEME Atlas of Anatomy. General Anatomy and Musculoskeletal System. Illustrations by Voll M and Wesker K. © Thieme 2020) **(d)** Radiograph of sacrum (anteroposterior view).

the dorsal sacral foramina. The lateral crest lateral to dorsal sacral foramina on either side is formed by the fusion of processes of the sacral vertebrae. The upper wider part of the lateral surface of sacrum formed by the vertebrae carries L-shaped articular surfaces for articulation with the corresponding surfaces of the iliac bones with which they articulate to form sacroiliac joints. On the sacrum, the rough areas (tuberosities) posterior to the auricular surfaces are joined with the corresponding ilium by a slope upward and medially are wedged between the hip bones and slung from them by ligaments. The weight of the body transmitted to the sacrum tends to drive it downward. This prevents the tightening of the posterior sacroiliac ligaments which draw the two hip bones firmly against the sacrum, increasing the rigidity of the sacroiliac joints by tight fitting of their irregular surfaces.

The large transverse process of the fifth lumbar vertebra may sometimes be fused to the lateral part of the sacrum unilaterally or bilaterally, leading to a clinical condition called sacralization of the fifth lumbar vertebra. On the other hand, the first sacral vertebra may be partly or completely separated from the remainder of the sacrum, leading to a condition called lumbarization.

Coccyx

The coccyx is also called tail bone. It is composed of four or five fused coccygeal vertebrae. This bone is triangular in shape. Its upper surface articulates with the apex of sacrum. The tip of coccyx lies at the level of the upper border of the symphysis. During clinical examination, the coccyx is palpable in the depth of natal cleft (**Fig. 9.2**).

Hip Bone

It is described in detail on pages 2,3, and 4 in, Chapter 1.

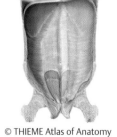
Introduction

The anterior abdominal wall is a soft musculoaponeurotic structure confined to the anterolateral aspects of the abdomen. It consists of nine layers from superficial to deep. These are skin Camper's fascia, Scarpa's fascia (two layers of superficial fascia in the lower part of abdomen), external oblique muscle, internal oblique muscle, transversus abdominis muscle, fascia transversalis, extraperitoneal tissue, and parietal peritoneum).

Surface Landmarks (Figs. 10.1 and 10.2)

1. Xiphoid process forms the upper limit of the anterior abdominal wall in the midline and lies in the subcostal angle.

2. Costal margin on either side of xiphoid process is formed by the fusion of 7th to 10th costal cartilages.

3. Iliac crest can be felt at the lateral end of the lower limit of anterior abdominal wall and can be traced forward to the anterior superior iliac spine.

4. Pubic symphysis forms the lower limit of the anterior abdominal wall in the midline.

5. Inguinal fold extends between anterior superior iliac spine and pubic tubercle. Deep to it lies inguinal ligament. It demarcates the junction between abdomen and thigh (**Fig. 10.1**).

Nine Regions of the Anterior Abdominal Wall

For the purpose of description during clinical examination, the anterior abdominal wall is divided into nine regions by two right and left vertical planes and two transpyloric and transtubercular horizontal planes (**Fig. 10.2**). These correspond with the 9 regions of abdominal cavity (**Fig. 10.2**).

1. *Right and left vertical planes* pass through the midinguinal points, that is, point on each inguinal ligament midway between anterior superior iliac spine and pubic symphysis. They correspond to midclavicular planes.

2. *Upper horizontal plane*, that is, transpyloric plane, passes horizontally midway between the jugular notch of the sternum and pubic symphysis at the level of lower border of L1 vertebra.

3. *Lower horizontal plane*, that is, transtubercular plane, passes horizontally through the tubercles of the iliac crests at the level of upper part of L5 vertebra.

4. Deep to inguinal ligament at the midinguinal point, the external iliac artery escapes from abdomen to continue as femoral artery. The pulsations of femoral artery can be felt at this point.

5. When the finger is run medially on the inguinal ligament to the pubic tubercle, the round spermatic cord covering it can be felt in male.

6. Superficial inguinal ring/aperture in the aponeurosis of external oblique is located immediately superolateral to the pubic tubercle.

7. A slight median groove on anterior abdominal wall extends between xiphoid process and pubic symphysis.

8. Deep to it lies linea alba, a fibrous raphe formed by the interlocking of the aponeurosis of three flat muscles on each side of the anterior abdominal wall.

9. Umbilicus, a scar, lies in the linea alba nearer to the pubis than the xiphoid process.

10. Linea semilunaris, a slight groove, is visible at the lateral edge of each rectus abdominis.

11. Murphy point is a point where linea semilunaris crosses the costal margin at the ninth costal cartilage. The fundus of gallbladder lies deep to it on the right side.

12. Three zig-zag horizontal grooves are seen crossing the rectus abdominis between the umbilicus and pubic symphysis. They are formed as tendinous intersections with the rectus abdominis muscle.

13. Umbilicus is a prominent scar lying below the midpoint of linea aspera.

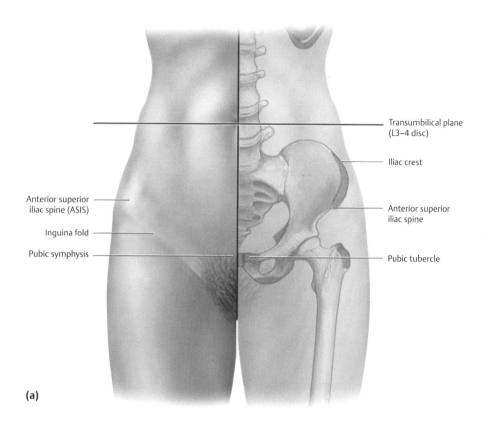

(a)

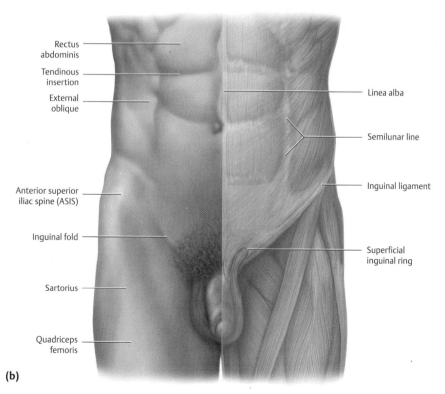

(b)

Fig. 10.1 Palpable structures in the abdomen and pelvis (anterior view). **(a)** Bony prominences. **(b)** Musculature. (From Gilroy AM et al. Atlas of Anatomy. Third Edition. 2016. Based on: Schuenke M., Schulte E, Schumacher U. THIEME Atlas of Anatomy. Illustrations by Voll and M. Wesker K. © Thieme 2020.)

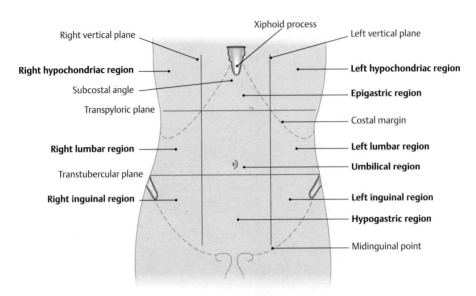

Fig. 10.2 Nine regions of the abdomen (labelled in bold).

14. Linea aspera is a linear groove that extends in the middle from xiphoid process to the pubic symphysis.

15. Linea semilunaris extend from pubic tubercle to the tip of ninth costal cartilage with slight lateral convexity. It corresponds to the lateral mansion of rectus abdominis.

Dissection and Identification

1. Make a vertical incision "A" in skin along the midline from the xiphoid process to the pubic symphysis encircling the umbilicus i.e. making sure that it encircles umbilicus on each side. The incision should not cut umbilicus in any event. Make another skin incision "B" from pubic symphysis, first up to pubic tubercle and then along the fold of groin to the anterior superior iliac spine. If the thorax has not been dissected, make a horizontal incision "C" and continue it posteriorly up to the posterior axillary line (**Fig. 10.3**).

2. Reflect skin flaps, leaving behind the superficial fascia on the anterior abdominal wall. Cut the fascia transversely from anterior superior iliac spine to the midline. Raise fascia and identify its fatty (Camper) and membranous (Scarpa) layers. Insert a finger deep to membranous layer and note the ease with which the membranous layer separates from the aponeurosis of external oblique muscle. Note that the membranous layer is fused with fascia lata of the thigh just inferior to the inguinal ligament.

3. Locate the superficial inguinal ring immediately superolateral to the pubic tubercle. Note the spermatic cord (in male) or round ligament of uterus (in female) emerging through it. Pass a finger along the spermatic cord medial to the body of the pubis.

4. Identify the anterior cutaneous branch of the iliohypogastric nerve piercing the external oblique aponeurosis a little superior to the superficial inguinal ring.

5. Divide the superficial fascia vertically in midline and in posterior axillary line up to the iliac crest. Reflect it and identify the anterior and lateral cutaneous branches of nerves emerging from the anterior and lateral parts of the abdominal wall, respectively.

6. Remove the membranous layer of fascia from the surface of the external oblique muscle and its aponeurosis. Care must be taken while doing so in superior part where the aponeurosis is

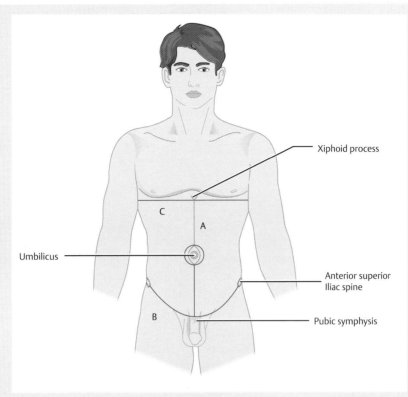

Fig. 10.3   Skin incisions to reflect the skin from anterior abdominal wall.

thin and easily removed and also in the anteroinferior part where the aponeurosis presents a triangular deficiency called superficial inguinal ring. Identify the medial and lateral crura forming the boundaries of the ring.

7. Note the origin of the external oblique muscles to the lower eight ribs, interdigitating with serratus anterior and latissimus dorsi. Separate the upper six digitations from the ribs. Divide the muscle vertically up to the iliac crest in front of this but avoid damage to the lateral cutaneous branches of nerves which pierce it close to the iliac crest.

8. Reflect the upper part of the external oblique forward to expose the internal oblique and its aponeurosis anterior to rectus abdominis. Cut the external oblique aponeurosis vertically lateral to the line of fusion and turn the muscle and aponeurosis down. Continue the cut backward medial to the superficial inguinal ring up to the pubis. Examine the internal oblique and inguinal ligament. Note the attachment of the internal oblique to the lateral part of the inguinal ligament.

9. Lift up the spermatic cord/round ligament of uterus to note the deep fibers of the inguinal ligament passing posteriorly to the pectin pubis. They constitute the lacunar ligament.

10. Remove fascia from the surface of internal oblique and note that some fibers of internal oblique pass onto the spermatic cord. These form loops which extend down the cord and testis and then turn upward toward the pubis. When these fibers contract, the testis is elevated toward the superficial inguinal ring.

11. Elevate the internal oblique and cut its attachments to the inguinal ligament, iliac crest, and costal margin carefully avoiding damage to the nerves of the anterior abdominal wall lying deep to it. Cut the muscle vertically from the iliac crest to the 12th costal cartilage. Strip the muscle forward from the transversus abdominis and the nerves between the two. Note that

this is difficult superiorly due to the presence of dense fascia between the muscles and is impossible inferiorly due to fusion of the arching aponeuroses of the two muscles forming the conjoint tendon/falx inguinalis.

12. Remove the fascia from the surface of transversus abdominis and clean the vessels and nerves present on its surface. Note the continuity of lateral cutaneous branches with these nerves.

13. Open the rectus sheath by giving vertical incision along the middle of the muscle. Reflect the flaps medially and laterally, by dividing its attachments to the tendinous intersections present in the anterior part of the rectus muscle. Elevate the muscle to expose the intercostal and subcostal nerves entering the sheath and piercing the muscle. Identify the mode of the rectus sheath formation.

14. Identify the fusion of the aponeurosis of rectus abdominis with that of the internal oblique, passing posterior to rectus abdominis above the arcuate line (fold of Douglas) and anterior to it below the arcuate line.

15. Identify the pyramidalis muscle, if present, in front of the lower part of rectus abdominis muscle. Note it is a small attachment to the upper surface of pubic symphysis and upper surface of pubis inferiorly, and linea alba superiorly. It is supplied by the subcostal nerve.

16. Divide the rectus abdominis muscle transversely in the middle and reflect its parts up and down cutting the intercostal nerves as they enter it. Trace superior and inferior epigastric arteries passing longitudinally deep to the muscle within the rectus sheath. Identify the arcuate line and note the inferior epigastric artery entering the rectus sheath anterior to it.

17. Now cut the remaining ribs in the midaxillary line and turn down the sternum, costal cartilages, and anterior parts of the ribs. Separate pleura and fascia from the back of the sternum and upper surfaces of the exposed portion of diaphragm. Its slips are attached to the xiphoid process. Identify the slips from the transversus abdominis beside those of the diaphragm. Note the continuity of transversus abdominis with transversus thoracis. Find the musculophrenic and superior epigastric branches of the internal thoracic/internal mammary arteries.

18. Cut the slips of origin of the diaphragm in front of the midaxillary line and cut transversus abdominis vertically up to the iliac crest, avoiding damage to the underlying transversalis fascia and peritoneum deep to it.

19. Turn the remains of the anterior abdominal wall, sternum, costal cartilages, and ribs downward, separating transversalis fascia from peritoneum.

20. Reflect the peritoneum downward with the anterior abdominal wall, cutting the falciform ligament which passes from the median part of the supraumbilical portion of anterior abdominal wall to the liver. Note ligamentum teres of the liver in its free posterior border.

21. Identify five ill-defined peritoneal folds on the posterior surface of the reflected lower, anterior abdominal wall. The five folds seen are: one lateral and one medial on each side and one median fold. They are formed by inferior epigastric vessels, lateral umbilical ligament (obliterated umbilical artery), and remnant of urachus, respectively. Note the attachment of obliterated urachus (median umbilical ligament) with the apex of the urinary bladder.

22. Now strip off the peritoneum from the posterior aspect of infraumbilical portion of the anterior abdominal wall and reconfirm the five ligaments extending from the umbilicus.

23. Identify the attachments of transversus abdominis and conjoint tendon and trace the continuity of the fascia transversalis enveloping the spermatic cord as the internal spermatic fascia.

Superficial Fascia

The superficial fascia of abdomen contains a variable amount of fat which gradually increases in the inferior half of the abdomen, specially below umbilicus.

In the inferior half of the anterior abdominal wall, the superficial fascia is composed of two layers:

1. A superficial fatty layer—*Camper fascia* which is continuous with the superficial fascia over the rest of the body.

2. A deep fibrous membranous layer—*Scarpa fascia* which fades above and laterally but fuses below the inguinal ligament with fascia lata and extends into: the penis as a tubular sheath forming deep fascia of penis; the wall of the scrotum forming dartos; and the perineum posteriorly where it is referred to as Colles fascia. At this site, it is fused with perineal body and posterior margin of the perineal membrane, as well as with pubic arch laterally, forming the superficial perineal space (**Fig. 10.4**).

If the penile urethra ruptures in the superficial perineal space, there is extravasation of urine in this space, which extends into spaces of scrotum and penis and lower part of anterior abdominal

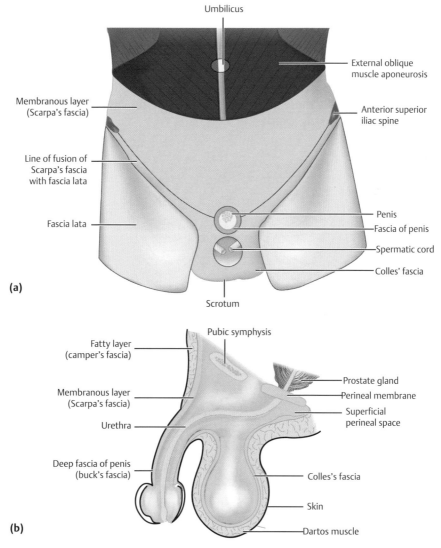

Fig. 10.4 Arrangement of two layers of superficial fascia in **(a)** lower part of the anterior abdominal wall and **(b)** perineal region.

wall but cannot extend into the thigh because of the attachment of Scarpa fascia with the fascia lata. Clinically, it presents as circumscribed swelling of peritoneum, scrotum, and lower part of anterior abdominal wall. In the female, the superficial perineal space splits in the median plane by vulva.

Cutaneous Nerves

The skin and muscles of the abdominal wall are innervated by the anterior rami of the lower five intercostal, subcostal, iliohypogastric (L1), and ilioinguinal (L1) nerves (i.e., T7 to L1 spinal segments) (**Fig. 10.5**).

These nerves are arranged with the same plane as the upper intercostal nerves except that the ilioinguinal nerve lacks a lateral cutaneous branch and its anterior branch traverses through the superficial inguinal ring.

The anterior cutaneous branch pierces the anterior wall of the rectus sheath a little lateral to the median plane. The anterior cutaneous branch of the 10th thoracic nerve emerges adjacent to the umbilicus, while the 1st lumbar nerve emerges above the superficial ring (ilioinguinal nerve).

The lateral cutaneous branches emerge through the external oblique muscle. The branches of subcostal and iliohypogastric nerve appear close to the iliac crest and descend over it to supply the skin.

Cutaneous Vessels (Fig. 10.5)

The small arteries accompanying the lateral cutaneous branches of the nerves arise from the posterior intercostal arteries, while those accompanying the anterior cutaneous branches arise from the superior and inferior epigastric arteries.

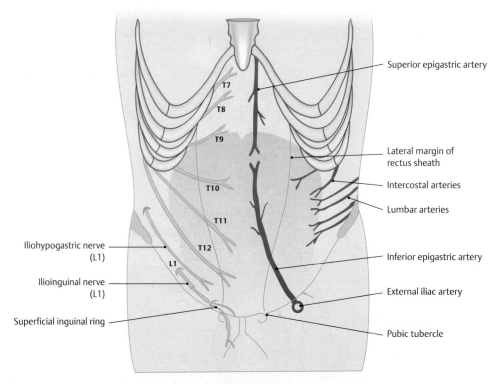

Fig. 10.5   Cutaneous nerves and vessels of anterior abdominal wall.

Below the umbilicus, the skin and superficial fascia of anterior abdominal wall are supplied by three small branches from each femoral artery. The superficial, external pudendal artery runs medially to supply the scrotum (or labium majus) and penis. The superficial epigastric artery runs superomedially across the inguinal ligament as far as the umbilicus. The superficial, circumflex iliac artery runs toward the anterior superior iliac spine to supply the adjacent abdominal wall and skin of the groin.

Superficial Veins

- *Below the umbilicus*, the superficial veins drain venous blood into the great saphenous vein in the groin.
- *Above the umbilicus*, the superficial veins venous blood into the axillary vein in the axilla. These two sets of veins anastomose freely with each other and with small veins which drain venous blood from the umbilicus into liver alongside the ligamentum teres (obliterated umbilical vein).

▮ Clinical Note

In obstruction of the superior or inferior vena cavae, these veins may be distended as an alternative channels for venous return.

If the venous drainage through the liver is blocked, backflow may occur to the umbilicus from the liver. This leads to the dilatation and tortuosity of veins, radiating from the umbilicus like spokes of a wheel producing a clinical sign called *caput medusae*.

Muscles of the Anterior Abdominal Wall

The muscles of anterior abdominal wall comprise three flat muscles: external oblique, internal oblique, and transversus abdominis, and two vertical muscles: rectus abdominis and pyramidalis on either side of the midline (**Figs. 10.6** and **10.7; Video 10.1**). The flat muscles lie on either side of abdomen.

The flat muscles are muscular posterolaterally and aponeurotic anteromedially. They are arranged in three layers. From superficial to deep, these are external oblique, internal oblique, and transversus abdominis.

As in the intercostal space, the neurovascular structures pass in the neurovascular plane between the intermediate and deep muscle layers, that is, internal oblique and transversus muscle layers.

The origin, insertion, nerve supply, and actions of anterior abdominal wall are provided in **Table 10.1**.

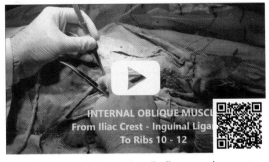

Video 10.1 Abdominal wall—flat muscles, rectus sheath, and linea alba.

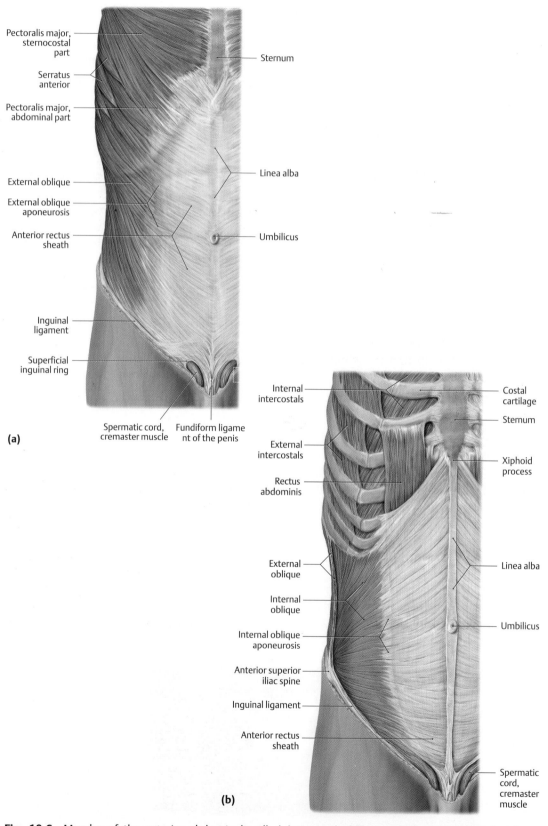

Fig. 10.6 Muscles of the anterior abdominal wall. **(a)** External oblique muscles. **(b)** Internal oblique muscles. (From Schuenke M, Schulte E, Schumacher U. THIEME Atlas of Anatomy. General Anatomy and Musculoskeletal System. Illustrations by Voll M and Wesker K. © Thieme 2020)

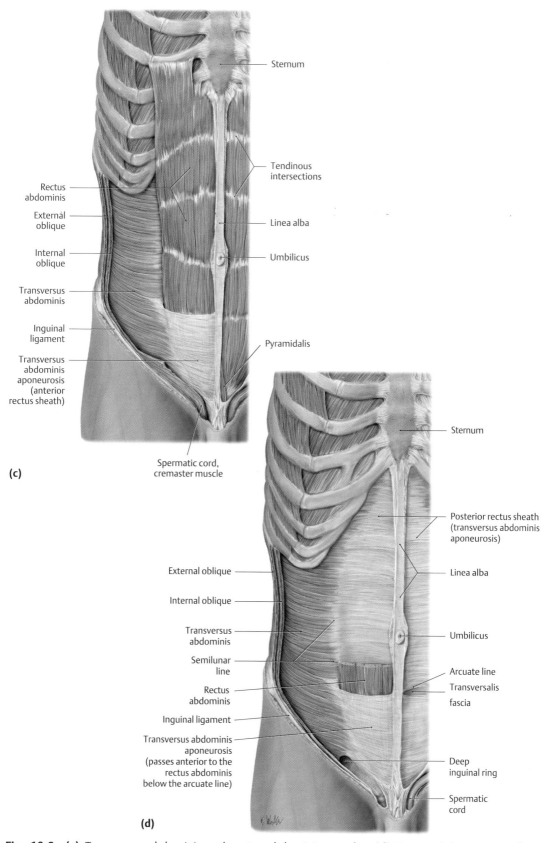

Fig. 10.6 **(c)** Transversus abdominis and rectus abdominis muscles. **(d)** Rectus abdominis muscle is *removed*. (From Schuenke M, Schulte E, Schumacher U. THIEME Atlas of Anatomy. General Anatomy and Musculoskeletal System. Illustrations by Voll M and Wesker K. © Thieme 2020)

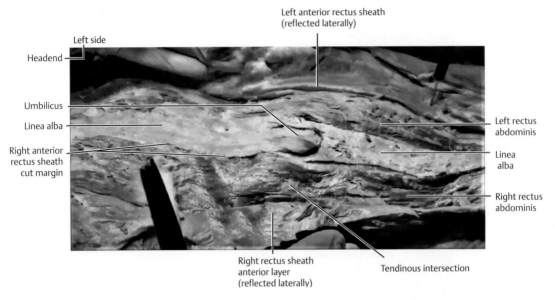

Fig. 10.7   Rectus abdominis.

Table 10.1   Origin, insertion, nerve supply, and actions of muscles of anterior abdominal wall

Muscles	Origin	Insertion	Nerve supply	Action
External oblique	By eight fleshly slips from external surfaces of 5th to 12th ribs	Linea alba, pubic tubercle and anterior half of iliac crest	Lower five intercostal and subcostal nerve	Compresses and supports abdominal viscera; flexes and rotates trunk
Internal oblique	Thoracolumbar fascia, anterior two-thirds of iliac crest and lateral two-thirds of inguinal ligament	Inferior borders of 10th to 12th ribs, linea alba and pectin pubis via conjoint tendon[a]	Lower six thoracic nerves and first lumbar nerve	Compresses and supports abdominal viscera; flexes and rotates trunk
Transversus abdominis	Internal surfaces of 7th to 12th costal cartilages, thoracolumbar fascia, anterior two-thirds of iliac crest, and lateral third of inguinal ligament	Xiphoid process, linea alba with aponeurosis of internal oblique, pubic crest, and pectin pubis via conjoint tendon	Lower six thoracic nerves and first lumbar nerve	Compresses and supports abdominal viscera
Rectus abdominis	Lateral head from pubic symphysis and medial head from pubic crest	Xiphoid process and fifth, sixth, and seventh costal cartilages	Lower six or seven thoracic nerves	Flexes trunk and compresses abdominal viscera, stabilizes and controls tilt of pelvis
Pyramidalis (absent in 20% of cases) (lies anterior to rectus abdominis)	Anterior surface of pubis and pubic ligament	Linea alba	Subcostal nerve	Tensor linea alba

[a]The lower arched and parallel fibers of the aponeurosis of internal oblique and transversus abdominis do not reach the linea alba, but fuse to form the *conjoint tendon* which turns downward to be attached on pubic crest and pectin pubis (pectineal line).

Fascia Transversalis

The deep surface of rectus abdominis is covered by a fascial sheet called fascia transversalis. This fascial lining continues with the fascial sheet lining the abdominal and pelvic cavities. It is given different name at different sites, such as, diaphragmatic fascia on the diaphragm, iliac fascia on the iliopsoas muscle, renal fascia covering the kidney and pelvic fascia lining the pelvic cavity.

Rectus Sheath

The rectus sheath is an aponeurotic sheath that encloses the rectus abdominis muscle on either side of linea alba. It has anterior and posterior walls, and contains rectus abdominis, pyramidalis (if present), the superior and inferior epigastric vessels, and anterior rami of the lower six thoracic nerves (**Fig. 10.8**; **Video 10.2**).

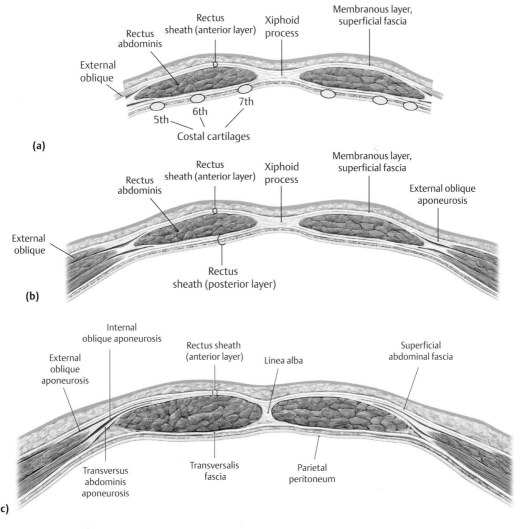

Fig. 10.8 Formation of rectus sheath at three different levels **(a)** Above the costal margin. **(b)** From costal margin to the arcuate line. **(c)** Inferior to arcuate line. (From Schuenke M, Schulte E, Schumacher U. THIEME Atlas of Anatomy. General Anatomy and Musculoskeletal System. Illustrations by Voll M and Wesker K. © Thieme 2020)

The sheath is made up from the aponeuroses of the three flat muscles of the anterior abdominal wall. The linea alba represents the fusion of the aponeuroses in the midline throughout the major part of the length of the rectus. Mostly the anterior wall of rectus sheath is formed by the aponeuroses of the external oblique and the anterior layer of the internal oblique, and the posterior wall is formed by the posterior layer of the internal oblique and transversus abdominis. The formation of the sheath from costal margin to pubic symphysis is as follows:

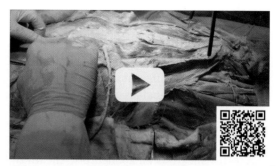

Video 10.2 Abdominal wall—rectus muscles, posterior rectus sheath, and vessels.

1. *Above the costal margin*: Only anterior wall of sheath is present and it is formed by the external oblique aponeurosis. The muscle lies directly on 7th, 6th, and 5th costal cartilages.

2. *Below costal margin and above arcuate lines:* Anterior wall of sheath is formed by aponeurosis of external oblique and anterior layer of aponeurosis of internal oblique. Posterior wall of sheath is formed by posterior layer of aponeurosis of internal oblique and aponeurosis of transverse abdominis.

3. *Above the pubic symphysis and below arcuate line,* i.e., about halfway between the umbilicus and pubic symphysis, only anterior wall is present and it is formed by aponeurosis of all three muscles, that is, external oblique, internal oblique, and transversus abdominis. The posterior wall is absent and rectus muscle lies directly on the fascia transversalis.

4. Midway between the umbilicus and pubic symphysis, the posterior wall of the sheath is a curved line with concavity facing downward. This is termed as "arcuate line/linea semicircularis/fold of Douglas."

   • The lateral border of the rectus—the linea semilunaris—can usually be identified in thin subjects. It crosses the costal margin in the transpyloric plane.
   • Three tendinous intersections firmly attach the anterior sheath wall to the muscle itself. They are situated at the level of the xiphoid, the umbilicus, and one between these two. These give the abdominal wall the "six-pack" appearance in muscular individuals.

Inguinal Canal

It is an oblique intramuscular passage parallel and immediately above the medial half of the inguinal ligament. It is approximately 4 cm long and allows passage to the spermatic cord (round ligament in the female) through the lower abdominal wall. It extends obliquely downward, forward and medially from the deep inguinal ring in a medial direction to the superficial inguinal ring (**Fig. 10.9**).

1. *Deep inguinal ring*: It is an opening in the transversalis fascia and lies halfway between the anterior superior iliac spine and the pubic tubercle. The inferior epigastric vessels pass medial to the deep ring.

2. *Superficial inguinal ring*: It is actually not a ring but a triangular slit-like defect in the external oblique aponeurosis above and medial to the pubic tubercle.

Wall of Inguinal Canal

Following are the walls of the inguinal canal:

1. *Anterior wall*: It is formed by the external oblique aponeurosis in the whole length of the canal. It is reinforced in its lateral third by the fleshy fibers of the internal oblique.

2. *Superior wall/roof*: It is formed by the arched fibers of internal oblique and transversus abdominis.

3. *Posterior wall*: It is formed by the transversalis fascia along its whole extent. In the medial two-thirds, it is reinforced by the conjoint tendon (the combined common insertion of the internal oblique and transversus into the pectineal line).

4. *Inferior wall*: It is formed by the grooved upper surface of the inguinal ligament.

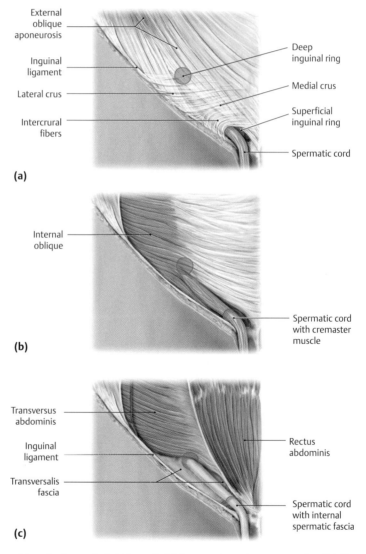

Fig. 10.9 Dissection of inguinal canal. **(a)** Superficial layer-external aponeurosis. **(b)** *Removed*: External oblique aponeurosis. **(c)** *Removed*: Internal oblique. (From Schuenke M, Schulte E, Schumacher U. THIEME Atlas of Anatomy. General Anatomy and Musculoskeletal System. Illustrations by Voll M and Wesker K. © Thieme 2020) *(Continued)*

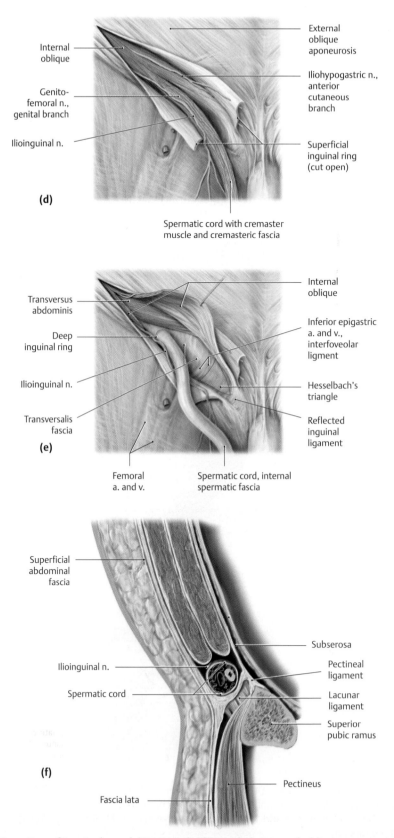

Fig. 10.9 Dissection of inguinal canal *(Continued)* **(d)** Divided: External oblique aponeurosis. **(e)** Divided: Internal oblique and cremaster. **(f)** Sagittal section through inguinoabdominal region. (Modified from Schuenke M, Schulte E, Schumacher U. THIEME Atlas of Anatomy. General Anatomy and Musculoskeletal System. Illustrations by Voll M and Wesker K. © Thieme 2020)

Contents of Inguinal Canal

The contents of the inguinal canal are:

1. Spermatic cord in male (or round ligament in the female).

2. Ilioinguinal nerve (L1).

Spermatic Cord

It is a cord like structure passing from testis to the deep inguinal ring in the anterior abdominal wall. Its lower part can be easily palpated within scrotum in living individuals. Its lower part can be easily palpated within scrotum in living individuals. It is the collection *vas deferens, nerves, blood, vessels (testicular artery and pampiniform plexus of veins) and lymph vessels.* The spermatic cord is covered by three layers of fascia which arise from the layers of the abdominal wall as the cord passes through the inguinal canal (**Figs. 11.10** and **11.2** in Chapter 11). From superficial to deep, these are:

1. *External spermatic fascia* from the external oblique aponeurosis.

2. *Cremasteric fascia and muscle* from the internal oblique aponeurosis.

3. *Internal spermatic fascia* from the transversalis fascia.

Contents of Spermatic Cord

The contents of spermatic cord include:

1. Ductus (vas) deferens.

2. Testicular artery, a branch of the abdominal aorta.

3. Pampiniform plexus of veins which coalesce to form the testicular vein at the deep inguinal ring.

4. Lymphatics from the testis and epididymis draining to the pre- and para-aortic nodes.

5. Autonomic nerves.

6. Remnants of processus vaginalis.

Nerves of Anterior Abdominal Wall

The nerves of the anterior abdominal wall comprise ventral rami of the lower six thoracic nerves and the first lumbar nerve (*iliohypogastric* and *ilioinguinal nerves*).

The lower five intercostal nerves leave the intercostal spaces between the slips of transversus abdominis arising from the costal cartilages and pass between the transversus and internal oblique. They run anteroinferiorly to enter the rectus sheath by piercing its posterior wall. They supply rectus abdominis, and emerge through the anterior wall of the sheath as anterior cutaneous branches. These nerves along with the subcostal, iliohypogastric, and ilioinguinal nerves supply the muscles of the anterior abdominal wall. The last three nerves pierce the transversus abdominis posteriorly to enter in the same plane as the others but differ from them in following aspects: (a) lateral cutaneous branches of the subcostal and iliohypogastric nerves pierce the oblique muscles close to the iliac crest and descend over it to the skin of gluteal region; (b) iliohypogastric nerve pierces the internal oblique close to the anterior superior iliac spine and becomes cutaneous by piercing the external oblique 2 to 3 cm superior to the superficial inguinal ring; (c) ilioinguinal nerve has no lateral cutaneous branch. It accompanies the spermatic cord or round ligament and emerges through the superficial inguinal ring to supply the skin on the anterior aspect of the thigh and external genitalia.

Arteries of the Abdominal Wall

The arteries of anterior abdominal wall include the superior and inferior epigastric arteries—branches of the internal thoracic and external iliac arteries, respectively—and the deep circumflex artery—a branch of the external iliac artery anteriorly. The two lower intercostal and subcostal arteries enter along the corresponding nerves into the neurovasculature of the abdominal wall.

The lumbar arteries enter the abdominal wall from the side.

1. *Superior epigastric artery*: It enters the rectus sheath deep to the costal cartilage and passes deep to rectus abdominis to anastomose with inferior epigastric artery.

2. *Musculophrenic artery*: It runs inferolaterally along the upper surface of the costal origin of diaphragm to the eighth intercostal space and supplies diaphragm and anterior abdominal wall.

3. *Inferior epigastric artery*: It arises from the external iliac artery just above the inguinal ligament. It runs upward and medially toward umbilicus, and at the lateral border of rectus abdominis it pierces fascia transversalis and passes deep to rectus abdominis to anastomose with the superior epigastric artery.

   The branches of inferior epigastric artery include pubic branch and cremasteric artery.

4. *Deep circumflex iliac artery*: It arises from external iliac artery close to inferior epigastric artery and runs deep to inguinal ligament toward the anterior superior iliac spine.

▌Clinical Notes

1. *Umbilical hernia*: It is protrusion of abdominal viscera through umbilicus. Congenital umbilical hernia occurs due to nonreturn of midgut loop back into the abdominal cavity. Acquired umbilical hernia occurs due to weakness of umbilical scar. In paraumbilical hernia, intestinal loop protrudes through linea alba around the umbilicus.

2. *Inguinal hernia*: It is the protrusion of loop of intestines into the inguinal canal. When protrusion occurs through the deep inguinal ring, it is called indirect inguinal hernia, and when the protrusion occurs through the posterior wall of the inguinal canal, it is called direct inguinal hernia (**Fig. 10.10**).

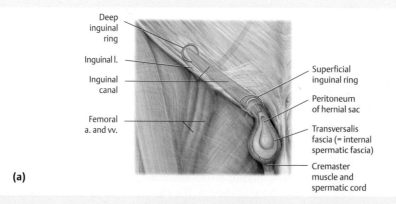

Fig. 10.10   Inguinal hernias. **(a)** Indirect inguinal hernia. (From Schuenke M, Schulte E, Schumacher U. THIEME Atlas of Anatomy. General Anatomy and Musculoskeletal System. Illustrations by Voll M and Wesker K. © Thieme 2020)

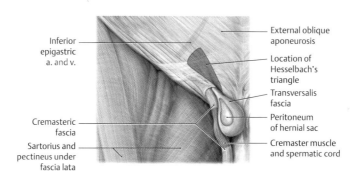

Inferior epigastric a. and v.

External oblique aponeurosis

Location of Hesselbach's triangle

Transversalis fascia

Peritoneum of hernial sac

Cremasteric fascia

Sartorius and pectineus under fascia lata

Cremaster muscle and spermatic cord

(b)

Fig. 10.10   Inguinal hernias. **(b)** Direct inguinal hernia. (From Schuenke M, Schulte E, Schumacher U. THIEME Atlas of Anatomy. General Anatomy and Musculoskeletal System. Illustrations by Voll M and Wesker K. © Thieme 2020)

- *Indirect inguinal hernia*: It usually occurs in younger males and is either congenital or acquired. The abdominal viscera protrude in the canal through deep inguinal ring. The protruded viscera are contained in the hernia sac—an outpouching of peritoneal membrane. The indirect inguinal hernias are located lateral to the inferior epigastric vessels.

- *Direct inguinal hernia*: It is always acquired and usually occurs in old age. In this, abdominal viscera protrude into the inguinal canal through its posterior wall medial to the inferior epigastric vessels.

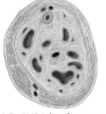
Introduction

The male external genital organs include penis, scrotum and its contents, and the spermatic cords (**Fig. 11.1**).

Dissection and Identification

1. First examine the pendulous sac (scrotum) of dark-colored rugose skin in the male cadaver. It is partitioned into two halves by the median scrotal septum lying in the midsagittal plane. Each half of the scrotum contains the testis, the epididymis, and the scrotal portion of the spermatic cord (**Fig. 11.1; Video 11.1**).

2. Make a vertical incision on each side of the scrotum, from the superficial inguinal ring to the inferior aspect of the scrotal sac. Reflect the skin from the underlying dartos muscle. Note the absence of fat in the superficial fascia. It contains dartos muscle and not the fat.

3. Lift the testis and spermatic cord from the scrotal sac. Observe that, inferiorly, each testis is connected to the wall of the scrotum by a scrotal ligament which is a remnant of the gubernaculum. Sever the scrotal ligament. Note the testis is surrounded by the coverings of the spermatic cord. Free the spermatic cord from the surrounding tissue and trace it to the superficial inguinal ring (**Video 11.2**).

4. Cut through the spermatic cord at the superficial inguinal ring and remove it along with the testis into a tray. Incise and try to separate the coverings of the spermatic cord, that is, external spermatic fascia, cremaster muscle and fascia, and internal spermatic fascia from outward to inward.

5. Separate various contents of the spermatic cord (**Fig. 11.2**). Identify the ductus (vas) deferens which is the posteriormost structure in the spermatic cord. It can be identified by its hard, cord-like texture. Find the artery to the vas deferens running on the surface of ductus

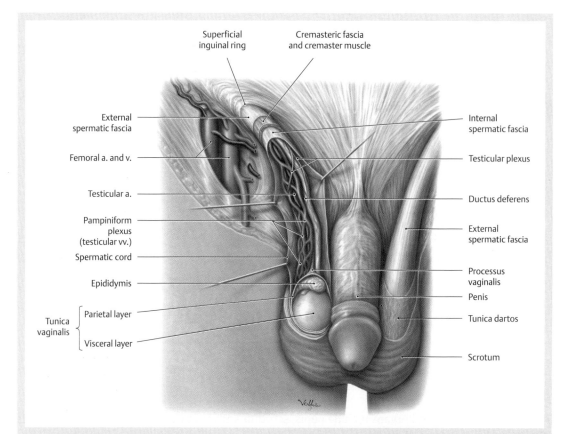

Fig. 11.1 Penis, scrotum, and spermatic cord. (From Schuenke M, Schulte E, Schumacher U. THIEME Atlas of Anatomy. General Anatomy and Musculoskeletal System. Illustrations by Voll M and Wesker K. © Thieme 2020)

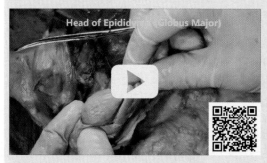

Video 11.1 Spermatic cord and testis.

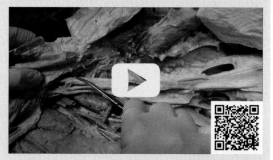

Video 11.2 Testis, epididymis, spermatic cord, ductus deferens, and clinical aspects.

deferens. Using blunt forceps, separate the ductus deferens from the surrounding pampiniform plexus of veins. Identify the testicular artery which can be differentiated from the veins due to its slightly thicker wall and tortuous course.

6. Note it is difficult to identify the nerves and lymphatics accompanying the blood vessels (or vas deferens) in the spermatic cord as they are too thin to dissect.

7. Observe that the anterolateral surface of the testis is covered by a serous membrane, the tunica vaginalis, which forms a closed sac. Open this sac by making a vertical incision along

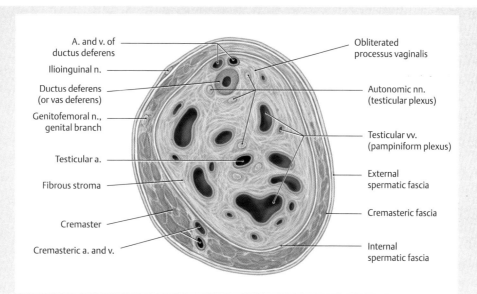

Fig. 11.2 Spermatic cord: Contents (cross-section). (From Schuenke M, Schulte E, Schumacher U. THIEME Atlas of Anatomy. General Anatomy and Musculoskeletal System. Illustrations by Voll M and Wesker K. © Thieme 2020)

the anterior surface of the outer (parietal) layer of the tunica vaginalis. Identify the cavity of the tunica vaginalis. Note that the inner layer of the tunica vaginalis covers the anterior and lateral surfaces of the testis and is tucked between the testis and epididymis to form the sinus of the epididymis. The visceral layer is continuous with the parietal layer near the posterior border of the testis.

8. On the posterosuperior aspect of the testis, identify the epididymis and its three parts, that is, head of the epididymis on the superior pole of the testis, body on the posterior aspect of the testis along its tail area, and tail of the epididymis located near the inferior pole of the testis.

9. Free the tail and body of the epididymis from the testis and note that the tail of epididymis is continuous with the ductus deferens.

10. At the superior pole of the testis, cut and reflect the tunica vaginalis which joins the testis with the head of the epididymis. Identify the efferent ductules which pass from the testis to the head of the epididymis.

11. Make a transverse cut through the testis and examine the structures with the help of a magnifying lens. On the surface of the testis, identify the thick fibrous tunica albuginea, which encloses the testis. Identify the fibrous bands called septae that radiate from the posterior aspect of the testis, called mediastinum testis. These septae divide the testis into the lobules called the seminiferous tubules.

12. Cut through the skin along the dorsum of the penis and reflect it. Observe the fundiform ligament, the extension of the membranous layer of the superficial fascia of the anterior abdominal wall. Find the superficial dorsal vein along the same line as the skin incision. Reflect it to expose the deep dorsal vein with the dorsal arteries and nerves on each side of it.

13. Make a transverse section through the body of the penis and examine the cut surface.

Scrotum

The scrotum is a pendulous sac of dark-colored skin. The skin of the scrotum is thin, rugose, and contains many sebaceous glands. A longitudinal median raphe is visible in the midline on the surface which indicates the embryological line of fusion of two halves of the scrotum. Beneath the skin lies a thin layer of involuntary dartos muscle. The scrotum is divided internally by the continuation of dartos muscle—septum of scrotum—into right and left compartments. Each half of the scrotal sacs contains spermatic cord, the testis, and its epididymis.

The layers of scrotal wall, from superficial to deep, are as follows:

1. Skin.

2. Dartos muscle.

3. External spermatic fascia.

4. Cremasteric muscle and fascia.

5. Internal spermatic fascia.

Testis and Epididymis

Testis is a male gonad to produce sperms and testosterone. It is oval in shape and compressed from side to side. The testis is 3.75 cm long, 2.5 cm broad from before backward, and 1.8 cm thick from side to side. The testes are responsible for spermatogenesis, an essential requirement for procreation. Their descent to an extra-abdominal position favors optimal spermatogenesis as the ambient scrotal temperature is approximately 3°C lower than the body temperature (**Fig. 11.3; Video 11.2**).

The external features of testis comprise (a) two poles: upper and lower; (b) two borders: anterior and posterior; and (c) two surfaces: medial and lateral.

Structure: The testis is enclosed in a thick fibrous capsule called tunica albuginea which projects forward along the posterior border to form a thickened ridge—the mediastinum testis. The mediastinum is traversed by neurovascular structures of the testis and rete testis. The testis is divided

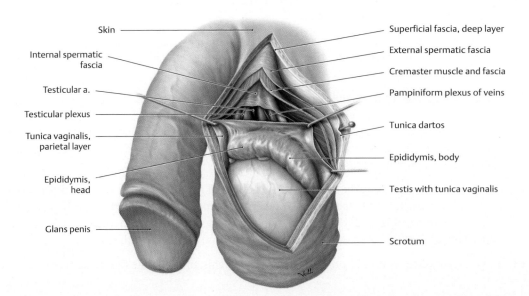

Fig. 11.3   Testis and epididymis in situ. (From Schuenke M, Schulte E, Schumacher U. THIEME Atlas of Anatomy. General Anatomy and Musculoskeletal System. Illustrations by Voll M and Wesker K. © Thieme 2020)

internally by a series of septa into approximately 200 lobules. Each lobule contains two to four seminiferous tubules, which anastomose into a plexus termed the *rete testis*. Each tubule is coiled when in situ, but when extended it measures approximately 60 cm. Thus, the overall length of seminiferous tubules is about 500 m. The interstitial cells responsible for the secretion of male sex hormones lie in the areolar tissue between the seminiferous tubules. Efferent ducts connect the rete testis to the epididymal head. Thus, they serve to transmit sperms from the testis to the epididymis (**Fig. 11.4**).

1. Tunica vaginalis is derived from the peritoneum. It is a double covering into which the testis is invaginated. It covers the epididymis with the exception of the posterior border.

2. Tunica albuginea is a tough fibrous capsule that envelops the testis.

3. The epididymis lies along the posterolateral and superior borders of the testis.

4. The upper poles of both the testis and epididymis bear an appendix testis and appendix epididymis (hydatid of Morgagni), respectively.

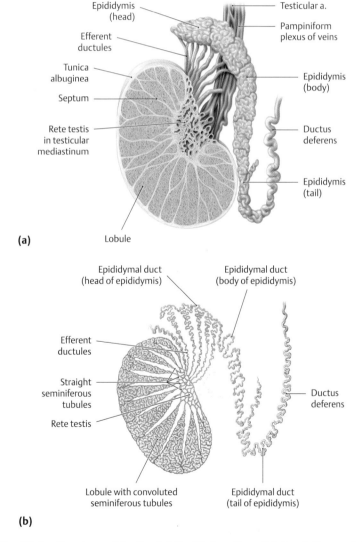

Fig. 11.4   Structure of testis. **(a)** Sagittal section. **(b)** Seminiferous tubules. (Modified from Schuenke M, Schulte E, Schumacher U. THIEME Atlas of Anatomy. Internal Organs. Illustrations by Voll M and Wesker K. © Thieme 2020)

Blood Vessels

It is from the testicular artery, a branch of the abdominal aorta. Venous drainage from the testis is to the pampiniform plexus of veins (**Fig. 11.5**), which lies within the spermatic cord, but coalesces to form a single vein at the deep inguinal ring. The left testicular vein drains to the left renal vein, whereas the right testicular vein drains directly to the inferior vena cava.

Lymphatic Drainage

It is to the para-aortic lymph nodes.

Nerve Supply

It is from T10 sympathetic fibers via the renal and aortic plexuses.

Epididymis

The epididymis is a comma-shaped structure that overlies the superior and posterolateral surfaces of the testis. It is an organ made up of highly coiled tube; the duct of epididymis acts as a reservoir of spermatozoa (refer to **Figs. 11.3** and **11.4**).

Its upper end, called the head, is enlarged and connected to the upper pole of the testis by efferent ductules. The middle part is called the body. The lower part is called the tail. The duct of epididymis is continuous with the vas deferens at the tail of the epididymis. The duct of epididymis is about 6 to 7 cm long.

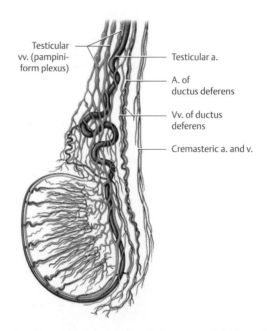

Fig. 11.5 Blood vessels of the testis (left lateral view). (From Schuenke M, Schulte E, Schumacher U. THIEME Atlas of Anatomy. General Anatomy and Musculoskeletal System. Illustrations by Voll M and Wesker K. © Thieme 2020)

Descent of the Testis (Fig. 11.6)

The testes develop in the abdominal cavity from the gonadal ridge in relation to the developing mesonephros, at the level of segments T10 to T12. Subsequently, they descend to reach the scrotum for spermatogenesis. It begins to descend during the second month of intrauterine life. The developing testis reaches iliac fossa by the third month, rests at the deep inguinal ring from the fourth to sixth month, traverses the inguinal canal during the seventh month, and reaches the superficial inguinal ring by the eighth month and the bottom of the scrotum by the ninth month.

Mechanism of Descent (Fig. 11.6)

The exact mechanism of descent of testis is not clear. Factors which contribute to the descent of testis are as follows:

1. Gubernaculums testis, a fibromuscular band which extends from the caudal pole of developing testis to the scrotum through inguinal canal. As it shortens relative to the growing fetus, the descent of testis occurs.

2. Increased intra-abdominal temperature.

3. Increased intra-abdominal pressure.

4. Male sex hormones produced by the testis.

5. Calcitonin gene-related peptide secreted by genitofemoral nerve.

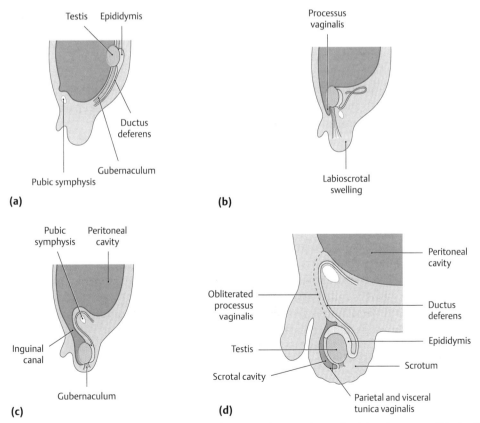

Fig. 11.6   Descent of the testis (left lateral view). **(a)** Second month of development. **(b)** Third month. **(c)** Birth. **(d)** After obliteration of the processus vaginalis of the peritoneum. (From Schuenke M, Schulte E, Schumacher U. THIEME Atlas of Anatomy. General Anatomy and Musculoskeletal System. Illustrations by Voll M and Wesker K. © Thieme 2020)

Dissection and Identification

1. Incise through and reflect the skin along the dorsum of penis, from the pubic symphysis to the end of prepuce and find the extension *Scarpa fascia* of the abdominal wall on to the penis. Identify fundiform ligament, an extension of the membranous layer of the superficial fascia of the abdominal wall on to the penis. Search the superficial fascia and follow it proximally to the superficial veins of the thigh. Deep to this vein is the deep fascia of the penis and suspensory ligament of the penis.

2. Divide the deep fascia of penis in line with the skin incision. Reflect it to expose the deep dorsal vein, with the dorsal arteries and nerves on either side. Cut a transverse section through the body of the penis, leaving the two parts connected by the skin on the urethral surface (**Fig. 11.7**).

Penis

The penis is a male organ of copulation. It provides passage to both urine and semen. It is mostly cylindrical and pendulors and lies in front of scrotum below the pubic symphysis. It is about 5 inch to 6 inch long in erect slate. It consists of two parts—the root and the body (**Fig. 11.7; Video 11.3**).

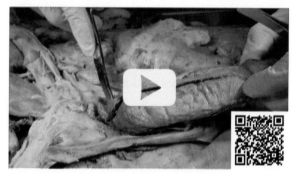

Video 11.3   Male genital organs—structural configuration.

Root: It is fixed and situated in the superficial perineal pouch. It consists of two crura and one bulb. Each crus is attached to the margin of pubic arch of respective side and is covered by ischiocavernosus muscle. The bulb is attached to the perineal membrane in the middle between the two crura and is covered by bulbospongiosus muscle. Its deep surface is pierced above its center by the urethra, which shows a dilatation (intrabulbar fossa).

Body: It is the free pendulous, elongated portion with enlarged cone-like distal end, the glans penis. This portion is covered by loose, hairless skin on all sides. Its ventral surface faces backward and downward, and dorsal surface faces forward and upward. It consists of three elongated masses of erectile tissue: two corpora cavernosa and one corpus spongiosum. The former are forward continuations of crura tapering and terminating under cover of glans penis. Each is surrounded by a strong fibrous envelop (tunica albuginea). Corpora spongiosum is forward continuation of the bulb of the penis; its end expands to form glans penis. It is traversed by urethra end to end and is also covered by a relatively thin tunica albuginea. The projecting margin at the base of glans penis is called corona glandis, which overhangs a constriction of the neck of the penis. The dilatation of urethra within glans penis is called navicular fossa. Prepuce (foreskin) is the fold of skin that can be retracted over glans. Frenulum is a median fold on the undersurface of glans. Preputial sac is the space between the glans and prepuce.

The penis is supported by the following two ligaments:

1. *Fundiform ligament*: It extends downward from linea alba and splits to enclose the penis.

2. *Suspensory ligament*: It lies deep and extends from pubic symphysis to the fascia on each side of the penis (**Fig. 11.8**).

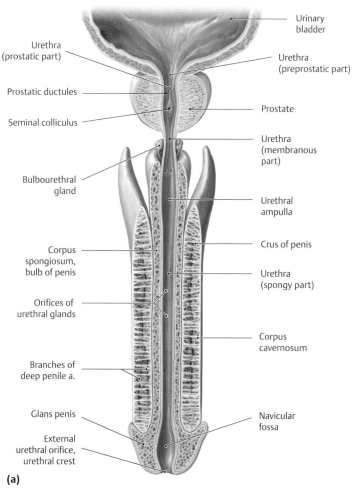

Urinary bladder

Urethra (prostatic part)

Urethra (preprostatic part)

Prostatic ductules

Prostate

Seminal colliculus

Urethra (membranous part)

Bulbourethral gland

Urethral ampulla

Corpus spongiosum, bulb of penis

Crus of penis

Urethra (spongy part)

Orifices of urethral glands

Corpus cavernosum

Branches of deep penile a.

Glans penis

Navicular fossa

External urethral orifice, urethral crest

(a)

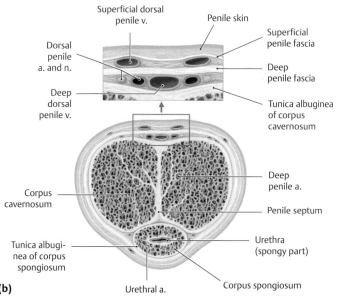

Superficial dorsal penile v.

Penile skin

Superficial penile fascia

Dorsal penile a. and n.

Deep penile fascia

Deep dorsal penile v.

Tunica albuginea of corpus cavernosum

Corpus cavernosum

Deep penile a.

Penile septum

Tunica albuginea of corpus spongiosum

Urethra (spongy part)

Urethral a.

Corpus spongiosum

(b)

Fig. 11.7 Penis. **(a)** Longitudinal section. (From Schuenke M, Schulte E, Schumacher U. THIEME Atlas of Anatomy. Internal Organs. Illustrations by Voll M and Wesker K. © Thieme 2020) **(b)** Cross-section through the shaft of the penis. (Modified from Schuenke M, chulte E, Schumacher U. THIEME Atlas of Anatomy. General Anatomy and Musculoskeletal System. Illustrations by Voll M and Wesker K. © Thieme 2020)
(Continued)

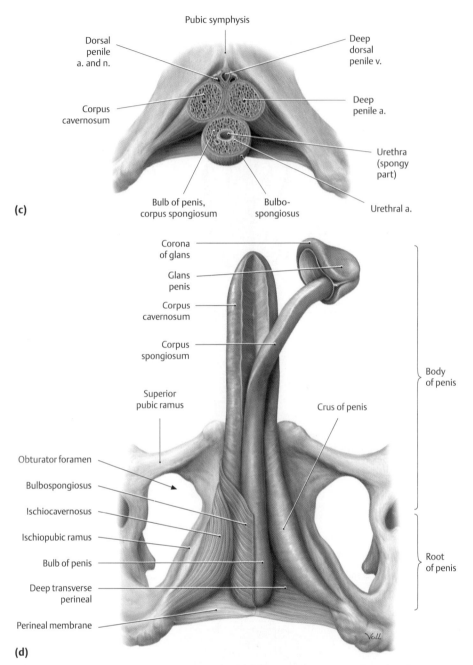

(c)

(d)

Fig. 11.7 *(Continued)* **(c)** Cross-section through the root of the penis. **(d)** Inferior view. (From Schuenke M, Schulte E, Schumacher U. THIEME Atlas of Anatomy. General Anatomy and Musculoskeletal System. Illustrations by Voll M and Wesker K. © Thieme 2020)

Arterial Supply

The penis is a highly vascular organ and is supplied by three branches of internal pudendal artery— deep artery of penis (in corpus cavernosum), dorsal artery of penis on dorsum, (deep to deep fascia), and artery of the bulb and superficial external pudendal artery (to the skin and fascia) (**Fig. 11.7** and **11.8**).

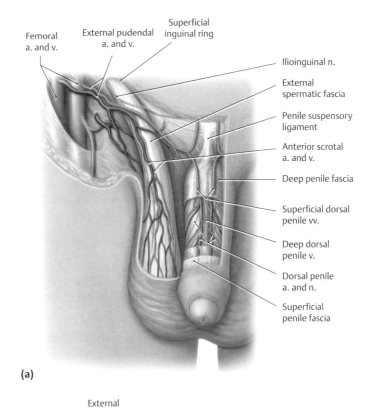

Femoral a. and v.

External pudendal a. and v.

Superficial inguinal ring

Ilioinguinal n.

External spermatic fascia

Penile suspensory ligament

Anterior scrotal a. and v.

Deep penile fascia

Superficial dorsal penile vv.

Deep dorsal penile v.

Dorsal penile a. and n.

Superficial penile fascia

(a)

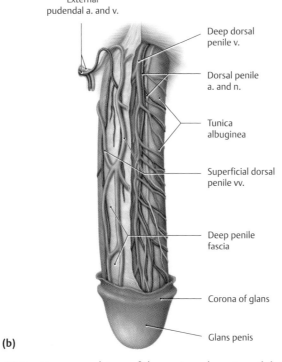

External pudendal a. and v.

Deep dorsal penile v.

Dorsal penile a. and n.

Tunica albuginea

Superficial dorsal penile vv.

Deep penile fascia

Corona of glans

Glans penis

(b)

Fig. 11.8 Neurovasculature of the penis and scrotum. **(a)** Anterior view. *Partially removed*: Skin and fascia. **(b)** Dorsal vasculature of the penis. (From Schuenke M, Schulte E, Schumacher U. THIEME Atlas of Anatomy. General Anatomy and Musculoskeletal System. Illustrations by Voll M and Wesker K. © Thieme 2020)

Venous Drainage

The veins of the penis do not correspond to the arteries (**Fig. 11.8**). These are the following:

1. Superficial dorsal vein drains the prepuce and skin of the penis.

2. Deep dorsal vein drains glans penis and corpora cavernosa.

Lymphatic Drainage

Lymph from the skin of the penis, including the prepuce, drains into superficial inguinal lymph nodes, while the lymph from the glans penis drains into deep inguinal nodes called *gland of Cloquet*. It is located in femoral canal.

Nerve Supply

Somatic innervation of penis is derived from dorsal nerves of penis to the skin of the body, prepuce, and glans.

1. Parasympathetic innervation is derived from pelvic splanchnic nerves through cavernous nerves, which arise from prostatic nerve plexuses. The cavernous nerves supply vasodilator fibers to blood vessels in erectile masses.

2. Sympathetic innervations derived from L1 segment of spinal cord reach through the inferior hypogastric plexus.

▋Clinical Notes

1. *Undescended testis (cryptorchidism)*: In this condition, testis fails to descend in scrotum. It may be present anywhere in its normal path of descent, such as iliac fossa, deep inguinal ring, inguinal canal, or superficial inguinal ring. The undescended testis fails to produce normal spermatozoa (spermatogenesis) and is prone to malignant change.

2. *Hydrocele*: It is the accumulation of fluid in the tunica vaginalis of testis. Often first noticed as swelling of Scrotum. In children, it is usually congenital, while in adults, it usually occurs due to inflammation or injury.

3. *Varicocele*: It is dilatation and tortuosity of veins forming pampiniform plexus. It mostly occurs on the left side as venous return through left testicular vein is prone to obstruction because the long left testicular vein enters the left renal vein at the right angle. Further, it may be compressed by a loaded colon and tumors of left kidney. Clinically, it presents as scrotal swelling which disappears in the supine position and reappears in the erect posture. The spermatic cord feels like a bag of worms.

CHAPTER

12   Loin

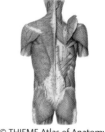

Learning Objectives

At the end of the dissection of loin, students should be able to identify the following:

- Extent of loin.
- Three layers of thoracolumbar fascia.
- Muscles enclosed between the layers of thoracolumbar fascia.
- Boundaries of lumbar triangle.

Introduction

The lower part of the back, between the lowest rib and the iliac crest on either side of the vertebral column, is termed as "loin."

Dissection and Identification

1. Turn the cadaver into the prone position. Now trace the lower part of the latissimus dorsi muscle to the iliac crest.

2. Expose the free, posterior border of the external oblique muscle.

3. Identify the lumbar triangle bounded by the edges of latissimus dorsi and external oblique muscles and the iliac crest (**Fig. 12.1**).

4. Reflect the remains of external oblique muscle anteriorly and latissimus dorsi inferiorly, to expose the thoracolumbar fascia. Note the attachment of the posterior part of the internal oblique to it.

5. Remove the remnants of latissimus dorsi.

6. Detach the serratus posterior inferior from the posterior layer of the thoracolumbar fascia. Cut this layer vertically from the level of the last rib to the iliac crest. Cut it transversely at the upper and lower ends of the cut. Reflect the layer to expose erector spinae. Pull this muscle medially, and trace the middle layer anterior to it. See its attachments. Cut it along its superior, medial, and inferior attachments and reflect it laterally.

7. Identify the quadratus lumborum muscle and push it medially to expose the anterior layer of thoracolumbar fascia.

8. Run your finger over the posterior surface of the anterior layer of the thoracolumbar fascia.

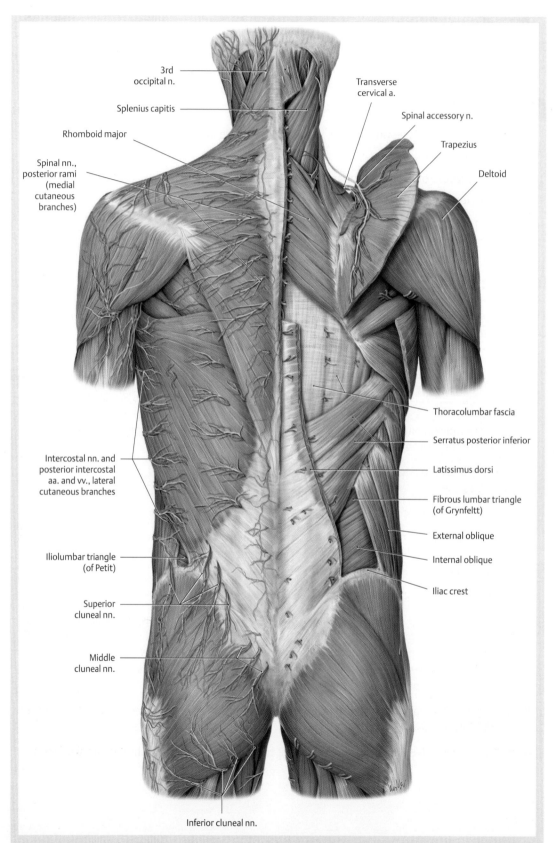

Fig. 12.1 Neurovasculature of the back and lumbar triangle. (From Schuenke M, Schulte E, Schumacher U. THIEME Atlas of Anatomy. General Anatomy and Musculoskeletal System. Illustrations by Voll M and Wesker K. © Thieme 2020)

Lumbar Triangle (of Petit)

It is bounded by latissimus dorsi, external oblique, and iliac crest. Its floor is formed by internal oblique.

Thoracolumbar Fascia

The whole of the back of the body is covered by the deep fascia. However, its thickness and strength is variable in different regions (**Fig. 12.2**).

In the *neck*, it is strong, dense, and forms part of the general investing layer of deep cervical fascia. Below the neck region, it is relatively thin and covers the superficial muscles which connect the upper limb with the trunk.

In the *lower thoracic, lumbar*, and *sacral regions*, it is well developed and very strong and lies deep to the superficial muscles of the back. It is termed as "thoracolumbar fascia." It binds the erector spinae, the long extensor muscle of the vertebral column to the posterolateral surfaces of the vertebral bodies. It also encloses the quadratus lumborum muscle in the lumbar region.

In the *lumbar region*, it is very strong and gives origin to the internal oblique and transversus abdominis muscles. Medially, thoracolumbar fascia splits into three layers: from deep to superficial, these are posterior, middle, and anterior.

1. Posterior layer passes behind the erector spinae and is attached to the tips of the spines of the lumbar vertebrae. It is this very layer which extends upward into the thoracic and cervical regions and downward into the sacral region.

   In the thoracic region, it forms a thin lamina which is attached to the spines of the thoracic vertebrae and the angles of the ribs. It lies deep to trapezius, rhomboids, and serratus posterior superior extending upward into the cervical region.

   In the sacral region, it stretches from the sacral spines to the ilium and sacrotuberous ligaments and fuses with the periosteum on the back of the sacrum and coccyx below the attachment of erector spinae on the sacrum.

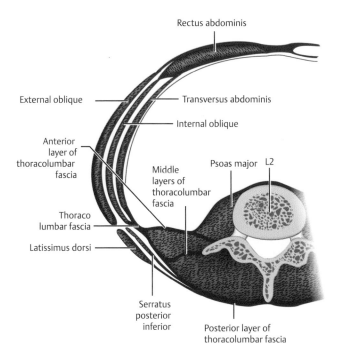

Fig. 12.2   Layers of thoracolumbar fascia as seen in a horizontal section through abdominal wall at the level of L2 vertebra.

2. Middle layer passes medially between the erector spinae and quadratus lumborum to the tips of the transverse processes of lumbar vertebrae.

3. Anterior layer passes in front of quadratus lumborum and gets attached to the anterior surfaces of the transverse processes of lumbar vertebrae. In this way, the quadratus lumborum gets enclosed between the anterior and middle layers. The quadratus lumborum muscle is attached to the anterior surfaces of the lumbar transverse processes and extends from the 12th rib above to the iliolumbar ligament and iliac crest below. Thus, the middle and anterior layers end above and below by being attached to the same structures as quadratus lumborum, posterior and anterior to it, respectively.

The anterior layer is a thin, thickened tendinous strip called *lateral arcuate ligament*. It extends from the tip of the first lumbar transverse process to the 12th rib and gives origin to the fibers of the diaphragm. The subcostal nerve and vessels pass from the thorax into the posterior abdominal wall posterior to the lateral arcuate ligament.

■ Clinical Notes

1. *Exposure of kidney from behind*: Knowledge of the anatomy of the loin region is essential for exposure of kidney from behind that is the retroperitoneal approach. It is indicated when peritoneal cavity is likely to be involved, such as inflammatory renal disease.

2. *Renal/ureteric colic*: Pain due to impaction of stone in ureter classically begins in loin and radiates to groin (for details, see page 205, Chapter 18).

3. *Lumbar hernia*: It may occur in the region of lumbar triangle.

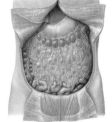

© THIEME Atlas of Anatomy

Introduction

The abdominal cavity is the largest cavity of the body. It is completely filled with the abdominal viscera such as stomach, intestines, liver, pancreas, spleen, kidneys, suprarenal glands and their associated ducts, blood, and lymph vessels.

The kidneys and suprarenal glands lie on the posterior abdominal wall enclosed in the fascial lining. The other viscera that lie anterior to them are more or less surrounded by the peritoneal cavity.

Dissection and Identification

1. Make diagonal incision from a point slightly to the left of the umbilicus, to the anterior superior iliac spine on both sides.

2. Pull the inferior triangular part of anterior abdominal wall inferiorly to examine the inner aspect of the anterior abdominal wall.

3. Identify five folds of the peritoneum located on the inner aspect of the lower part of the anterior abdominal wall that is median umbilical fold, medial umbilical folds, and lateral umbilical folds. The median umbilical fold which runs superiorly from the apex of the bladder to the umbilicus is formed by the underlying median umbilical ligament which is a remnant of the fetal urachus. The paired medial umbilical folds cover the underlying medial umbilical ligaments which are the remnants of the fetal umbilical arteries. The lateral umbilical folds overlie the inferior epigastric vessels (**Fig. 13.1**).

4. Now, identify the paired peritoneal fossae which lie between the peritoneal folds in the lower part of the inner surface of the anterior abdominal wall. Note the supravesical fossae, between the median umbilical fold and the medial umbilical folds, medial inguinal fossae, between the medial umbilical folds and the lateral umbilical folds, and lateral inguinal fossae, just lateral to the lateral inguinal folds and containing the deep inguinal rings.

5. Just superior to the midpoint of the inguinal ligament, identify the deep inguinal ring which is covered by the parietal peritoneum.

6. Remove the peritoneum and extraperitoneal adipose tissue around the deep inguinal ring to expose the transversalis fascia. Confirm the location of the deep inguinal ring just lateral to the inferior epigastric artery and vein.

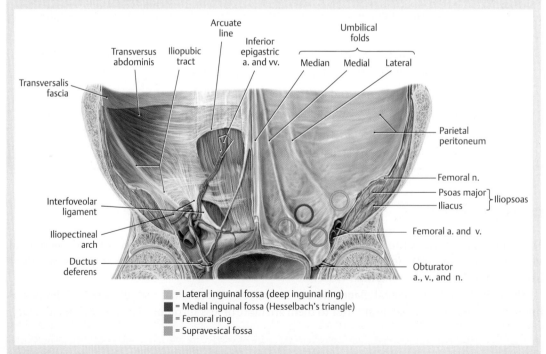

Fig. 13.1   Features on the inner aspect of the lower part of the anterior abdominal wall. (Modified from Schuenke M, Schulte E, Schumacher U. THIEME Atlas of Anatomy. General Anatomy and Musculoskeletal System. Illustrations by Voll M and Wesker K. © Thieme 2020)

7. In the male, identify the ductus deferens and the associated blood vessels and nerves that pass through the deep inguinal ring into the abdominal cavity. In the female, identify the round ligament of the uterus with associated vessels.

8. Make a vertical incision in the posterior wall of the rectus sheath from the xiphoid process just slightly left of the linea alba to the level of the umbilicus. Make another incision along the left costal margin to the midaxillary line and reflect the flap of the anterior abdominal wall laterally. Put your hand deep to the anterior abdominal wall along the vertical incision directed upward and to the right and feel the peritoneal fold extending from the anterior abdominal wall and diaphragm and to the liver. This is falciform ligament. Identify the round ligament of the liver (ligamentum teres) from the umbilicus to liver along the lower free border of falciform ligament.

9. Next, sever the attachment of the falciform ligament of the liver from the internal surface of the anterior abdominal wall.

10. Cut along the right costal margin to the midaxillary line and reflect the right flap of anterior abdominal wall laterally.

11. Examine the abdominal viscera in situ. The space of the peritoneal cavity that has been opened is called the greater sac. This space is located between the parietal layer of peritoneum lining the inner surface of the abdominal wall and the visceral layer of peritoneum covering outer surface of the abdominal viscera (**Fig. 13.2**).

12. Without dissecting, examine the exposed abdominal viscera within the peritoneal cavity. Identify the liver which occupies the right upper quadrant; attachment of falciform ligament dividing the liver into right and left lobes.

13. Identify the stomach which lies in the upper left quadrant and whose anterior surface is partially covered by liver. Reach around the left side of the stomach with your right hand and palpate the spleen behind the stomach.

14. Identify the peritoneal fold attached to the greater curvature of stomach and covering most of the viscera in the abdominal cavity.

15. Reflect the greater omentum superiorly and identify the structures which it partially covers. On the right side of the abdominal cavity, identify the caecum and the ascending colon. Observe the transverse colon span horizontally across the abdominal cavity and is attached to the greater omentum. On the left side, observe the sigmoid colon. Usually, the descending colon is covered by the coils of jejunum and ileum located in the central region of abdominal cavity.

16. Cut through the greater omentum 2 to 3 cm away from its attachment to the stomach to open the omental bursa (lesser sac). Put your hand into the bursa and explore its boundaries as it lies behind the stomach and lesser omentum.

17. Pull the liver superiorly to expose the lesser omentum which extends from the abdominal part of the esophagus, lesser curvature of the stomach, and first part of the duodenum to the porta hepatis on the inferior surface of the liver.

18. The lesser sac communicates through the epiploic foramen (foramen of Winslow) with the greater sac. The epiploic foramen lies behind the free margin of lesser omentum. Hold the free margin of the lesser omentum between the fingers and thumb of your left hand and palpate the structures lying between its two layers, that is bile duct in front and to the right, hepatic artery in front and to the left, and portal vein posteriorly.

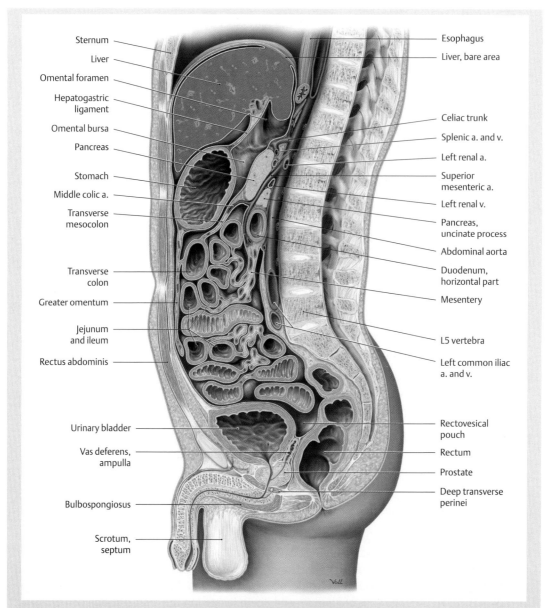

Fig. 13.2 Midsagittal section through abdominal cavity view (from left side) to show the disposition of abdominal viscera. (From Schuenke M, Schulte E, Schumacher U. THIEME Atlas of Anatomy. Internal Organs. Illustrations by Voll M and Wesker K. © Thieme 2020)

Peritoneum

The peritoneum is a tough layer of elastic areolar tissue. It is lined by simple squamous epithelium. The peritoneum forms a closed sac which is invaginated by abdominal viscera. Consequently, the peritoneum is divided into two layers: (1) an outer or parietal layer and (2) an inner or visceral layer.

Parietal Peritoneum

It lines the internal surface of the abdominal wall. Its blood and nerve supply are the same as those of the overlying body wall. The parietal peritoneum is innervated by somatic nerves and hence sensitive to pain when cut.

Visceral Peritoneum

It surrounds the mobile parts of the intra-abdominal gut completely except for a narrow strip where it passes as a double-layered fold (mesentery) to the posterior abdominal wall. The nerve supply and blood supply of visceral peritoneum are same as those of the underlying viscera. It is innervated by autonomic fibers and hence insensitive to pain when cut. However, visceral peritoneum evokes pain when viscera is stretched, distended, or undergoes ischemia.

Functions of peritoneum include movements of viscera, protection of viscera, absorption and dialysis, healing power, and adhesions and storage of fat.

Divisions of the Peritoneal Cavity

The peritoneal cavity is divided into two parts: (1) a large greater sac and (2) a much smaller lesser sac. The whole of the peritoneal cavity forms greater sac except for its small extension which passes between the stomach and the posterior abdominal wall. It is termed as "lesser sac" or "omental bursa." The two sacs communicate with each other through a foramen epiploicum (foramen of Winslow).

Peritoneal Folds and Pouches

As a result of invagination of peritoneal cavity by abdominal viscera, a number of peritoneal folds, pouches, spaces, and recesses are formed.

The location and extent of greater sac of peritoneum are well appreciated by tracing the vertical and horizontal disposition of peritoneum.

Vertical disposition: The vertical disposition of peritoneum is given in **Fig. 13.3**.

Horizontal disposition: The horizontal disposition of peritoneum above the transverse colon, that is the supracolic compartment, is given in **Fig. 13.4**, while that below the transverse colon, that is the infracolic compartment, is given in **Fig. 13.5**.

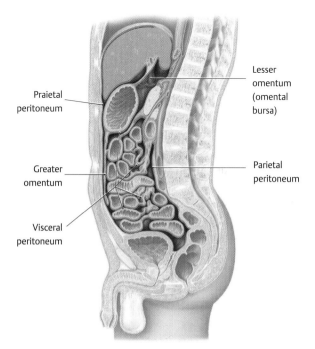

Fig. 13.3   Vertical disposition of peritoneum. (From Schuenke M, Schulte E, Schumacher U. THIEME Atlas of Anatomy. Internal Organs. Illustrations by Voll M and Wesker K. © Thieme 2020)

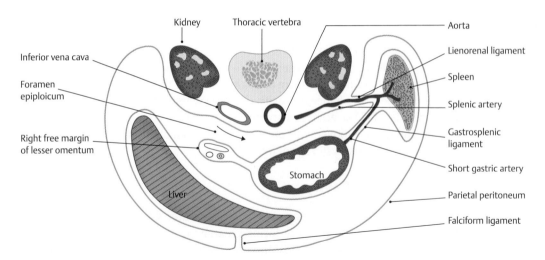

Fig. 13.4   Horizontal disposition of peritoneum above the transverse colon.

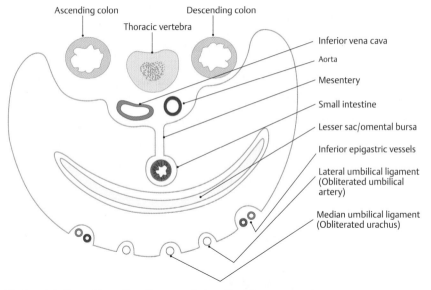

Fig. 13.5   Horizontal disposition of peritoneum below the transverse colon.

Greater Omentum (Fig. 13.6)

It is a large fold of peritoneum hanging down from greater curvature of stomach like an apron and covering the loops of intestines. It is made up of four layers of peritoneum. The anterior two layers descend from greater curvature of stomach and fold back to ascend as posterior two layers to the posterior abdominal wall. The fourth layer is partially fused to the upper aspect of transverse colon and mesocolon (**Fig. 13.6; Video 13.1**).

The contents of greater omentum include the following:

1. Right and left gastroepiploic vessels just below the greater curvature of the stomach.

2. It is often laden with fat.

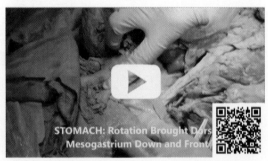

Video 13.1   Peritoneal cavity—greater sac, lesser sac, and greater omentum.

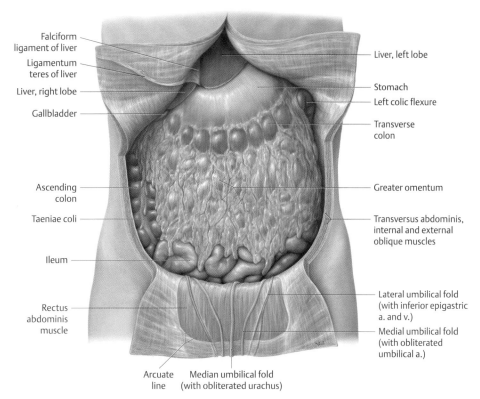

Falciform ligament of liver

Ligamentum teres of liver

Liver, right lobe

Gallbladder

Ascending colon

Taeniae coli

Ileum

Rectus abdominis muscle

Liver, left lobe

Stomach

Left colic flexure

Transverse colon

Greater omentum

Transversus abdominis, internal and external oblique muscles

Lateral umbilical fold (with inferior epigastric a. and v.)

Medial umbilical fold (with obliterated umbilical a.)

Arcuate line

Median umbilical fold (with obliterated urachus)

Fig. 13.6 Greater omentum (anterior abdominal wall retraction). (From Schuenke M, Schulte E, Schumacher U. THIEME Atlas of Anatomy. Internal Organs. Illustrations by Voll M and Wesker K. © Thieme 2020)

The greater omentum serves the following functions:

1. As a storehouse of fat.

2. It protects the peritoneal cavity against infection.

3. It limits the spread of infection by moving to the site of infection and sealing it off from the surrounding areas. For this very reason, the greater omentum is also termed as "*policemen of the abdomen*".

Lesser Omentum

It is a fold of peritoneum between the lesser curvature of the stomach and the first 2 cm of the duodenum below and to the liver above.

The right free margin of the lesser omentum contains (a) hepatic artery proper, (b) portal vein, and (c) bile duct.

Along the lesser curvature of the stomach, it contains (a) right gastric vessels, (b) left gastric vessels, (c) gastric group of lymph nodes, and (d) branches from the gastric nerves.

Mesentery

It is a broad, fan-shaped fold of peritoneum which suspends the small intestine from the posterior abdominal wall (**Fig. 13.7**).

It has two borders: attached border and free border. The attached border (root of the mesentery) is 15 cm long. It is directed obliquely downward and to the right from the duodenojejunal flexure on the left side of vertebra L2 to the right sacroiliac joint.

The free or intestinal border is 6 m long and is attached to the jejunum and ileum. It is thrown into pleats like that of a miniskirt.

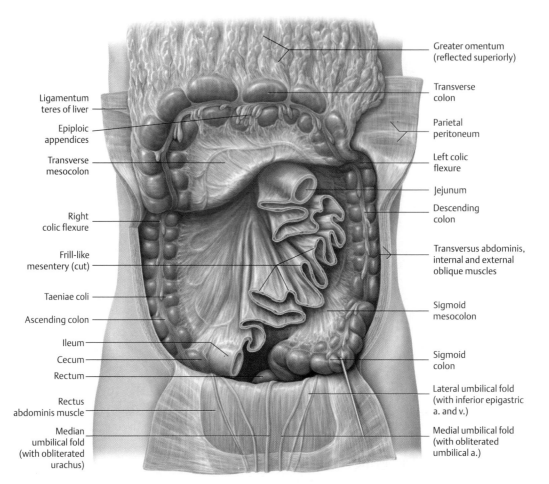

Greater omentum
(reflected superiorly)

Transverse
colon

Ligamentum
teres of liver

Epiploic
appendices

Transverse
mesocolon

Right
colic flexure

Frill-like
mesentery (cut)

Taeniae coli

Ascending colon

Ileum

Cecum

Rectum

Rectus
abdominis muscle

Median
umbilical fold
(with obliterated
urachus)

Parietal
peritoneum

Left colic
flexure

Jejunum

Descending
colon

Transversus abdominis,
internal and external
oblique muscles

Sigmoid
mesocolon

Sigmoid
colon

Lateral umbilical fold
(with inferior epigastric
a. and v.)

Medial umbilical fold
(with obliterated
umbilical a.)

Fig. 13.7 Mesenteries (reflected greater omentum and transverse colon). (From Schuenke M, Schulte E, Schumacher U. THIEME Atlas of Anatomy. Internal Organs. Illustrations by Voll M and Wesker K. © Thieme 2020)

The contents of mesentery are as follows:

1. Jejunal and ileal branches of the superior mesenteric artery and accompanying veins.

2. Autonomic nerve plexuses.

3. Lymphatics or lacteals.

4. Lymph nodes (100–200).

5. Fat.

Mesoappendix

It is a small, triangular fold of peritoneum which suspends the transverse colon from the upper part of the posterior abdominal wall, where it is attached to the head and body of pancreas. It contains the middle colic vessels, nerves, lymph nodes, and lymphatics.

Transverse Mesocolon

It is a large, horizontal, double-layered fold of peritoneum which suspends transverse colon from the posterior abdominal wall (**Fig. 13.7**).

Sigmoid Mesocolon

It is a triangular fold of peritoneum which suspends the sigmoid colon from the pelvic wall. The root of sigmoid mesocolon is V-shaped with apex over the left ureter, left limb on left external iliac artery, and right limb on pelvic surface of sacrum, extending downward and medially up to S3 vertebra (**Fig. 13.7**).

Peritoneal Recess and Pouches (Video 13.2)

Lesser Sac (Omental Bursa)

It is essentially a diverticulum of peritoneal cavity behind the stomach (**Fig. 13.8**). It communicates with greater sac through epiploic foramen. The omental bursa in situ is shown in **Fig. 13.9**.
   The boundaries of lesser sac are as follows:

1. *Anterior*: Caudate lobe of liver, lesser omentum, stomach, and anterior layers of greater omentum.

2. *Posterior*: Posterior two layers of greater omentum and stomach bed.

3. *Right*: Reflection of peritoneum from diaphragm to right caudate lobe, floor of epiploic foramen and also the reflection of peritoneum from head and neck of pancreas to the posterior surface of the first part of duodenum, and right free margin of greater omentum.

4. *Left*: Gastrophrenic ligament, splenic pedicle (gastrosplenic and lienorenal ligaments).

5. *Superior*: Reflection of peritoneum from esophagus onto diaphragm, upper end of fissure for ligamentum venosum, and upper border of caudate lobe of liver.

6. *Inferior*: Continuation of anterior and posterior layers of greater omentum below the transverse colon. Omentum at its lower margin, which gets obliterated in adults below the level of transverse colon (**Fig. 13.10**).

Lesser sac presents the following three recesses:

1. Superior recess, behind lesser omentum and liver.

2. Inferior recess, below with the lower part of greater omentum.

3. Splenic recess, between gastrosplenic and lienorenal ligaments (**Fig. 13.11**).

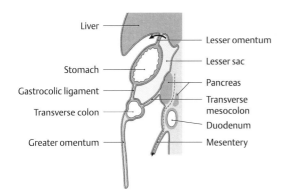

Fig. 13.8 Location of lesser sac or omental bursa (blue coloured area). (From Schuenke M, Schulte E, Schumacher U. THIEME Atlas of Anatomy. Internal Organs. Illustrations by Voll M and Wesker K. © Thieme 2020)

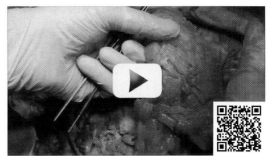

Video 13.2 Peritoneal cavity—Foramen of Winslow.

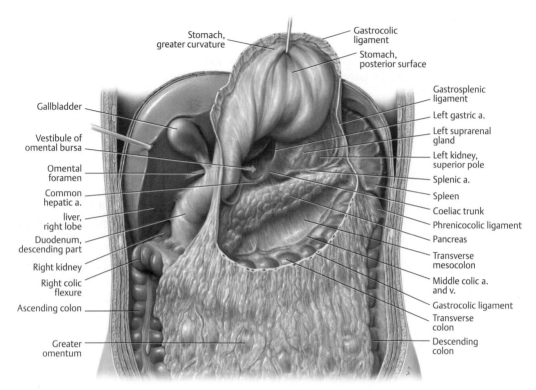

Fig. 13.9   Omental bursa in situ. (From Schuenke M, Schulte E, Schumacher U. THIEME Atlas of Anatomy. Internal Organs. Illustrations by Voll M and Wesker K. © Thieme 2020)

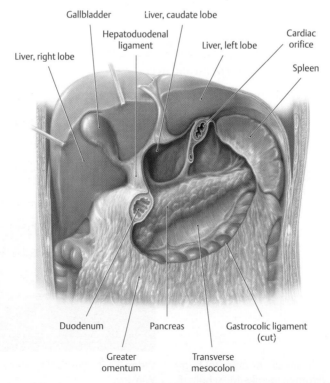

Fig. 13.10   Boundaries of the lesser sac (omental bursa). (From Schuenke M, Schulte E, Schumacher U. THIEME Atlas of Anatomy. Internal Organs. Illustrations by Voll M and Wesker K. © Thieme 2020)

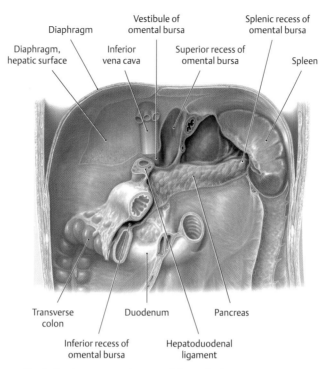

Fig. 13.11 Posterior wall of the lesser sac (omental bursa) showing its recesses. (From Schuenke M, Schulte E, Schumacher U. THIEME Atlas of Anatomy. Internal Organs. Illustrations by Voll M and Wesker K. © Thieme 2020)

Epiploic/Omental Foramen (Foramen of Winslow)

The boundaries of epiploic/omental foramen are as follows:

1. *Anterior*: Right free margin of lesser omentum containing portal vein, hepatic artery, and bile duct.

2. *Posterior*: Inferior vena cava, right suprarenal gland, and the level of T12 vertebra.

3. *Superior*: Caudate process of caudate lobe of liver.

4. *Inferior*: First part of duodenum and horizontal part of hepatic artery.

Greater and lesser sacs of peritoneum communicate with each other through epiploic foramen (**Fig. 13.8**, see arrow)

Hepatorenal Pouch (Morison's Pouch)

It is located on the posteroinferior surface of liver in front of the right kidney.
Following are the boundaries of hepatorenal pouch:

1. Anterior:
   - Inferior surface of the right lobe of liver.
   - Gallbladder.
2. Posterior:
   - Right suprarenal gland.
   - Upper part of the right kidney.
   - Second part of the duodenum.
   - Hepatic flexure of the colon.

- Transverse mesocolon.
- Part of the head of the pancreas.

3. Superior:
- Inferior layer of the coronary ligament.

4. Inferior:
- Opens into the general peritoneal cavity.

Rectouterine Pouch (Pouch of Douglas)

It is located in the pelvis between the rectum and uterus. This pouch is the most dependent part of the peritoneal cavity, where the body is in erect position and most dependent part of the pelvic cavity in the supine position.

The boundaries of rectouterine pouch are the following:

1. *Anterior*: Uterus and the posterior fornix of the vagina.

2. *Posterior*: Rectum.

3. *Inferior (floor)*: Rectovaginal fold of peritoneum.

▌ Clinical Notes

1. *Peritonitis*: It is the inflammation of peritoneum. It may be localized or generalized. The generalized peritonitis may be fatal after abdominopelvic surgery.

2. *Internal hernia*: It is the herniation of intestinal loop into lesser sac through foramen epiploicum. If it gets strangulated, the reduction of hernia is not possible by enlarging the epiploic foramen because of its important relations. The reduction is done by aspirating the swollen bowel loop and pushing it from within the lesser sac.

3. *Subphrenic abscess*: The hepatorenal pouch (Morrison pouch) is the commonest site of abscess formation postoperatively because it is the most dependent part of abdominal cavity proper in supine position, as it is continuous with the epiploic foramen to the left and right paracolic gutter below. The abscess may form here secondary to cholecystitis, perforated duodenal ulcer, and appendicitis.

4. *Pelvic abscess*: The rectouterine pouch is the commonest site of pelvic abscess because it is the most dependent part of peritoneal cavity in the true pelvis. The pus can be drained either through rectum or posterior vaginal wall.

14

Abdominal Part of Esophagus, Stomach, Celiac Trunk, and Spleen

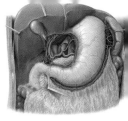

© THIEME Atlas of Anatomy

At the end of the dissection of the abdominal part of esophagus, stomach, celiac trunk and spleen, students should be able to identify the following:

- Celiac trunk, its vertebral level, relations, and branches, veins corresponding to the branches of the celiac trunk, and where they drain.
- Abdominal part of esophagus, note its location, relations, nerve, and vascular supply.
- Stomach and its size, shape, location, borders, surface, curvatures, notches, parts, and peritoneal relations.
- Structures forming the stomach bed.
- Arteries supplying the stomach and the corresponding veins.
- Pyloric sphincter and cardiac end of the stomach, the characteristics of the gastric canal, and parts of the stomach.
- Lymph nodes draining the stomach.

Dissection and Identification

1. Pull the liver upward to expose the lesser omentum. Peel off the anterior layer of lesser omentum to expose structures present within it. Using blunt forceps, clean and identify the vessels along the lesser curvature of the stomach. Identify the gastric branches of both the right and left gastric arteries along the anterior and posterior aspects of the lesser curvature of the stomach. Trace the branches of left gastric artery (**Fig. 14.1**) toward the abdominal part of the esophagus which they supply. Trace the right gastric artery to its origin from hepatic artery proper (**Video 14.1**).

2. Identify the epiploic foramen (foramen of Winslow) which lies posterior to the free edge of the lesser omentum extending between the first part of duodenum and porta hepatis. Clean and identify the structures that lie in the free margin of the lesser omentum. To the left, identify the common hepatic artery and trace it and the common bile duct which lies to its right, toward the porta hepatis. Displace the artery and the bile duct to expose the portal vein that lies posterior to them.

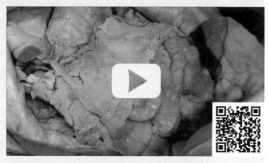

Video 14.1 Overview of abdominal organs.

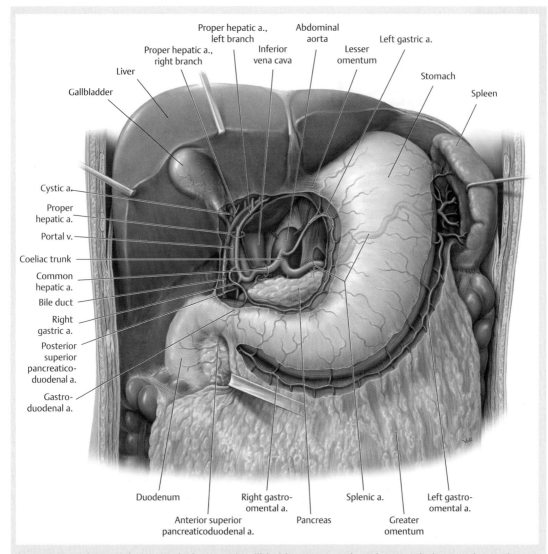

Fig. 14.1   Celiac trunk: Stomach, liver, and gallbladder. (From Schuenke M, Schulte E, Schumacher U. THIEME Atlas of Anatomy. Internal Organs. Illustrations by Voll M and Wesker K. © Thieme 2020)

3. Follow the common hepatic artery downward to the upper border of duodenum where it gives off gastroduodenal artery which passes inferiorly, posterior to the first part of the duodenum. Reflect the stomach superiorly and follow the gastroduodenal artery to its terminal branches, the right gastroepiploic artery, and the superior pancreaticoduodenal artery.

4. Using blunt dissection, clean the right and left gastroepiploic arteries, which lie along the greater curvature of the stomach. Identify the multiple gastric branches supplying the stomach and the omental branches supplying the greater omentum from both the right and left gastroepiploic arteries.

5. The junction between the stomach and duodenum is a narrow opening surrounded by thick circular muscle fibers forming pyloric sphincter. Feel the thickening between your fingers and thumb and put two ligatures on either side of the pyloric sphincter and cut the stomach between the ligatures immediately to the right of the pylorus. Divide the right gastric and right gastroepiploic vessels and turn the stomach upward and to the left to expose the omental bursa (**Fig. 14.2**; **Video 14.2**).

6. Remove the peritoneum from the posterior wall of the bursa and examine the posterior relations of the stomach on the posterior abdominal wall forming "stomach bed," that is, the pancreas, part of left kidney, left suprarenal gland, and left crus of the diaphragm.

7. Identify the celiac trunk (**Fig. 14.2**), a short, thick artery that arises from the anterior aspect of the abdominal aorta just below the diaphragm and above the L1 vertebra. Note the paired celiac ganglia on either side of the celiac trunk and the dense network of nerve fibers, celiac plexus around it, and its branches.

8. Remove the nerve fibers surrounding celiac trunk and its branches and examine the origin of its three branches: left gastric, common hepatic, and splenic.

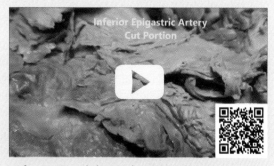

Video 14.2 Abdominal viscera—an overview.

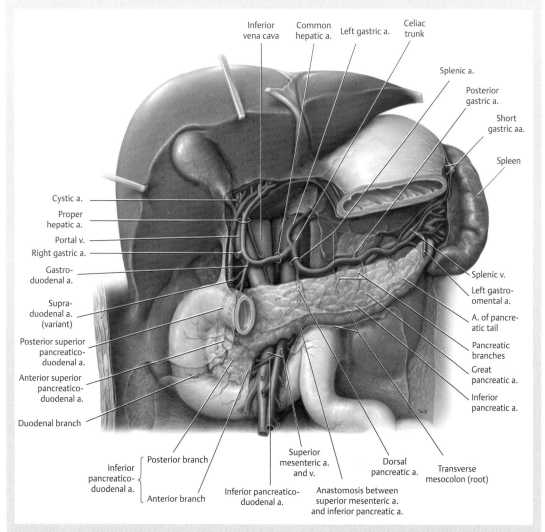

Fig. 14.2 Celiac trunk: Pancreas, duodenum, and spleen. (From Schuenke M, Schulte E, Schumacher U. THIEME Atlas of Anatomy. Internal Organs. Illustrations by Voll M and Wesker K. © Thieme 2020)

Follow the left gastric artery upward toward the cardiac orifice of the stomach. The rest of its course and branches have been dissected earlier.

9. Identify the spleen and examine its relationship to the visceral organs which contact its surface. Review the relationship of the hilum of the spleen to the tail of the pancreas. The end of the tail of the pancreas passes within the lienorenal ligament and contacts the hilum of the spleen. Mobilize the spleen and identify the splenic artery and vein (**Fig. 14.2**).

10. Cut the splenic vessels close to the hilum and remove the spleen by cutting rest of the lienorenal ligament, taking care to leave the tail of the pancreas. Identify the two surfaces of the spleen and the visceral surface. The diaphragmatic surface is smooth and rounded. The visceral surface is subdivided into three areas: the gastric surface, the renal surface, and the colic surface. Note the superior border of the spleen is notched.

11. Now, follow the splenic artery (**Fig. 14.2**) which pursues a tortuous course along the superior border of the pancreas. Note that, along its course, it gives numerous short pancreatic branches. Trace the artery across the front of the left kidney into the lienorenal ligament as it passes to the hilum of the spleen. Before entering the spleen, the artery divides into three or four splenic arteries. Note its branches: the left gastroepiploic artery and short gastric arteries.

12. Strip off the peritoneum from the anterior and posterior surfaces of the stomach close to the cardiac end and find the branches of the anterior and posterior vagal trunks supplying the respective surfaces of the stomach. The nerves can be identified by a gentle traction on the vagal trunks from the thoracic side of the diaphragm.

13. Remove the stomach by cutting through the abdominal part of the esophagus, left gastric vessels, and gastrophrenic and gastrosplenic ligaments.

14. Make an incision through the wall of the stomach along the entire length of the greater curvature. Open it and remove any food content by washing under running water. Observe the mucosal folds, called rugae, project into the lumen of the stomach.

15. Note that the pyloric sphincter bulges the mucous membrane into the pyloric part and narrows the opening to a small hole. Strip the mucous membrane from a part to expose the inner muscular coat.

Abdominal Part of Esophagus

It enters the abdomen through the esophageal opening of the diaphragm (**Fig. 14.3**) at the level of vertebra T10, slightly to the left of the median plane. Abdominal part of esophagus is only about 1.25 cm long.

The esophageal opening transmits the anterior and posterior vagal trunks, esophageal branches of the left gastric artery, and the accompanying veins.

The abdominal part of esophagus is one of the major sites of portosystemic anastomosis. The lower end of esophagus acts as physiological sphincter as a result of precise neuromuscular coordination.

Stomach

The stomach is the most distensible part of the gastrointestinal tract. It lies obliquely in the upper left part of the abdomen, occupying the epigastric, umbilical, and left hypochondriac regions, mostly under cover of the left costal margin (**Figs. 14.3–14.5**).

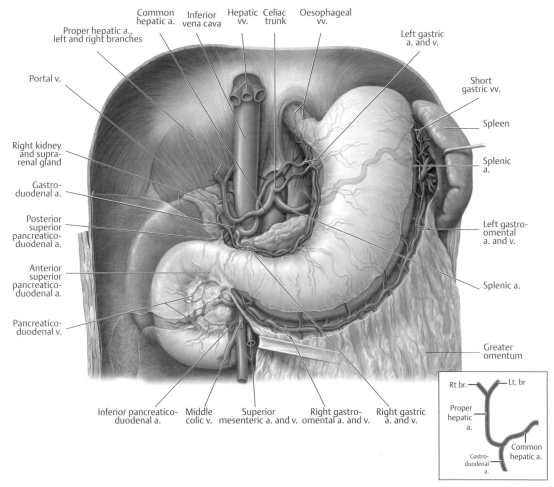

Fig. 14.3 Abdominal part of esophagus and stomach. (Modified from Schuenke M, Schulte E, Schumacher U. THIEME Atlas of Anatomy. Internal Organs. Illustrations by Voll M and Wesker K. © Thieme 2020) Figure in the insert shows common hepatic artery and its branches.

External Features (Fig.14.4)

The stomach is usually "J" shaped when empty and presents two orifices or openings, two curvatures or borders, and two surfaces.

Two Orifices

1. *Cardiac orifice* lies below the left of the costal cartilage 2.5 cm away from sterna margin at the level of T11 vertebra.

2. *Pyloric orifice* lies 1.25 cm to the right of median plane at the level of L1 vertebra.

Two Curvatures

1. *Lesser curvature* is concave along the right border of stomach and provides attachment to lesser omentum.

2. *Greater curvature* is convex along the left border of stomach to which greater omentum is attached.

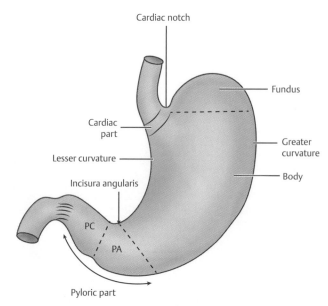

Fig. 14.4   External features of stomach. Abbreviations: PA, Pyloric antrum; PC, Pyloric canal.

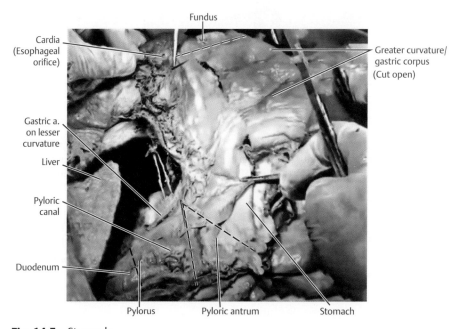

Fig. 14.5   Stomach.

Two Surfaces

The *anterosuperior surface* faces forward and upward, while *posteroinferior surface* faces backward and downward.

Subdivisions (Fig. 14.4)

The stomach is subdivided into four parts: *cardia, fundus, body,* and *pylorus*. The incisura angularis is a notch on the lesser curvature inferiorly. The *cardia/cardiac* part lies near the inferior oesophageal orifice. The *fundus* lies above the transverse line passing through the cardiac notch to the greater curvature. The body lies below the horizontal line passing through the cardiac notch and above the oblique line passing from incisura angularis to the greater curvature of stomach. The pyloric part lies distal to body upto duodenum.

Relations

Peritoneal Relations

At the lesser curvature, the two layers of peritoneum lining the anterior and posterior surfaces of the stomach meet to form the lesser omentum. Similarly, along the greater curvature the two layers of peritoneum meet to form the greater omentum. Near the fundus, the two layers of peritoneum meet to form the gastrosplenic ligament. Near the cardiac end, the peritoneum on the posterior surface is reflected on to the diaphragm to form the gastrosplenic ligament.

Visceral Relations

1. *Anterior surface*: It is related to the liver, diaphragm, and anterior abdominal wall.
2. *Posterior surface*: It is related to structures forming the *stomach bed*, such as:
   - Diaphragm.
   - Left kidney.
   - Left suprarenal gland.
   - Pancreas.
   - Transverse mesocolon.
   - Splenic flexure of colon.
   - Spleen.

All of these are separated from the stomach by the cavity of the lesser sac, except spleen which is separated by the greater sac.

Blood Vessels and Nerves

Blood Supply

The rich arterial supply to the stomach is exclusively from all the three branches of the celiac trunk. The venous drainage is to the portal system (**Fig. 14.3**).

Lymphatic Drainage

The lymph vessels run along the blood vessels to the small lymph node lying beside them. The main lymph nodes, such as pancreaticosplenic and pyloric, lie on the posterior abdominal wall near the pancreas (**Fig. 14.6**).

Nerve Supply

The parasympathetic nerve supply is by the anterior and posterior vagal trunks which arise from the esophageal plexus and enter the abdomen through the esophageal hiatus. Hepatic branches of the anterior vagus pass to the liver, while celiac branch of the posterior vagus passes to the celiac ganglion. The anterior and posterior vagal trunks run along the lesser curvature of stomach as the anterior and posterior nerves of Latarjet from which terminal branches arise to supply the stomach. The vagi provide a motor and secretory supply to the stomach (**Fig. 14.7**).

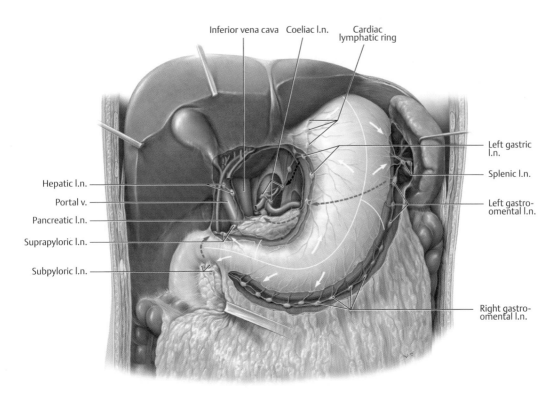

Fig. 14.6 Lymphatic drainage of stomach. (From Schuenke M, Schulte E, Schumacher U. THIEME Atlas of Anatomy. Internal Organs. Illustrations by Voll M and Wesker K. © Thieme 2020)

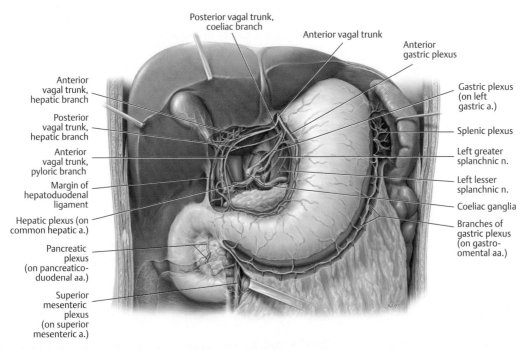

Fig. 14.7 Innervation of anterior stomach. (From Schuenke M, Schulte E, Schumacher U. THIEME Atlas of Anatomy. Internal Organs. Illustrations by Voll M and Wesker K. © Thieme 2020)

Interior of the Stomach

1. Thick mucosa lining is thrown into longitudinal folds along the lesser curvature and is irregular elsewhere.

2. Presence of a large number of small depressions in the mucous membrane is called gastric pits.

3. Lumen along the lesser curvature is called gastric canal (canal of Magenstrasse).

Celiac Trunk (refer to Figs. 14.2 and 14.3)

This short arterial trunk arises from the aorta at the level of T12/L1 and after a short course divides into three terminal branches: left gastric, splenic, and common hepatic.

1. *Left gastric artery*: This small branch passes upward to supply the lower esophagus by branches which ascend through the esophageal hiatus in the diaphragm. It then descends in the lesser omentum along the lesser curvature of the stomach.

2. *Splenic artery*: It is the largest branch of celiac trunk. It runs a tortuous course along the superior border of the pancreas in the posterior wall of the lesser sac to reach the hilum of the spleen through the lienorenal ligament. The splenic artery gives off short gastric arteries which supply the stomach fundus and a left gastroepiploic artery which runs in the gastrosplenic ligament and greater omentum to supply the greater curvature of the stomach.

3. *Common hepatic artery*: It runs to the right toward the first part of the duodenum in the posterior wall of the lesser sac. It then ascends between the layers of the right free border of the lesser sac to reach the porta hepatis. Before reaching the porta hepatis, it divides into right and left hepatic arteries, and from the right branch the cystic artery is usually given off. Before it ascends toward porta hepatis, the hepatic artery gives rise to gastroduodenal and right gastric arteries. The gastroduodenal artery passes behind the first part of the duodenum and then branches further into superior pancreaticoduodenal and gastroepiploic arteries. The right gastroepiploic artery runs along the lower part of the greater curvature to supply the stomach.

Spleen

The spleen is the largest mass of lymphoid tissue in the body. It is a wedge-shaped organ lying high up in the left hypochondrium behind stomach, below the left hemidiaphragm, which, in addition to pleura, separates it from the 9th ,10th, and 11th ribs.

It is about the size of a clenched fist. On an average, it is 1 inch (2.5 cm) thick, 3 inch (7.5 cm) broad, and 5 inch (12.5 cm) long, and weighs 7 ounce.

External Features (Fig. 14.8)

The spleen presents two ends, three borders, two poles, and two surfaces.

1. Anterior end or extremity is expanded and looks like a border. It is directed downward and forward and extends up to the midaxillary line.

2. Posterior end or extremity is rounded. It is directed upward, backward, and medially to lie on the upper pole of the left kidney.

3. Superior border is characteristically notched near the anterior end.

4. Inferior border is rounded.

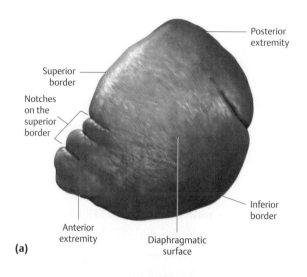

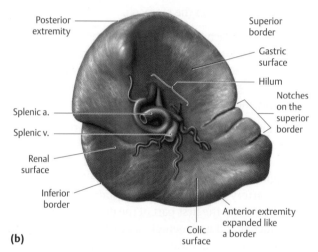

Fig. 14.8 External features of spleen. **(a)** Costal surface. **(b)** Visceral surface. (Modified from Schuenke M, Schulte E, Schumacher U. THIEME Atlas of Anatomy. Internal Organs. Illustrations by Voll M and Wesker K. © Thieme 2020)

5. Intermediate border is low ridge at the junction of gastric and renal impressions.

6. Diaphragmatic surface is convex and smooth, while the visceral surface is concave and irregular.

7. The diaphragmatic surface is related to diaphragm which separates it from the left costodia-phragmatic recess and 9th, 10th, and 11th ribs.

8. The visceral surface presents the hilum and bears the following impressions:
   - Gastric impression, for the fundus of the stomach.
   - Renal impression for the left kidney.
   - Colic impression for the splenic flexure of the colon and pancreatic impression for the tail of pancreas.

The *hilum* lies on the lower part of the gastric impression along the intermediate border of the spleen. The gastrosplenic and lienorenal ligament are attached to the hilum. The gastrosplenic ligament contains short gastric arteries. The tail of pancreas lies in lienorenal ligament and may reach the hilum.

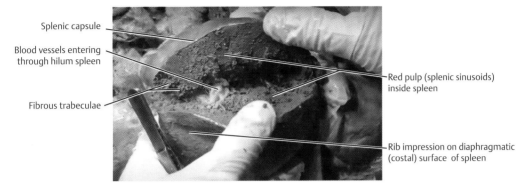

Splenic capsule

Blood vessels entering through hilum spleen

Fibrous trabeculae

Red pulp (splenic sinusoids) inside spleen

Rib impression on diaphragmatic (costal) surface of spleen

Fig. 14.9   Spleen.

Structure and Function

Structurally, spleen is a highly vascular reticuloendothelial organ. It consists of thick fibroelastic capsule from which trabeculae extend into the pulp of the spleen (**Fig. 14.9**). The spleen is made of red pulp and white pulp. The white pulp consisting of lymphoid follicles is scattered throughout the richly vascularized sinusoids forming the red pulp. The spleen plays an important role in the development of immunity and its removal increases the susceptibility of individual to infection.

Blood Supply

The arterial supply is from splenic artery (**Fig 14.8b**), a branch of celiac trunk. The venous drainage occurs through splenic vein into the portal vein.

▌ Clinical Notes

1. *Esophageal varices*: It is the dilatation, tortuosity, and lengthening of veins in the lower end of esophagus. Their rupture causes hematemesis. These veins are the communicating channels between the portal and caval systems (portacaval anastomosis) and get involved in portal hypertension.

2. *Gastric ulcers*: They commonly occur along the lesser curvature of stomach because it is subjected to maximum insult by spicy food and irritable liquids.

3. *Splenomegaly*: It is the enlargement of spleen which may occur due to a number of diseases such as malaria, chronic myeloid leukemia, and cirrhosis of liver. The enlarged spleen, especially if massive, projects downward and medially toward the right iliac fossa, and notches on its anterior border can be easily palpated.

15 Duodenum, Pancreas, and Portal Vein

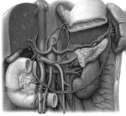

© THIEME Atlas of Anatomy

Learning Objectives

At the end of the dissection of duodenum and pancreas, students should be able to identify the following:

- Duodenum in situ and trace its extent from the pylorus to duodenojejunal flexure. Note its parts, flexures, length, shape, location, and vertebral levels.
- Peritoneal reflections, folds, and recesses related to duodenum.
- Relations of duodenum with pancreas, bile duct, and portal vein.
- Suspensory ligament of duodenum (ligament of Treitz).
- Supraduodenal, superior pancreaticoduodenal, and inferior pancreaticoduodenal vessels; anterior and posterior pancreaticoduodenal anastomoses.
- Plicae circulares and major and minor duodenal papillae in the interior of the duodenum.
- Pancreas in situ. Note its parts, borders, surfaces, and relations.
- Trace the peritoneal reflections on the pancreas.
- Main and accessory pancreatic ducts. Note the herringbone pattern of the main pancreatic duct.
- Blood supply, lymphatic drainage, and innervation of duodenum and pancreas.
- Portal vein and its main tributaries, namely, superior mesenteric, splenic, and inferior mesenteric veins. Trace the termination of portal vein and enumerate the sites of portacaval anastomoses.

Dissection and Identification

1. Remove the transverse colon and stomach, and identify the duodenum encircling the head of the pancreas. Note the four parts of duodenum: first, second, third, and fourth. Note that with the exception of its first part, the whole of duodenum is retroperitoneal.

2. Observe the structures related to different parts of the duodenum. Cut the peritoneum along the lateral side of the descending (second) part of the duodenum and reflect the duodenum to the left to expose the structures lying posterior to it.

3. Remove the peritoneum surrounding the fourth part of the duodenum and observe the inferior mesenteric vein lateral to it. Try to find a slender fibromuscular band (suspensory ligament of Treitz) extending from the superior aspect of duodenojejunal flexure to the right crus of the diaphragm.

4. Open the duodenum along its entire length by cutting along its convex surface. Clean the interior to see the mucosal surface. Observe that the first part of the duodenum is smooth without mucosal folds. The remaining parts of the duodenum have large circular mucosal folds.

5. On the medial wall of the second (descending) part of the duodenum, identify the major duodenal papilla, located at the upper end of the longitudinal fold of the duodenum. At the apex

of the major (greater) duodenal papilla, identify the small opening of the hepatopancreatic ampulla (ampulla of Vater), through which the main pancreatic duct and common bile duct empty into the duodenum.

6. Approximately 2 cm superior to the greater duodenal papilla, try to locate the opening of the accessory pancreatic duct (duct of Santorini) on the minor (lesser) duodenal papilla.

7. Define the extent of pancreas lying horizontally across the posterior abdominal wall. Note the four parts of pancreas from right to left: head, neck, body, and tail.

8. Note that the head of the pancreas is the flattened and enlarged portion that rests within the C-curve of the duodenum. A tongue-like process from the most inferior portion of the head is the uncinate process, which "hooks" to the left and lies posterior to the superior mesenteric vessels.

9. Lift the tail and the body of the pancreas from the posterior abdominal wall and examine the structures lying immediately posterior to them. Trace the splenic vein as it runs posterior to the tail, body, neck, and head of the pancreas. Note that the splenic vein receives the inferior mesenteric vein and ends posterior to the neck of the pancreas by joining the superior mesenteric vein to form the portal vein.

10. Free the horizontal (third) part of the duodenum and the uncinate process of the pancreas from the posterior abdominal wall. Turn the second part of the duodenum and the head of the pancreas to the left. Look for the bile duct and posterior pancreaticoduodenal vessels. Note the bile duct lies in a groove on the posterior surface of the head of pancreas. Find its union with the pancreatic duct close to the duodenum.

11. Using a probe and forceps, remove the stroma from the posterior surface of the pancreas to expose the grayish white pancreatic ducts. Observe that the large main pancreatic duct begins in the tail of the pancreas and ends at the hepatopancreatic ampulla that opens on the greater duodenal papilla in the second part of the duodenum. Along its course, it receives numerous smaller pancreatic ducts at right angle, forming a "herringbone pattern."

12. Note that the accessory pancreatic duct begins within the head of the pancreas, superior to the main pancreatic duct and opens on the summit of the lesser duodenal papilla.

Duodenum

The duodenum is the first part of the small intestine which is the widest and most fixed. It joins the stomach to the jejunum. It is approximately 25 cm long and curves around the head of pancreas. Its primary function is the absorption of digested products. It is located in the epigastric and umbilical region astride the vertical column (**Fig. 15.1**). Despite its relatively short length, the surface area for absorption is greatly enhanced by the mucosa being thrown into folds bearing villi, which are visible only at a microscopic level. With the exception of the first 2.5 cm, the duodenum is a retroperitoneal organ.

Parts

The C-shaped duodenum is divided into four parts (**Fig. 15.2**; **Video 15.1**):

1. *First (superior) part* (5 cm): It passes upward, backward, and to the right from pylorus.

2. *Second (descending) part* (7.5 cm): It begins at the superior duodenal flexure and descends around the head of the pancreas up to the lower border of L3 vertebra.

3. *Third (horizontal) part* (10 cm): It passes horizontally across the vertebral column. This part is crossed anteriorly by the root of the mesentery and superior mesenteric vessels.

4. *Fourth (ascending) part* (2.5 cm): It passes upward to the left on the vertebral column and terminates as the duodenojejunal junction. The duodenojejunal junction is 2 to 3 cm to the left of median plane. It is demarcated by a peritoneal fold stretching from this junction to the right crus of the diaphragm covering the suspensory ligament of Treitz. The terminal part of the inferior mesenteric vein lies adjacent to the duodenojejunal junction and serves as a useful landmark to the surgeons.

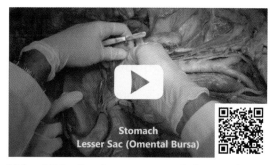

Video 15.1   Duodenum: parts, relations, and vasculature.

Blood supply: It is by superior and inferior pancreaticoduodenal arteries which run between duodenum and the pancreatic head. The superior pancreaticoduodenal artery arises from the celiac

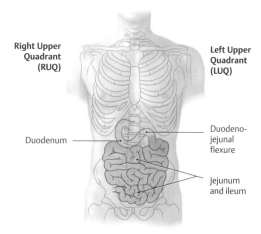

Fig. 15.1   Location of duodenum (anterior view). (From Schuenke M, Schulte E, Schumacher U. THIEME Atlas of Anatomy. Internal Organs. Illustrations by Voll M and Wesker K. © Thieme 2020)

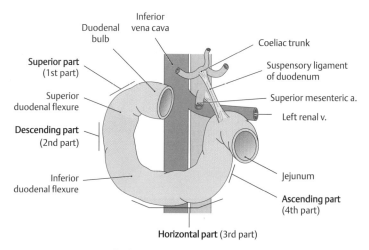

Fig. 15.2   Parts of duodenum. (From Schuenke M, Schulte E, Schumacher U. THIEME Atlas of Anatomy. Internal Organs. Illustrations by Voll M and Wesker K. © Thieme 2020)

trunk through gastroduodenal artery, while inferior pancreaticoduodenal artery arises from the superior mesenteric artery (see **Fig. 14.2**).

Interior of the Duodenum

In the midsection, the interior of duodenum presents a small eminence on the posteromedial aspect of the mucosa called *major duodenal papilla*. The common opening of the bile duct and main pancreatic duct (duct of Wirsung) is present on its summit. This common opening is guarded by the sphincter of Oddi. A smaller accessory pancreatic duct (duct of Santorini) opens into the duodenum at a small distance above on the summit of minor duodenal papilla (**Fig. 15.3**).

Pancreas

The pancreas is a soft, elongated gland lying across the upper part of posterior abdominal wall from duodenum to the hilum of the spleen. It is mostly—a retroperitoneal organ and lies roughly along the transpyloric plane. It has a head, neck, body, and a tail. The head is bound laterally by the curved duodenum and the tail extends to the hilum of the spleen in the lieno-renal ligament. The superior mesenteric artery and vein first pass behind the pancreas, then anterior to the uncinate process and the third part of the duodenum to enter the root of the mesentery of the small intestine (**Figs. 15.4 and 15.5; Video 15.2**).

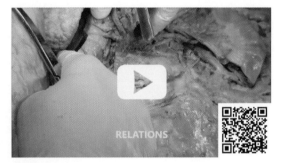

Video 15.2   Pancreas.

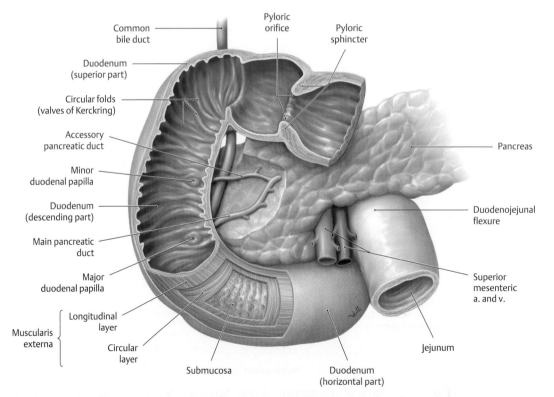

Fig. 15.3   Interior of duodenum. (From Schuenke M, Schulte E, Schumacher U. THIEME Atlas of Anatomy. Internal Organs. Illustrations by Voll M and Wesker K. © Thieme 2020)

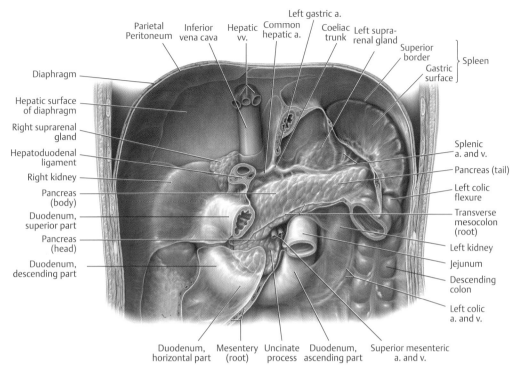

Fig. 15.4 Pancreas and spleen in situ. (Modified from Schuenke M, Schulte E, Schumacher U. THIEME Atlas of Anatomy. Internal Organs. Illustrations by Voll M and Wesker K. © Thieme 2020)

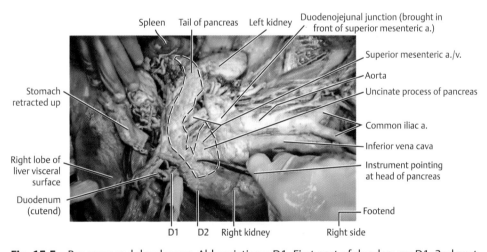

Fig. 15.5 Pancreas and duodenum. Abbreviations: D1, First part of duodenum; D1, 2nd part of duodenum.

Relations

The inferior vena cava, aorta, celiac plexus, left kidney (and its vessels), and left adrenal gland form posterior pancreatic relations. In addition, the portal vein is formed behind the neck of pancreas by the union of the splenic and superior mesenteric veins. The lesser sac and stomach form anterior pancreatic relations.

Structure

The pancreas is an exoendocrine gland. The exocrine part consists of acini which secrete a number of enzymes that break down proteins, carbohydrates, and fat in the alkaline conditions of the duodenum. The endocrine part consists of islets of Langerhans, made up of minute cells such as alpha cells and beta cells. They secrete insulin and glucagon directly into the blood stream to control the blood sugar level.

Ducts of Pancreas (Fig 15.6)

1. *Main pancreatic duct (duct of Wirsung)* courses the length of the gland near its posterior surface ultimately draining pancreatic secretions into the ampulla of Vater, together with the common bile duct, and thence into the second part of the duodenum. It is easily identified by its white color and "herringbone" appearance.

2. *Accessory duct (duct of Santorini)* drains the uncinate process of the pancreas and opens slightly proximal to the ampulla into the second part of the duodenum about 8 to 10 cm distal to pylorus (**Fig. 15.6**).

Vessels and Lymph Nodes

The arterial supply of the pancreatic head is derived from the superior and inferior pancreaticoduodenal arteries. The remaining portion is supplied by the splenic artery coursing along the upper border of the body of the pancreas which it supplies by a large branch called *arteria pancreatica magna* and numerous smaller unnamed branches.

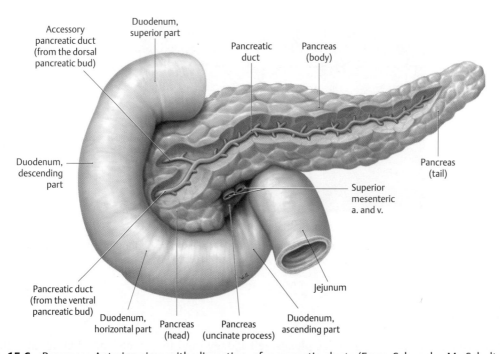

Fig. 15.6 Pancreas: Anterior view with dissection of pancreatic duct. (From Schuenke M, Schulte E, Schumacher U. THIEME Atlas of Anatomy. Internal Organs. Illustrations by Voll M and Wesker K. © Thieme 2020)

The *veins* from pancreas drain into splenic, superior mesenteric, and portal veins.

The *lymph nodes* draining the pancreas which lie along the superior border of pancreas are called *pancreaticosplenic nodes* and along the superior and inferior pancreaticoduodenal arteries (**Fig. 15.7**).

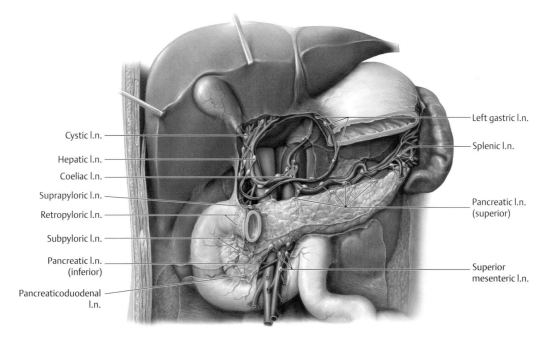

Fig. 15.7 Lymphatic drainage of stomach, liver, spleen, pancreas, and duodenum. (From Schuenke M, Schulte E, Schumacher U. THIEME Atlas of Anatomy. Internal Organs. Illustrations by Voll M and Wesker K. © Thieme 2020)

Portal Vein (Fig. 15.8)

The portal vein is a large vein (about 8 cm long) which receives blood from abdominal and pelvic parts of the alimentary canal except the lower part of the rectum and anal canal, and also from spleen, pancreas, and gallbladder. It transports blood to the liver which ultimately drains into the inferior vena cava through the hepatic veins (**Fig. 15.8**). The portal vein delivers nutrients from small intestine to the liver.

The portal vein is formed behind the neck of the pancreas by the union of the superior mesenteric and splenic veins at the level of L2 vertebra (**Fig. 15.9**). It then passes behind the first part of the duodenum in front of the inferior vena cava. Now it ascends toward the porta hepatis in the right free margin of the lesser omentum forming the anterior boundary of epiploic foramen (foramen of Winslow). At the porta hepatis, it divides into right and left branches. The right branch is shorter and wider than the left branch. It receives cystic vein before entering into the right lobe of the liver. The left branch is longer and narrower than the right. Just before entering the left lobe of the liver, it receives paraumbilical veins in ligamentum teres and ligamentum venosum.

The tributaries of portal vein include splenic vein, superior mesenteric vein, left gastric vein, right gastric vein, superior pancreaticoduodenal vein, cystic vein, and paraumbilical veins. The veins that correspond to the branches of the celiac trunk and superior mesenteric arteries drain into the portal

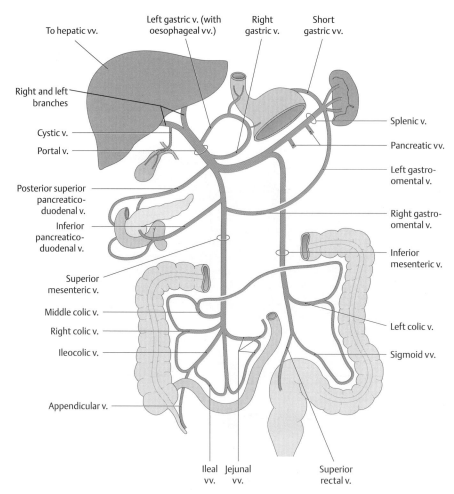

Fig. 15.8 Portal vein distribution. (From Schuenke M, Schulte E, Schumacher U. THIEME Atlas of Anatomy. Internal Organs. Illustrations by Voll M and Wesker K. © Thieme 2020)

vein or one of its tributaries. The inferior mesenteric vein drains into the splenic vein (for further details see **Fig. 15.8** and **Video 15.3**).

Portosystemic (Portacaval) Anastomosis

At a number of sites, communications occur between the portal and systemic circulations to form important routes for collateral circulation in portal obstruction. For example, when the direct pathway through the liver becomes

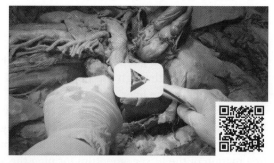

Video 15.3   Portal vein.

obstructed (such as in cirrhosis), the pressure within the portal vein rises, and under these circumstances, the portosystemic anastomoses form an alternative route for the blood to take. The important sites of portosystemic anastomosis are as follows:

1. *Lower esophagus*: Formed by tributaries of the left gastric (portal) and esophageal (systemic) veins.

2. *Anal canal*: Formed by the superior rectal (portal) and middle and inferior rectal (systemic) veins.

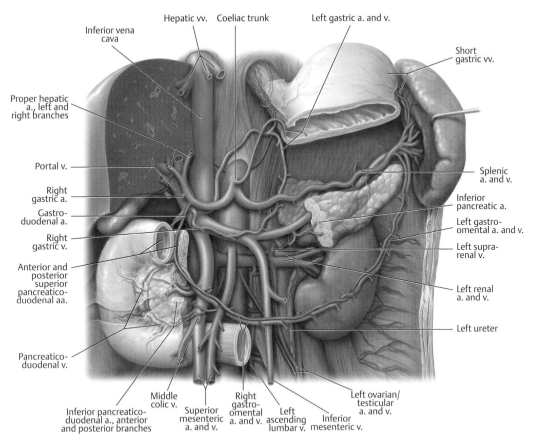

Fig. 15.9   Portal vein, pancreas, and spleen. (From Schuenke M, Schulte E, Schumacher U. THIEME Atlas of Anatomy. Internal Organs. Illustrations by Voll M and Wesker K. © Thieme 2020)

3. *Bare area of the liver*: Formed by the small veins of the portal system and the phrenic veins (systemic).

4. *Umbilical region*: Formed by small paraumbilical veins which ultimately drain into the portal vein and the superficial veins of the anterior abdominal wall (systemic).

5. *Posterior abdominal wall*: Formed by veins of retroperitoneal organs (portal) and retroperitoneal veins (systemic).

▮ Clinical Notes

1. *Duodenal ulcers*: They commonly occur in the first part of duodenum because it receives acidic chyme from the stomach. The duodenal ulcer is seen as a triangular shadow (duodenal cap/bulb) in barium meal X-ray abdomen (**Fig. 15.10**).

2. *Carcinoma head of pancreas*: It is common and, if occurs, compresses the bile duct to cause persistent obstructive jaundice. The surgical resection of carcinoma is difficult because of important relations of head of pancreas.

3. *Portal hypertension*: It occurs when pressure within the portal vein rises above 40 mm Hg, usually due to obstruction of portal vein in alcoholic cirrhosis. This leads to splenomegaly, esophageal varices, hemorrhoids, etc.

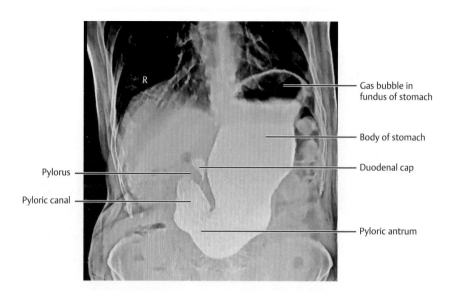

Fig. 15.10 Barium meal x-ray abdomen showing stomach and duodenal cap. Image courtesy Dr. Ravindra Goyal, MD, Dhanvantri CT Scan and MRI Centre, Haridwar, Uttrakhand, India.

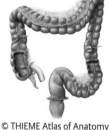
Small Intestine

Dissection and Identification

1. Reflect the transverse colon and mesocolon upward. Pull the loops of small intestine, the jejunum, and the ileum, inferiorly and to the left so that the right surface of the mesentery is exposed. By blunt dissection, remove the right layer of the mesentery along its attachment along the posterior abdominal wall from the duodenojejunal junction to the ileocecal junction (**Video 16.1**).

2. Remove the fat from the mesentery to expose the superior mesenteric vessels and their branches and tributaries (jejunal and ileal) in the mesentery. Note that the arteries supply the jejunum and ileum by a series of anastomotic arterial loops or arcades. Observe that the number of arterial arcades increases from the jejunum to the ileum. In the jejunum, there is one/two level(s) of arterial arcades with long intestinal branches (vasa recta), whereas in the ileum there are four to five levels of arterial arcades with short vasa recta. Also, note that there is an increase in the amount of fat in the distal portion of the mesentery.

3. Follow the trunk of the superior mesenteric artery upward to its origin from the abdominal aorta, posterior to the neck of the pancreas. Follow it distally and note that it passes anterior to the uncinate process of the pancreas, crosses anterior

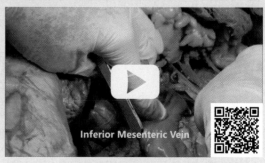

Inferior Mesenteric Vein

Video 16.1 Small intestine and its mesentery.

to the horizontal part of the duodenum, and enters the root at the mesentery.

4. Find the other branches of the superior mesenteric artery, that is, inferior pancreaticoduodenal artery, middle colic artery, right colic artery, and ileocolic artery arising from its right side (**Video 16.2**).

5. Observe that the middle colic artery divides within the transverse mesocolon into a right branch and a left branch. The right colic artery runs retroperitoneally toward ascending colon and divides into ascending and descending branches. Finally, the terminal branch of the superior mesenteric artery, the ileocolic artery, runs downward and toward the right and gives branches to ileum, cecum, and appendix.

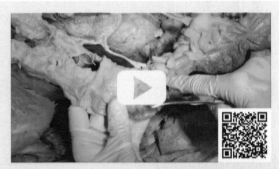

Video 16.2   Superior mesenteric artery and its distribution.

6. Reflect the loops of small intestine superiorly and to the right. Palpate the underlying abdominal aorta and then remove the peritoneum that covers its surface. Identify the inferior mesenteric artery as it arises from the anterior aspect of the abdominal aorta posterior to the horizontal part of duodenum.

7. Note that as the inferior mesenteric artery passes inferiorly and to the left, it gives off several branches.

8. Clean the branches and observe that the left colic artery runs retroperitoneally to the left toward descending colon and divides into ascending branch and descending branch. The sigmoidal arteries enter the root of the sigmoid mesocolon and supply the sigmoid colon. The superior rectal artery is the continuation of inferior mesenteric artery and it passes into the pelvic cavity.

9. Tie a pair of ligatures around the jejunum close to the duodenojejunal flexure and another around the ileum close to cecum. Cut across the jejunum and ileum between each pair of ligatures, respectively, and remove them by cutting the mesentery close to the intestine. Wash out the intestine with water and cut few inches of pieces of jejunum and ileum close to the ends.

10. Open the lumen by giving a longitudinal cut and observe the circular mucosal folds, called plicae circulares, on the internal surface of the jejunum and ileum. The plicae circulares in the proximal jejunum are more pronounced and more numerous than they are in the ileum.

11. Note that in the distal ileum, along the antimesenteric border, oval-shaped submucosal aggregates of lymphatic nodules called Peyer patches are visible and are often palpable.

12. Identify the inferior mesenteric vein and its tributaries. The inferior mesenteric vein joins the splenic vein or the superior mesenteric vein, usually posterior to the body of the pancreas.

General Features

The small intestine is about 6 m long and extends from pylorus to the ileocecal junction. It comprises the duodenum, jejunum, and ileum. A large internal surface area of the small intestine facilitates absorption of digested products. The small intestine (jejunum and ileum) is suspended from the posterior abdominal wall by its mesentery, which provides considerate mobility to it. The jejunum constitutes the upper two-fifths of the mobile part, while ileum constitutes the lower two-fifths. The origin (root) of the mesentery measures approximately 15 cm and passes from the duodenojejunal flexure to the right sacroiliac joint. It contains superior mesenteric vessels, lymphatics, and autonomic nerves. The distal border is obviously of the same length as the small intestine. Although no obvious distinction appears between the jejunum and ileum, certain characteristics help distinguish between them, such as the following (**Fig. 16.1**):

1. Loops of jejunum tend to occupy the umbilical region, whereas the ileum occupies the lower abdomen and pelvis (**Fig. 16.2**).

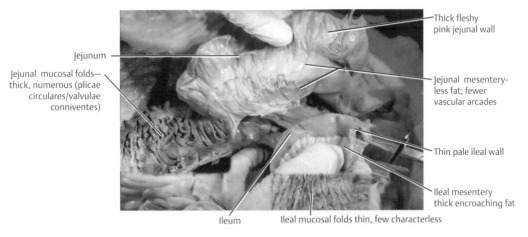

Fig 16.1 Jejunum and ileum.

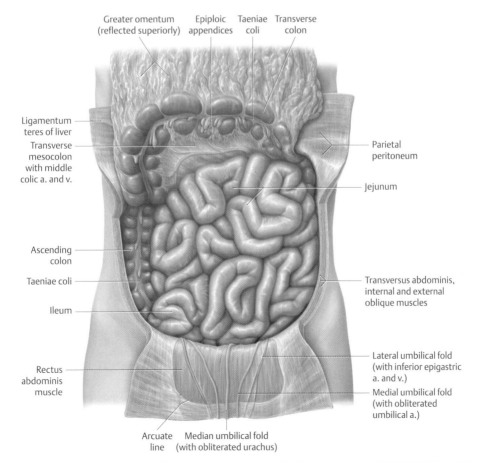

Fig. 16.2 Jejunum and ileum in situ. (From Schuenke M, Schulte E, Schumacher U. THIEME Atlas of Anatomy. Internal Organs. Illustrations by Voll M and Wesker K. © Thieme 2020)

2. Circular folds—the plicae circulares—are more prominent in the jejunum than in the ileum (**Fig. 16.3**).

3. Diameter of the jejunum is greater than that of the ileum.

4. Mesentery to the jejunum is thicker than that to the ileum.

5. Mesentery of jejunum presents windows due to less fat deposition.

6. Jejunum presents one to two arterial arcades with fewer and longer vasa recta, whereas ileum presents three to six arterial arcades with more and shorter vasa recta.

7. Peyer patches are present in ileum, while they are absent in jejunum.

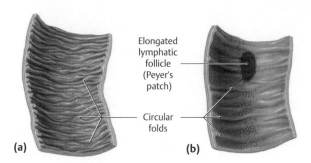

Fig. 16.3   Interior of small intestine. **(a)** Jejunum. **(b)** Ileum. (From Schuenke M, Schulte E, Schumacher U. THIEME Atlas of Anatomy. Internal Organs. Illustrations by Voll M and Wesker K. © Thieme 2020)

Blood Supply of the Small Intestine

Superior Mesenteric Artery

It arises from the front of abdominal aorta at the level of L2 vertebra about 0.5 cm below the celiac trunk. It passes over the third part of the duodenum to enter the root of the mesentery and pass toward the right iliac region on the posterior abdominal wall. The jejuna and ileal branches arise, divide, and reanastomose within the mesentery to produce arcades. Vasa recta (end-artery vessels) arise from the arcades to supply the gut wall (**Figs. 16.4** and **16.5**).

Branches

Origin of the branches of superior mesenteric artery is described in the following text.
The following branches arise from the right side of the artery:

1. Inferior pancreaticoduodenal.

2. Middle colic.

3. Right colic.

4. Ileocolic arteries.

The jejunal and ileal branches arise from the left side of the artery.

1. *Inferior pancreaticoduodenal artery*: It arises on the duodenum and passes upward and to the right to form arcades with the superior pancreaticoduodenal artery to supply duodenum and the head and uncinate process of the pancreas.

2. *Middle colic artery*: It arises at the lower border of the pancreas and then turns forward into the transverse mesocolon to divide into right and left branches. These branches anastomose with

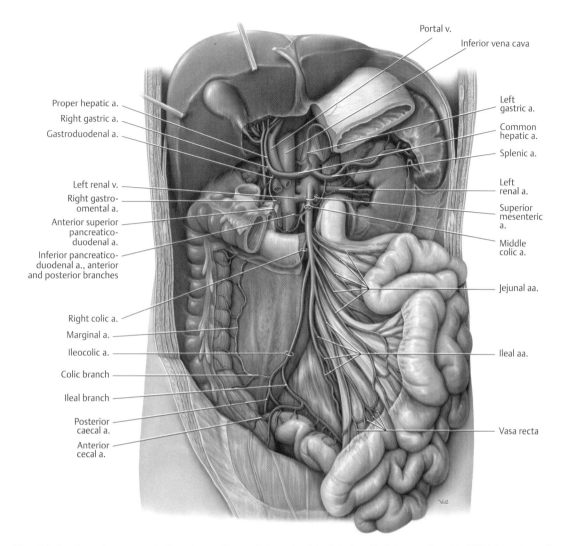

Fig. 16.4 Superior mesenteric artery. (From Schuenke M, Schulte E, Schumacher U. THIEME Atlas of Anatomy. Internal Organs. Illustrations by Voll M and Wesker K. © Thieme 2020)

each other close to the transverse colon to form part of the marginal artery. The marginal artery of Drummond runs along ascending, transverse, and descending parts of the colon and receives the branches of the other colic arteries. Branches from the marginal artery pass to the colon.

3. *Right colic artery*: It arises near the middle of superior mesenteric artery. It runs to right behind the peritoneum and passes across the structures of the posterior abdominal wall to join the marginal artery near the superior end of the ascending colon.

4. *Ileocolic artery*: It is the longest branch. It passes downward and to the right to divide into ascending and descending branches. Its ascending branch is the beginning of the marginal artery, while its descending branch supplies the colon, cecum, appendix vermiformis, and the terminal part of the ileum. It anastomoses with the last ileal branch of the superior mesenteric artery.

5. *Appendicular artery*: It enters the lowest part of the mesentery and passes posterior to the terminal part of the ileum into the mesentery of the appendix.

6. *Jejunal and ileal branches*: They are 12 to 15 in number and enter the mesentery of the small intestine. They branch and anastomose with each other to form a series of arterial arcades from which further branches form a second, and in the lower part of the mesentery, a third and even a fourth tier of arcades. They send branches to each side of the small intestine.

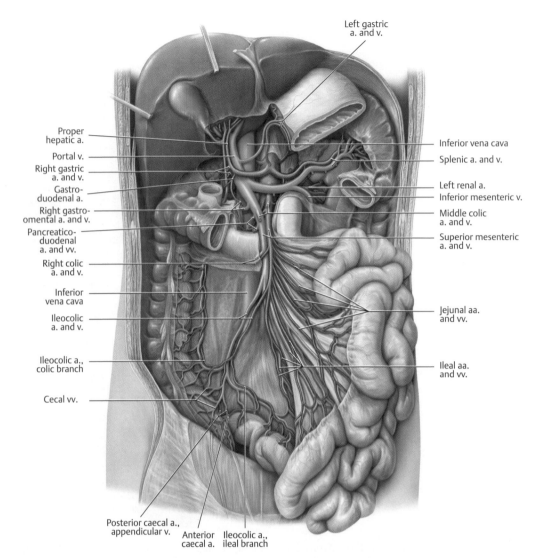

Fig. 16.5 Superior and inferior mesenteric veins. (From Schuenke M, Schulte E, Schumacher U. THIEME Atlas of Anatomy. Internal Organs. Illustrations by Voll M and Wesker K. © Thieme 2020)

Superior Mesenteric Vein

It is the major/formative tributary of the portal vein and drains the venous blood from distal portion of GIT. It lies immediately to the right of the superior mesenteric artery. Superiorly, it deviates to the right to join the splenic vein and form the portal vein posterior to the neck of pancreas. It drains venous blood from the territory of the artery. Its tributaries include right gastroepiploic and pancreaticoduodenal veins and, occasionally, the inferior mesenteric vein (**Fig. 16.5**).

Inferior Mesenteric Artery (Video 16.3)

It arises from the front of the abdominal aorta at the level of L3 vertebra posterior to the horizontal part of the duodenum (**Fig. 16.6**). It supplies

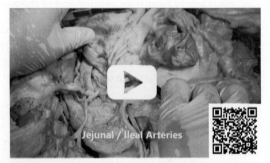

Video 16.3 Distribution of Inferior mesenteric artery in hindgut—high-definition clinical demonstration.

the intestine from the left part of the transverse colon to the anal canal. It descends on the left of aorta, posterior to the peritoneum. On the middle of the left common iliac artery it continues as superior rectal artery after giving rise to the sigmoidal arteries (**Fig. 16.7**).

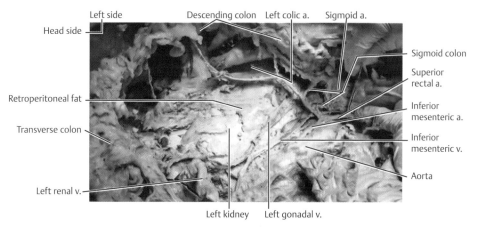

Fig. 16.6　Colon and inferior mesenteric vessels.

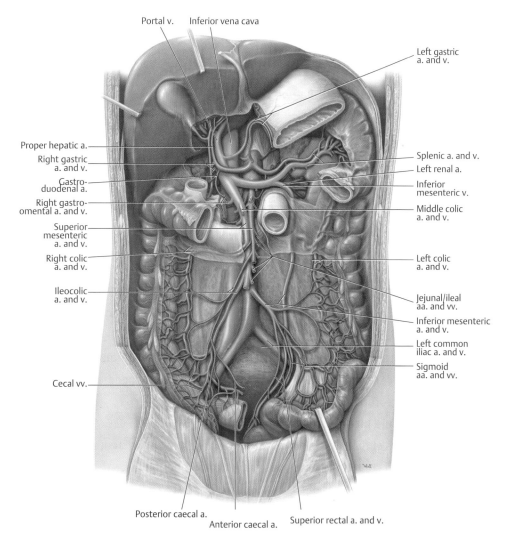

Fig. 16.7　Inferior mesenteric artery and vein. (From Schuenke M, Schulte E, Schumacher U. THIEME Atlas of Anatomy. Internal Organs. Illustrations by Voll M and Wesker K. © Thieme 2020)

Branches

1. *Left colic artery*: It arises a short distance below the duodenum and passes to the left where it divides into ascending and descending branches which form part of the marginal artery. Its ascending branch crosses the lower pole of the left kidney and joins the middle colic part of the marginal artery, thus helping to supply the left flexure and left part of the transverse colon. Its descending branch supplies the descending colon and anastomoses with the sigmoid arteries.

2. *Sigmoid arteries* (two or three in number): They run inferiorly and to the left. They anastomose with each other and continue with the marginal artery to supply the descending colon in the left iliac fossa and the sigmoid colon. The lowest sigmoid artery anastomoses with the superior rectal artery by a small branch.

3. *Superior rectal artery*: It is a continuation of inferior mesenteric artery at the pelvic brim. It enters the lesser pelvis and divides into right and left branches.

Inferior Mesenteric Vein

It is the upward continuation of the superior rectal vein. It ascends lateral to the inferior mesenteric artery, and receives tributaries corresponding to the branches of this artery. The vein then passes lateral to the duodenojejunal flexure (**Figs. 16.5** and **16.7**).

Lymph Nodes of the Mesentery of Small Intestine

Numerous lymph nodes lie between the two layers of the mesentery and gradually increase in diameter toward the root. The lymph vessels of small intestine are called lacteals due to their white coloration because they contain milky white emulsion of fat. These vessels finally converge at the root of the mesentery to form intestinal trunk which drains into the large lymphatic sac, the cisterna chyli.

Large Intestine

Learning Objectives

At the end of dissection of large intestine, the student should be able to identify:

- Various parts of large intestine.
- Peritoneal reflections and recesses related to the ileocaecal junction.
- Relations of caecum and note the features of ileocaecal and appendicular orifices.
- Position, gross features of appendix.
- Mesoappendix and blood vessels.
- External features of the large intestine and compare them with that of small intestine.
- Attachments and contents of transverse and sigmoid mesocolon.
- Hepatic and splenic flexures of colon.
- Blood vessels supplying the colon. Discuss the formation of marginal artery of Drummond.
- Various groups of colic lymph nodes.

Dissection and Identification

1. Examine the parts of the large intestine, which include cecum, vermiform appendix, ascending colon, transverse colon, descending colon, sigmoid colon, rectum, and anal canal. The rectum and anal canal lie within the pelvic cavity and will be studied during the dissection of the pelvis (**Video 16.4**).

2. Note the three distinctive features of large intestine that distinguish it from the small intestine. These are the presence of taeniae coli, epiploic appendages, and haustrations (or sacculations).

3. The taeniae coli are three narrow distinct longitudinal bands of smooth muscle which run along the entire length of the cecum and colon. The three taeniae coli converge at the base of the vermiform appendix on the cecum. Follow the three taeniae coli from the cecum to the sigmoid colon.

4. Observe that due to the shorter length of the taeniae coli, the wall of the large intestine between the bands pouches out into a series of sacculations called the "haustrations." Note the appendices epiploicae, the fat-filled outpouchings of the visceral peritoneum.

5. Turn the cecum upward to uncover the structures posterior to it. On the lateral surface of the cecum, make a longitudinal incision through its wall. On the internal medial wall of the cecum, identify the ileocecal orifice and the orifice of the vermiform appendix. Determine the position of the vermiform appendix in the cadaver. In most cases, the vermiform appendix is an intraperitoneal structure, and its distal segment hangs free into the iliac fossa or pelvic cavity.

6. Put a pair of ligatures at the junction of descending colon and sigmoid colon. Cut across the colon between the two ligatures and remove the colon and cecum in one piece by cutting the peritoneum and blood vessels close to them. Wash the colon and observe the external features.

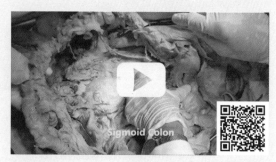

Video 16.4   Large intestine.

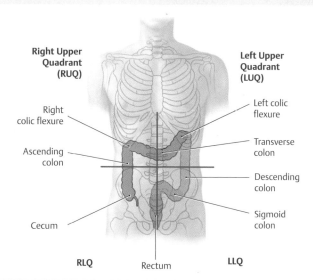

Fig. 16.8   Location and parts of large intestine. (From Schuenke M, Schulte E, Schumacher U. THIEME Atlas of Anatomy. Internal Organs. Illustrations by Voll M and Wesker K. © Thieme 2020)

General Features

The large intestine is about 1.5 m long and extends from cecum in the right iliac fossa to the anus in the perineum. It surrounds the centrally placed loops of small intestine. It is much shorter than the small intestine and decreases in diameter from the cecum to the descending colon (**Fig. 16.8**).

The large intestine consists of the cecum and vermiform appendix, ascending colon, transverse colon and descending colon, sigmoid colon, rectum, and anal canal.

Cardinal Features of Large Intestine

The cecum, ascending colon, transverse colon and descending colon, and sigmoid colon have similar characteristic features called cardinal features. These are appendices epiploicae, taeniae coli, and sacculations (**Fig. 16.9**).

1. *Appendices epiploicae*: These are fat-filled peritoneal tags present over the surface of cecum and colon.

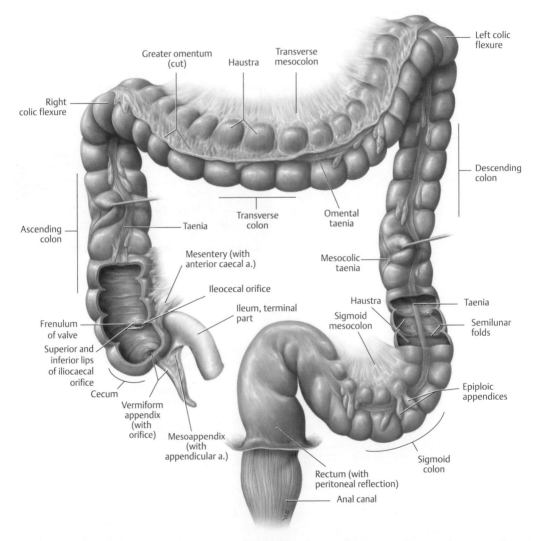

Fig. 16.9 Cardinal features of large intestine. (From Schuenke M, Schulte E, Schumacher U. THIEME Atlas of Anatomy. Internal Organs. Illustrations by Voll M and Wesker K. © Thieme 2020)

2. *Taeniae coli*: These are three ribbon-like flattened bands of longitudinal muscle coat. They course from base of appendix to the rectosigmoid junction.

3. *Sacculations*: These are dilatations in the wall of cecum and colon between the taeniae. The sacculations take place because taeniae are shorter than the bowel itself.

Cecum (L. cecum = blind) (Fig. 16.9)

It is the dilated blind end (commencement) of the large intestine in the right iliac fossa. It is approximately 6 cm in length and 7.5 cm in width (i.e., it has more width than length). Superiorly, it joins the ascending colon and terminal part of the ileum. It lies on the iliacus and psoas muscles. The genitofemoral, femoral, and lateral cutaneous nerves and testicular or ovarian vessels also form its posterior relations. Generally, the cecum is almost surrounded by peritoneum but is often attached by it to iliac fossa laterally and medially, forming a wide retrocecal peritoneal recess. The interior of cecum presents two orifices, ileocecal orifice and orifice of appendix. The first is guarded by upper and lower lips whose ends unite to form right and left cecal frenula. The appendicular orifice is guarded inferiorly by small semicircular fold called valve of Gerlach.

Ascending Colon (Fig. 16.9)

It is 12 to 120 cm long and extends upward from cecum to the inferior aspect of the right lobe of the liver where it turns sharply to the left to form right/hepatic flexure. The peritoneum covers the front and sides of the ascending colon and binds it to the posterior abdominal wall. It is separated from the anterior abdominal wall by greater omentum.

Transverse Colon (Fig. 16.9)

It is usually the longest (40–50 cm) and mobile part of the colon. It extends between the right (hepatic) and left (splenic) flexures and forms a dependent loop between them, whose lowest part may reach well below the umbilicus in the erect position. The transverse colon is suspended from posterior abdominal wall by the transverse mesocolon. This is fused to the posterior surface of the greater omentum. The left colic flexure (splenic flexure) lies at the junction of transverse colon and descending colon.

Descending Colon (Fig. 16.9)

It is about 25 cm long and extends downward from left colic flexure to the pelvic brim, where it becomes continuous with the sigmoid colon. It is covered by peritoneum on the front and sides.

Sigmoid Colon (Pelvic Colon) (Fig. 16.9)

It varies in length from 15 to 80 cm. It extends from pelvic brim on the left side to third piece of sacrum where it continues as rectum. It is suspended from pelvic wall by a fold of peritoneum called sigmoid mesocolon.

The sigmoid mesocolon has an inverted "V"-shaped attachment. Just lateral to the inverted "V," a pocket-like extension of peritoneal cavity called intersigmoid peritoneal recess passes upward, posterior to the root of mesocolon. The left ureter lies behind this recess. The inferior mesenteric artery divides near the apex of inverted "V"; the superior rectal artery enters the right limb and left sigmoidal arteries enter the left limb.

Vermiform Appendix

The appendix is a narrow blind tube arising from posteromedial aspect of the cecum (**Fig. 16.9**). It presents a worm-like appearance. It varies enormously in length but in adults is 5 to 15 cm long. The base of the appendix is attached to the posteromedial surface of cecum 2 to 3 cm inferolateral to the ileocecal junction. The surface marking for the base of the appendix is represented by McBurney point. The base of the appendix is fixed but the remaining part may lie in a number of positions. However, in most cases, the appendix lies in the retrocecal position. The characteristic features of the appendix are as follows:

1. It has a small mesentery that descends behind the terminal ileum.

2. It is supplied by the appendicular artery (a branch of the ileocolic), which courses within its mesentery. In cases of appendicitis, there is thrombosis of the appendicular artery. When this happens, gangrene and perforation of the appendix inevitably take place.

3. The lumen of appendix is relatively wide in infants but gradually narrows throughout life, often becoming obliterated in the elderly; hence, appendicitis is rare in the infants.

4. The taeniae coli of the cecum converge at the base of appendix.

5. The bloodless fold of Treves (ileocecal fold) is a small peritoneal reflection passing from the anterior terminal ileum to the appendix.

Blood Supply of the Large Intestine

1. The cecum and appendix are supplied by ileocolic artery.

2. The ascending colon and right colic flexure are supplied by ileocolic and right colic arteries.

3. The transverse colon is mainly supplied by middle colic artery but its right and left flexures are also supplied by right and left colic arteries.

4. The descending colon is supplied by left colic and upper sigmoidal branches of inferior mesentery artery (**Fig. 16.10**).

Lymph Nodes of the Large Intestine

Small lymph nodes lie along the marginal artery called paracolic lymph nodes. The lymph draining through these nodes passes to the nodes lying along the ileocolic, right colic, middle colic and left colic arteries which are called intermediate colic nodes. From these nodes, it passes to the lymph nodes lying along the superior and inferior mesenteric arteries. The lymph vessels from nodes along the superior mesenteric artery pass to the intestinal trunk in the root of mesentery, whereas those draining the lymph nodes along the inferior mesenteric artery enter into lumbar lymph nodes. Ultimately, from both these the lymph reaches cisterna chyli (**Fig. 16.11**).

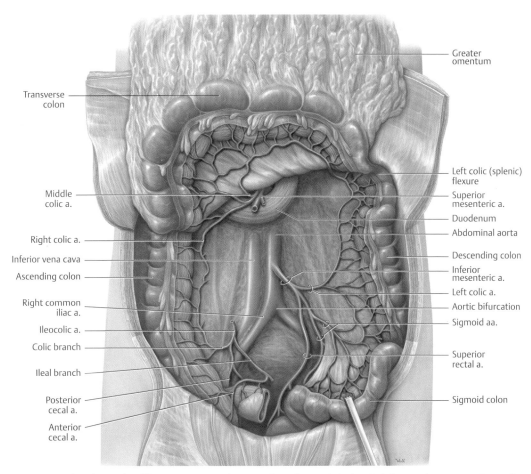

Greater omentum

Transverse colon

Left colic (splenic) flexure

Middle colic a.

Superior mesenteric a.

Duodenum

Abdominal aorta

Right colic a.

Descending colon

Inferior vena cava

Inferior mesenteric a.

Ascending colon

Left colic a.

Right common iliac a.

Aortic bifurcation

Ileocolic a.

Sigmoid aa.

Colic branch

Ileal branch

Superior rectal a.

Posterior cecal a.

Anterior cecal a.

Sigmoid colon

Fig. 16.10 Blood supply of large intestine. (From Schuenke M, Schulte E, Schumacher U. THIEME Atlas of Anatomy. Internal Organs. Illustrations by Voll M and Wesker K. © Thieme 2020)

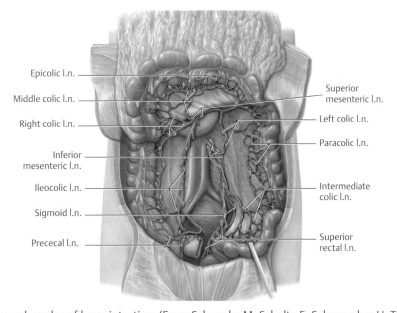

Epicolic l.n.

Superior mesenteric l.n.

Middle colic l.n.

Left colic l.n.

Right colic l.n.

Paracolic l.n.

Inferior mesenteric l.n.

Ileocolic l.n.

Intermediate colic l.n.

Sigmoid l.n.

Prececal l.n.

Superior rectal l.n.

Fig. 16.11 Lymph nodes of large intestine. (From Schuenke M, Schulte E, Schumacher U. THIEME Atlas of Anatomy. Internal Organs. Illustrations by Voll M and Wesker K. © Thieme 2020)

▌Clinical Notes

1. *Meckel diverticulum*: It is a persistent, proximal part of vitellointestinal duct. It is 2 inch (5 cm) long and occurs in 2% of cases. It is located about 2 feet proximal to the ileocecal junction.

2. *Typhoid ulcers*: These are ulcerations of Peyer patches of small intestine. They are vertical and mostly occur in the ileum.

3. *Appendicitis*: It is the inflammation of appendix which commonly occurs due to obstruction of its lumen by fecalith. Pain of appendicitis is usually referred to the umbilicus in initial stages but in later stages it is felt in the right iliac fossa on palpation with maximum tenderness being at the McBurney point.

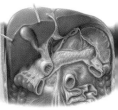
Dissection and Identification

1. Pull the liver downward and cut the anterior layers of the coronary and left triangular ligaments. Care should be taken not to cut inferior vena cava. The liver in situ is shown in **Fig. 17.1**.

2. Identify the inferior vena cava on the upper left posterior aspect of liver. Strip a bit of liver downward from it and note the hepatic veins entering into the inferior vena cava.

3. Separate the inferior vena cava if it is deeply buried into the liver.

4. Now cut the structures present in the right free margin of lesser omentum adjacent to the porta hepatis.

5. In this way, the liver is released from the abdominal cavity. Now take it out and put it in a dissection tray to study.

6. Identify the features on the posteroinferior surface of the liver.

7. Clear the structures within the porta hepatis and trace their entries to the liver (**Fig. 17.2**).

8. Give a longitudinal incision through the wall of the gallbladder and cystic duct.

9. Clean the interior of gallbladder and cystic duct with a jet of water and examine the features in the mucous lining.

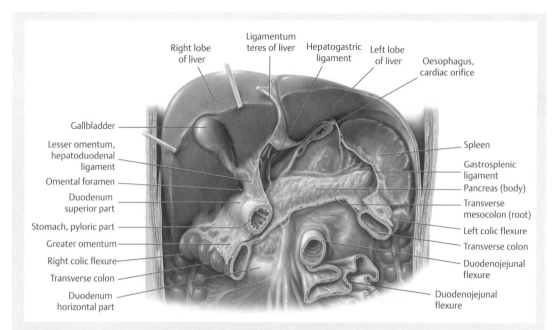

Fig. 17.1 Liver in situ. (Modified from Schuenke M, Schulte E, Schumacher U. THIEME Atlas of Anatomy. Internal Organs. Illustrations by Voll M and Wesker K. © Thieme 2020)

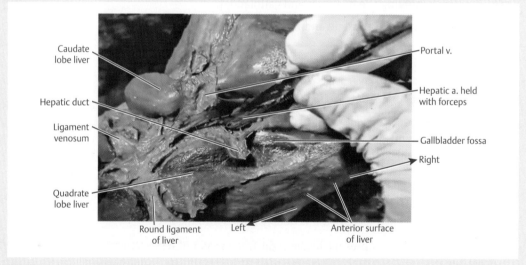

Fig. 17.2 Porta hepatis.

Liver

It is the largest gland in the body. It predominantly occupies the right hypochondrium but its left lobe extends into the epigastrium and part of the left hypochondrium in the abdominal cavity (**Fig. 17.3**). It is reddish brown in color, soft in consistency, and friable. It weighs around 1,600 g in males and 1,300 g in females.

The liver is wedge-shaped and presents two surfaces—diaphragmatic surface and posteroinferior surface. The two are separated from each other by a sharp inferior border. The diaphragmatic surface is divisible into anterior, superior, right, and posterior parts.

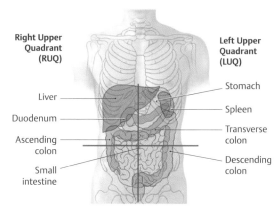

Fig. 17.3   Location of the liver (anterior view). (From Schuenke M, Schulte E, Schumacher U. THIEME Atlas of Anatomy. Internal Organs. Illustrations by Voll M and Wesker K. © Thieme 2020)

Lobes

Anatomically, the liver is divided into large right lobe and smaller left lobe. They are separated by the attachment of falciform ligament anterosuperiorly; on the posteroinferior surface, they are separated from each other by fissure for ligamentum venosum and ligamentum teres (**Fig. 17.4**; **Video 17.1**).

The right lobe is much larger than the left lobe and forms five-sixths of the liver. It contributes to all the five surfaces of the liver and presents the caudate and quadrate lobes. The posteroinferior surface of the liver presents an H-shaped arrangement of grooves and fossa. The boundaries of H are as follows:

1. Right anterior limb formed by fossa for gallbladder.

2. Right posterior limb formed by groove for inferior vena cava.

3. Left anterior limb formed by fissure for ligamentum teres.

4. Left posterior limb formed by ligamentum venosum.

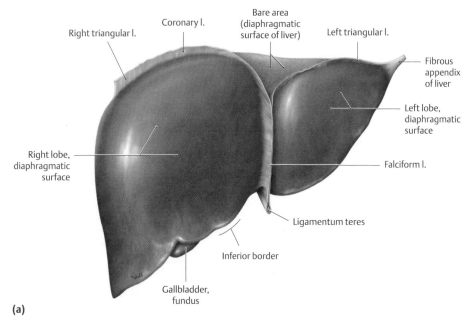

(a)

Fig. 17.4   Surfaces and lobes of the liver. **(a)** Anterior view. (From Schuenke M, Schulte E, Schumacher U. THIEME Atlas of Anatomy. Internal Organs. Illustrations by Voll M and Wesker K. © Thieme 2020) *(Continued)*

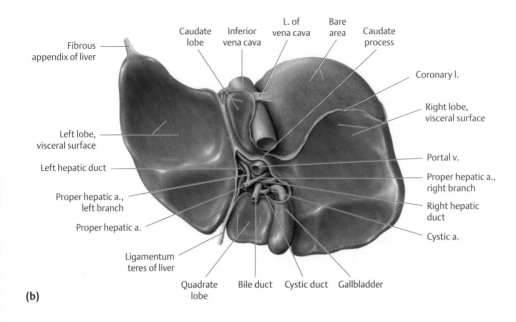

(b)

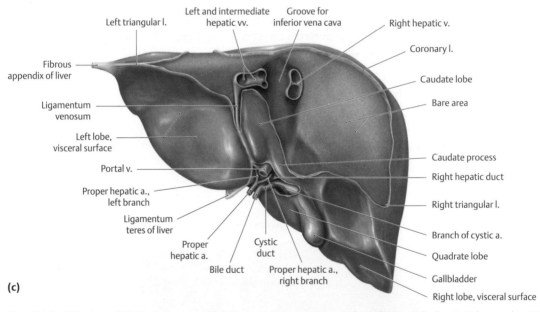

(c)

Fig. 17.4 *(Continued)* **(b)** Inferior view. **(c)** Posterior view. (From Schuenke M, Schulte E, Schumacher U. THIEME Atlas of Anatomy. Internal Organs. Illustrations by Voll M and Wesker K. © Thieme 2020)

The ligamentum teres is the fetal remnant of left umbilical vein which returns oxygenated blood from the placenta to the fetus. The *ligamentum venosum* is a fetal remnant of *ductus venosus* which partially bypasses the liver by transporting blood from left umbilical vein to the inferior vena cava.

On the posteroinferior surface, the part of the liver between groove for ligamentum venosum and groove for inferior vena cava is called *caudate lobe,*

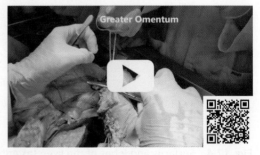

Video 17.1 Liver in situ.

while part of the liver between the groove for ligamentum teres and fossa for gallbladder is called *quadrate lobe*. Thus, anatomically right lobe of the liver includes caudate and quadrate lobes.

Peritoneal Relations

The liver is covered by peritoneum everywhere except for:

1. A triangular bare area, on the posterior surface of the right lobe, limited by upper and lower layers of the coronary ligament and by the right triangular ligament.

2. Groove for the inferior vena cava.

3. Fossa for the gallbladder (**Fig. 17.4**).

Relations

Superior surface: It is convex and related to pericardium in the middle and to diaphragm on either sides.

Anterior surface: It is triangular and slightly convex. It is related to the xiphoid process and anterior abdominal wall in the median plane and diaphragm on each side.

Posterior surface: It is concavoconvex and presents four features: bare area of the liver, groove for inferior vena cava, caudate lobe and fissure for ligamentum venosum, and groove for esophagus. The bare area is related to right suprarenal gland.

Inferior surface: It is irregular in shape and directed downward, backward, and to the left. The important features present on the surface include fissure for ligamentum teres, porta hepatis, quadrate lobe, and fossa for gallbladder. It presents various impressions produced by neighboring viscera, namely (**Fig. 17.5**):

1. Gastric impression on the inferior surface of the left lobe, inferior to esophageal groove.

2. Lesser omentum, pylorus, and first part of duodenum on the quadrate lobe.

3. Colic impression for the hepatic flexure of the colon, renal impression for the right kidney, and the duodenal impression for the second part of duodenum to the right of fossa for gallbladder.

Right lateral surface: It is convex; its upper one-third is related to the diaphragm, the pleura, and the lung, whereas the middle one-third to the diaphragm and the costodiaphragmatic recess of the pleura and the lower one-third to the diaphragm alone.

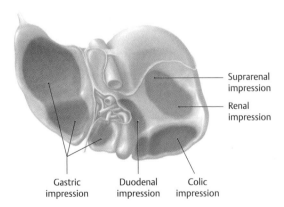

Suprarenal impression

Renal impression

Gastric impression   Duodenal impression   Colic impression

Fig. 17.5   Visceral relations of the liver. (From Schuenke M, Schulte E, Schumacher U. THIEME Atlas of Anatomy. Internal Organs. Illustrations by Voll M and Wesker K. © Thieme 2020)

Blood Supply

The liver is supplied by both hepatic artery and portal vein. It receives 20% of its blood through the hepatic artery and 80% through the portal vein.

Venous Drainage

The hepatic sinusoids drain into interlobular veins which join to form sublobular veins. The sublobular veins join to form right, left, and middle hepatic veins which finally drain the corresponding areas of the liver back into the inferior vena cava.

True Lobes of the Liver

On the basis of intrahepatic distribution of branches of hepatic artery, portal vein, and bile duct, the liver is divided into two physiological/true lobes by an imaginary sagittal plane (*Cantlie plane*) (**Fig. 17.6**). On the anterosuperior surfaces, it passes from cystic notch to the inferior vena cava, and on the posteroinferior surface, it passes from fossa for gallbladder to the groove for inferior vena cava. Each lobe is further divided into anterior and posterior parts called segments of the liver. Each segment is further divided into superior and inferior parts, thus forming subsegments of the liver.

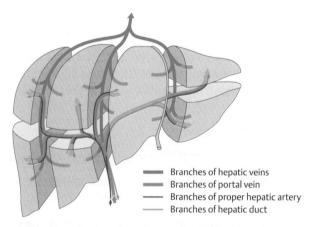

Branches of hepatic veins
Branches of portal vein
Branches of proper hepatic artery
Branches of hepatic duct

Fig. 17.6   Segmentation of the liver. (From Schuenke M, Schulte E, Schumacher U. THIEME Atlas of Anatomy. Internal Organs. Illustrations by Voll M and Wesker K. © Thieme 2020)

█ Clinical Notes

1. *Hepatitis*: It is the inflammation of the liver usually caused by infection or amoebiasis.

2. *Cirrhosis of the liver*: As a result of severe malnutrition or excessive intake of alcohol, the liver parenchyma undergoes degeneration which leads to fibrosis and shrinkage of the liver. Also see Clinical Notes on page 196.

Biliary Apparatus

The biliary apparatus comprise two parts: intrahepatic and extrahepatic. The intrahepatic part consists of bile canaliculi, bile ductules, and interlobular ducts. The interlobular ducts of right and left lobes of the liver unite to form right and left hepatic ducts, respectively.

The extrahepatic part consists of right and left hepatic ducts, common hepatic ducts, gallbladder, cystic duct, and common bile duct (**Fig. 17.7**).

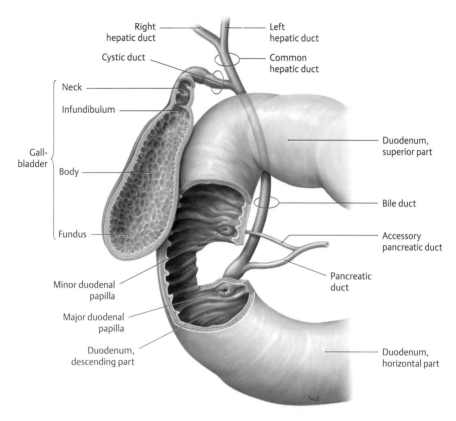

Fig. 17.7 Extrahepatic biliary apparatus. (From Schuenke M, Schulte E, Schumacher U. THIEME Atlas of Anatomy. Internal Organs. Illustrations by Voll M and Wesker K. © Thieme 2020)

Gallbladder

The gallbladder is a pear-shaped sac adherent to the undersurface of the right lobe of the liver (in fossa for gallbladder) (**Figs. 17.7–17.9**). The duodenum and transverse colon lie behind it. The shallow fossa for gallbladder extends from the right end of the porta hepatis to the inferior border of the liver. It is a reservoir of bile (30–60 mL capacity), which it concentrates.

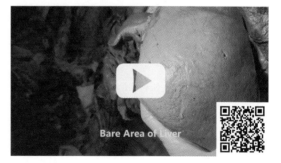

Video 17.2 Gallbladder and extrahepatic biliary apparatus.

The gallbladder is divided into fundus, body, infundibulum, and neck. The fundus is the most anterior and expanded part which projects beyond the inferior margin of the liver. On the surface, it corresponds to the tip of ninth costal cartilage. The neck is the narrow right portion of gallbladder. It shows a small projection on its right side called Hartmann pouch. The mucous lining of neck is folded spirally to form a *spiral valve* (**Video 17.2**).

Cystic Duct

The cystic duct is about 2 to 4 cm in length. It begins at the neck of the gallbladder and descends in the lesser omentum with the common hepatic duct, which it joins at an acute angle at a variable point to form the bile duct.

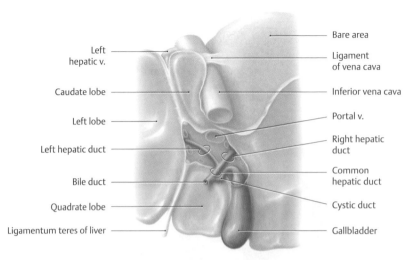

Fig. 17.8 Location of gallbladder (inferior view). (From Schuenke M, Schulte E, Schumacher U. THIEME Atlas of Anatomy. Internal Organs. Illustrations by Voll M and Wesker K. © Thieme 2020)

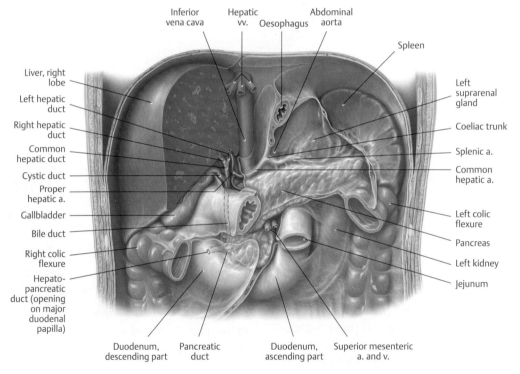

Fig. 17.9 Extrahepatic biliary tract in situ. (From Schuenke M, Schulte E, Schumacher U. THIEME Atlas of Anatomy. Internal Organs. Illustrations by Voll M and Wesker K. © Thieme 2020)

Bile Duct

The duct is formed by the union of the cystic and common hepatic ducts (vide supra). It is about 8 cm in length and has a diameter of about 6 mm. The bile duct courses downward and backward, sequentially in the free margin of the lesser omentum (*supraduodenal part*) behind the first part of the duodenum (*retroduodenal part*) and in the groove behind the head of pancreas (*infraduodenal part*). Near the middle of the left side of the second part of the duodenum, it comes close to the main pancreatic duct which it accompanies up to the wall of the duodenum (*intraduodenal part*).

The bile duct usually joins the main pancreatic duct (duct of Wirsung) and opens at the major duodenal papilla on the medial aspect of the interior of the second part of the duodenum; before opening the combined ducts, it presents a dilatation called *hepatopancreatic ampulla*. The terminal part of the bile duct is surrounded just above its junction with the main pancreatic duct by a ring of smooth muscle called sphincter choledochus (choledochus = bile duct) that is sphincter of bile duct.

Often a less-developed sphincter is found around the terminal part of the main pancreatic duct, the *sphincter pancreaticus.* A well-developed sphincter surrounds the hepatopancreatic ampulla, is called the sphincter of hepatopancreatic ampulla, or sphincter of Oddi (**Figs. 17.10** and **17.11**).

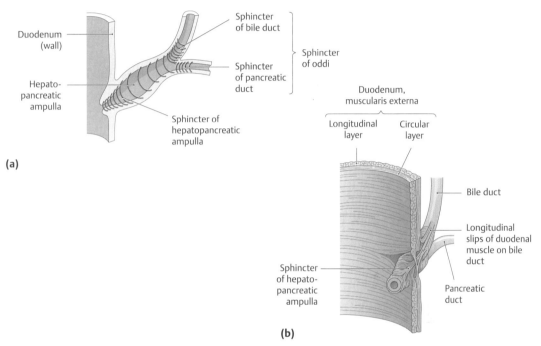

Fig. 17.10   Sphincters of the extrahepatic biliary apparatus. **(a)** Sphincters of the pancreatic duct, bile ducts, and hepatopancreatic ampulla. **(b)** Sphincter of hepatopancreatic ampulla in duodenal wall. (From Schuenke M, Schulte E, Schumacher U. THIEME Atlas of Anatomy. Internal Organs. Illustrations by Voll M and Wesker K. © Thieme 2020)

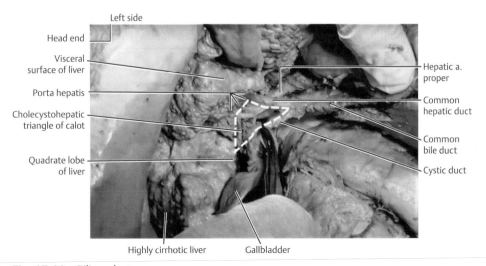

Fig. 17.11   Biliary ducts.

▌Clinical Notes

1. *Cirrhosis of the liver*: It is the fibrosis of the liver parenchyma. Parenchymal cells of the liver undergo degeneration following excessive alcoholic intake or severe infection and replaced by fibrous tissue. Clinically, it presents as portal hypertension leading to hemostasis, piles, etc.

2. *Calot triangle (cystohepatic triangle)*: It is bounded by cystic duct inferiorly, common hepatic duct medially, and inferior surface of the liver superiorly. It contains right hepatic artery, cystic artery, and cystic lymph node (node of Lund). During cholecystectomy, the cystic artery and cystic duct are clamped and cut. Locate the artery behind the lymph node.

3. *Cholelithiasis (gallstones)*: Bile is stored and concentrated in the gallbladder. Certain substances within the bile such as cholesterol may crystalize to form gallstones. The gallstones are made up of cholesterol, bile pigment, or both. When they impact cystic duct, biliary colic occurs, which typically radiates to the inferior angle of scapula.

4. The CT scan of upper abdomen can provide detailed information about the injuries and/or diseases of liver, pancreas, stomach, and spleen etc (**Fig. 17.12**).

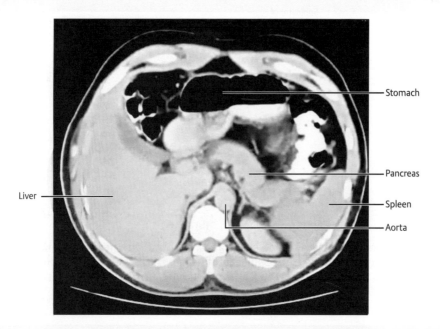

Fig. 17.12   CT scan of upper abdomen showing liver, stomach, and spleen etc. Image courtesy Dr. Ravindra Goyal, MD, Dhanvantri CT Scan and MRI Centre, Haridwar, Uttrakhand, India.

18 Kidney, Ureter, and Suprarenal Gland

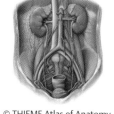

© THIEME Atlas of Anatomy

Dissection and Identification

1. Remove the pararenal fat in both paravertebral gutters between the level of the T12 and L3 vertebrae to expose the anterior layer of the renal fascia. Make a vertical incision through the renal fascia and remove the perirenal fat which surrounds the kidneys and suprarenal glands (**Video 18.1**).

2. Identify the right and left suprarenal glands. Observe they are located at the superior pole of the respective kidney. The inferior surface of the suprarenal gland contacts the upper pole of the kidney. Posteriorly, each suprarenal gland

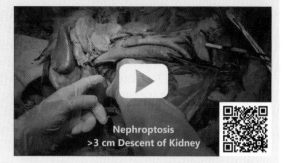

Nephroptosis
>3 cm Descent of Kidney

Video 18.1 Kidney.

rests against the lumbar part of the diaphragm. Note that the right suprarenal gland is triangular, whereas the left is semilunar in shape.

3. Find the arteries and veins of the suprarenal glands. There are three sets of arteries which supply each suprarenal gland: (a) superior suprarenal arteries, branches of the inferior phrenic artery, (b) middle suprarenal arteries arising directly from the aorta, and (c) inferior suprarenal arteries, arising from the renal arteries.

4. In contrast, there is only one suprarenal vein associated with each gland. Trace the right suprarenal vein to the inferior vena cava and the left suprarenal to the left renal vein into which they drain, respectively (**Fig. 18.1**).

5. Now, examine the bean-shaped kidneys and note that usually the right kidney is slightly lower than the left kidney. Follow the left renal vein from the inferior vena cava to the left kidney and note its tributaries (left inferior suprarenal vein and left testicular/ovarian vein). Displace the vein to expose the renal artery which lies posterior to it. Note that the most posterior structure at the hilum is the renal pelvis which continues below as ureter.

6. Turn the left kidney medially to expose the muscles, blood vessels, and nerves which are related to its posterior surface. Carry out the same dissection on the right side and note that the right inferior suprarenal vein and right testicular/ovarian vein drain into inferior vena cava.

7. Cut the left renal vessels and ureter and remove the kidney. To study the internal structure of a kidney, make a longitudinal incision through the entire length of a kidney from the lateral border toward the hilum of the kidney.

8. On the cut surface of the kidney, identify the following: cortex (outer), medulla containing renal pyramids (inner) and renal sinus (innermost), the space containing renal pelvis, major and minor calyces, blood vessels, and fat.

9. Note that the rounded renal papilla is located at the apex of each renal pyramid and contains the excretory ducts which empty into a minor calyx. A number of minor calyces converge to form three or four major calyces, which join to form the renal pelvis within the renal sinus.

Kidneys

Kidneys are bean-shaped solid organs (10–12 cm long) located on the posterior abdominal wall in paravertebral gutters, posterior to the peritoneum. They occupy epigastric, hypochondriac, lumbar, and umbilical regions (**Fig. 18.1**). The kidneys are largely responsible for removing excess water, salts, and waste products (viz., urea) from the body and maintain its pH. The kidneys are reddish brown in color; each kidney is about 11 cm long, 5 cm wide, and 2.5 cm thick. The left kidney is a little longer and narrower as compared to the right kidney; on an average, a kidney weighs about 150 g in males and 135 g in females (**Figs. 18.2–18.4**).

The kidney presents upper and lower poles, medial and lateral borders, and anterior and posterior surfaces. The upper pole is broad and closely related to the corresponding suprarenal gland. The lower pole is pointed. The anterior surface appears slightly irregular, whereas the posterior surface is flat. The lateral border is convex and medial border concave. Its middle, the medial border, shows a vertical cleft, the hilus or hilum, which transmits structures entering and leaving the kidney and leads to a space within the kidney called sinus of the kidney (**Fig. 18.3**).

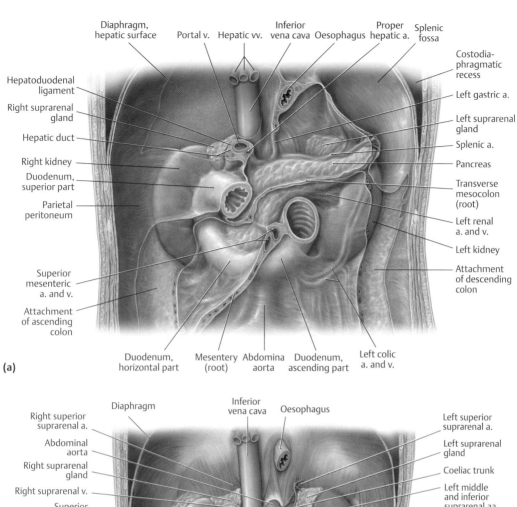

Fig. 18.1 Kidneys and suprarenal glands in situ. **(a)** *Removed*: Intraperitoneal organs, along with portions of the ascending and descending colon. **(b)** *Removed*: Peritoneum, spleen, and gastrointestinal organs, along with fat capsule (left side). *Retracted*: Esophagus. (From Schuenke M, Schulte E, Schumacher U. THIEME Atlas of Anatomy. Internal Organs. Illustrations by Voll M and Wesker K. © Thieme 2020)

Hilum

The structures seen in the hilum from anterior to posterior are as follows:

1. Renal vein.

2. Renal artery.

3. Renal pelvis, the expanded upper end of the ureter (**Fig. 18.3**).

Coverings of the Kidney

Each kidney is enclosed from superficial to deep by fibrous capsule, perirenal fat, and pararenal fat (**Fig. 18.5**).

Fibrous capsule is a thin membrane which closely invests the kidney and continues to line the renal sinus.

The *perirenal or perinephric fat* is a layer of adipose tissue lying outside the fibrous capsule. It fills up the extra space in the renal sinus.

The *pararenal or paranephric fat* is a variable amount of fat lying outside the renal fascia. It fills up the paravertebral gutter and provides a cushion for the kidney.

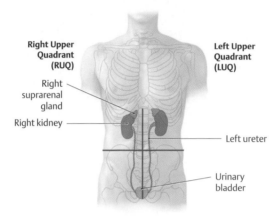

Fig. 18.2 Location of kidney and suprarenal glands. (From Schuenke M, Schulte E, Schumacher U. THIEME Atlas of Anatomy. Internal Organs. Illustrations by Voll M and Wesker K. © Thieme 2020)

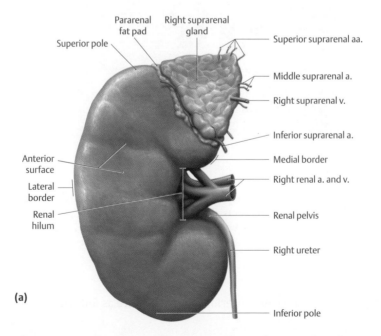

Fig. 18.3 Right kidney. **(a)** Anterior view. (From Schuenke M, Schulte E, Schumacher U. THIEME Atlas of Anatomy. Internal Organs. Illustrations by Voll M and Wesker K. © Thieme 2020)

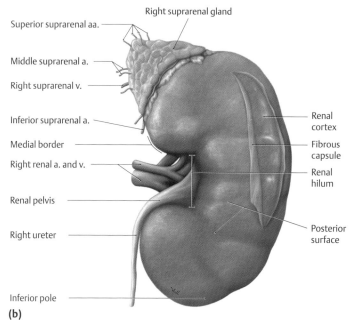

Superior suprarenal aa.

Middle suprarenal a.

Right suprarenal v.

Inferior suprarenal a.

Medial border

Right renal a. and v.

Renal pelvis

Right ureter

Inferior pole

Right suprarenal gland

Renal cortex

Fibrous capsule

Renal hilum

Posterior surface

(b)

Fig. 18.3 Right kidney. **(b)** Posterior view. (From Schuenke M, Schulte E, Schumacher U. THIEME Atlas of Anatomy. Internal Organs. Illustrations by Voll M and Wesker K. © Thieme 2020)

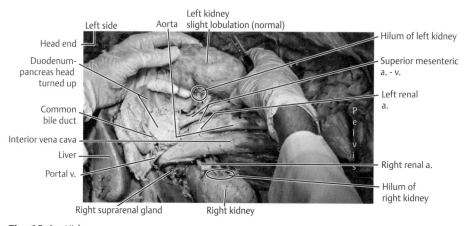

Left side

Head end

Duodenum-pancreas head turned up

Common bile duct

Interior vena cava

Liver

Portal v.

Right suprarenal gland

Aorta

Left kidney slight lobulation (normal)

Right kidney

Hilum of left kidney

Superior mesenteric a. - v.

Left renal a.

Pelvis

Right renal a.

Hilum of right kidney

Fig. 18.4   Kidneys.

Relations

Posterior: The posterior surfaces of each kidney are related to the following:

1. Diaphragm.

2. Psoas major.

3. Quadratus lumborum.

4. Transversus abdominis.

5. Subcostal vessels.

6. Subcostal, iliohypogastric, and ilioinguinal nerves (**Fig. 18.6**).

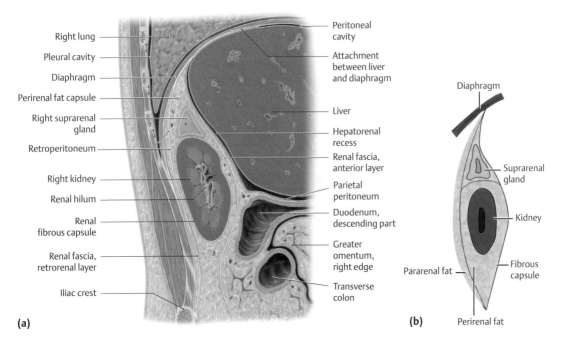

Fig. 18.5   (a) Right kidney in the renal bed. (From Schuenke M, Schulte E, Schumacher U. THIEME Atlas of Anatomy. Internal Organs. Illustrations by Voll M and Wesker K. © Thieme 2020). **(b)** Coverings of kidney.

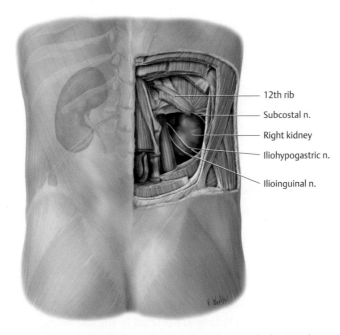

Fig. 18.6   Posterior relations of right kidney. (From Schuenke M, Schulte E, Schumacher U. THIEME Atlas of Anatomy. Internal Organs. Illustrations by Voll M and Wesker K. © Thieme 2020)

In addition, the right kidney is related to the 12th rib, whereas the left kidney to the 11th and 12th ribs.

Anterior: The anterior surface of the left kidney is related to the following (**Fig. 18.7**):

1. Left suprarenal gland.

2. Spleen.

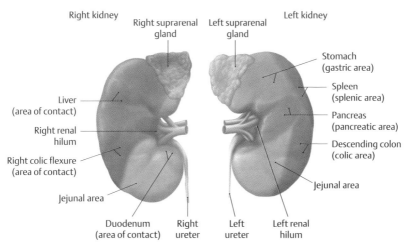

Fig. 18.7   Anterior relations of kidneys. (From Schuenke M, Schulte E, Schumacher U. THIEME Atlas of Anatomy. Internal Organs. Illustrations by Voll M and Wesker K. © Thieme 2020)

3. Stomach.

4. Pancreas.

5. Splenic vessels.

6. Splenic flexure and descending colon.

7. Jejunum.

The anterior surface of the right kidney is related to the following (**Fig. 18.7**):

1. Right suprarenal gland.

2. Liver.

3. Second part of duodenum.

4. Hepatic flexure of colon.

Structure of Kidney

On naked eye examination of a coronal section of the kidney, the cut surface presents:

1. An outer reddish brown cortex adjacent to the capsule.

2. An inner, pale medulla made up of about 10 dark conical masses, the renal pyramids. The apices pyramids form the renal papillae which indent the minor calyces.

3. A space, the renal sinus (**Figs. 18.8** and **18.9**).

The renal cortex covers the pyramid and extends between them as renal columns, thus dividing the cortex into:

1. Cortical arches or cortical lobules, which cap over the bases of the pyramids.

2. Renal columns, which extend between the pyramids.

Each pyramid along with the overlying cortex forms a lobe of the kidney. The renal sinus, a space extending into the kidney from the hilus, contains:

1. Branches of the renal artery.

2. Tributaries of the renal vein.

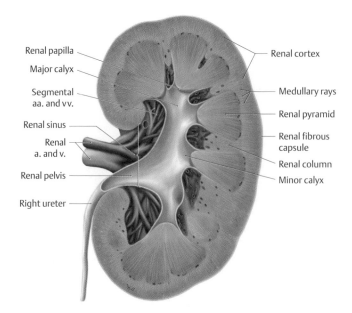

Fig. 18.8   Kidney internal features. (From Schuenke M, Schulte E, Schumacher U. THIEME Atlas of Anatomy. Internal Organs. Illustrations by Voll M and Wesker K. © Thieme 2020)

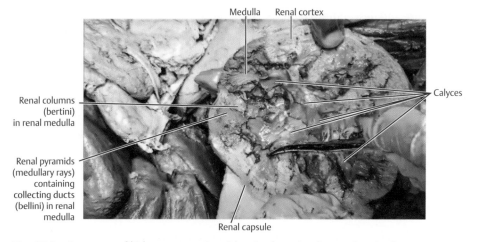

Fig. 18.9   Structure of kidney as seen in midsagittal section (posterior view).

3. Renal pelvis:
- 2 to 3 major calyces.
- 7 to 13 minor calyces.

Vessels of Kidney

The renal arteries arise from the aorta at the level of L2. Together, the renal arteries direct 25% of the cardiac output toward the kidneys. Each renal artery divides into five segmental arteries at the hilum, which, in turn, divide sequentially into lobar, interlobar, arcuate, and radial cortical branches. The radial cortical branches give rise to the afferent arterioles which pass to the glomeruli; from the glomeruli, efferent arterioles either form capillary plexus around the convoluted tubules or form straight arterioles further to become efferent arterioles. The differential pressures between the afferent and the efferent arterioles lead to the production of an ultrafiltrate, which then passes through and is modified by the nephron to produce urine.

The right renal vein passes behind the inferior vena cava, while the left renal vein is long as it courses in front of the aorta to drain into the inferior vena cava. The capillaries drain sequentially into interlobular veins, arcuate and interlobar veins and pass to the renal sinus to form tributaries of renal vein.

Ureter

The ureter is a narrow muscular tube (25 cm long and 5 mm wide) which provides passage to urine from kidney to the urinary bladder. It begins at the renal pelvis and descends along its medial margin of the kidney. It then passes downward and slightly medially on the psoas major muscle and enters the pelvis by crossing in front of the termination of common iliac artery. At the upper end, the ureter forms funnel-shaped dilatation called renal pelvis located in the renal sinus. In the pelvis, the ureter runs downward, and slightly backward and laterally, along the anterior part of the greater margin of the greater sciatic notch. Opposite the ischial spine, it turns forward and medially to reach the base of the urinary bladder. It enters the bladder wall obliquely (**Figs. 18.2** and **18.10**). The intravesical portion of ureter is tortuous (2 cm long) and produces sphincter-like effect. In males, the ureter is crossed superficially near its termination by the ductus deferens. In females, the ureter passes above the lateral fornix of the vagina but below the uterine artery (**Video 18.2**).

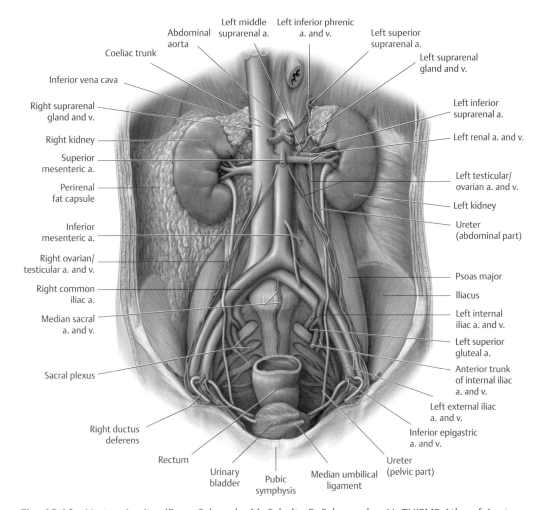

Fig. 18.10 Ureters in situ. (From Schuenke M, Schulte E, Schumacher U. THIEME Atlas of Anatomy. Internal Organs. Illustrations by Voll M and Wesker K. © Thieme 2020)

Constrictions

The ureter presents normal constrictions at the following three sites:

1. At the pelviureteric junction.
2. At the pelvic brim.
3. At the entry into the bladder wall.

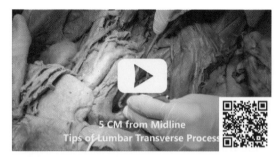

Video 18.2   Renal pelvis and ureter.

Blood Supply

As the ureter has both abdominal and pelvic parts, it receives blood supply from multiple sources:

1. Upper part receives direct branches from the renal vessels.
2. Middle part receives direct branches from the aorta and gonadal arteries.
3. Lower part receives branches from the inferior vesical, middle rectal, and uterine arteries.

Nerve Supply

Nerve supply is by sympathetic fibers from T10 to L1 segments and parasympathetic fibers from S2 to S4 segments.

Suprarenal (Adrenal) Glands (Video 18.3)

The suprarenal glands are important endocrine glands situated over the upper pole of the kidneys behind the peritoneum on the posterior abdominal wall (**Fig. 18.11**). The right gland lies behind the right lobe of the liver and immediately posterolateral to the inferior vena cava. The left gland is related anteriorly to the lesser sac and stomach.

Each gland measures about 50 mm in height, 30 mm in breadth, and 10 mm in thickness, and weighs about 5 g, which is about 1/3 of the kidney at birth and about 1/13 of kidney in an adult.

The right suprarenal gland is triangular/pyramidal in shape. It has an apex, a base, anterior and posterior surfaces, and anterior, medial, and lateral borders (**Fig. 18.12**).

The left gland is semilunar in shape. It has upper, narrow, and lower rounded ends. It has medial convex and lateral concave borders and anterior and posterior surfaces (**Fig. 18.12**).

Structure

The adrenal glands comprise an outer cortex and an inner medulla. The cortex is derived from mesodermal lining of the peritoneal cavity and is responsible for the production of steroid hormones (glucocorticoids, mineralocorticoids, and sex steroids). The medulla is derived from neural crest and acts as a part of the sympathetic nervous system. It receives sympathetic preganglionic fibers from the greater splanchnic nerves which stimulate the medulla to secrete noradrenaline and adrenaline into the

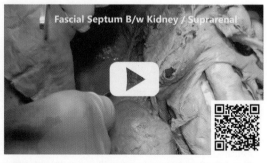

Video 18.3   Locations of Suprarenal glands.

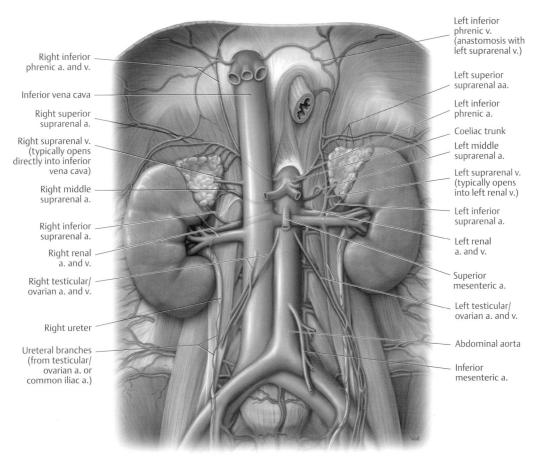

Fig. 18.11   Blood vessels of kidneys and suprarenal glands. (From Schuenke M, Schulte E, Schumacher U. THIEME Atlas of Anatomy. Internal Organs. Illustrations by Voll M and Wesker K. © Thieme 2020)

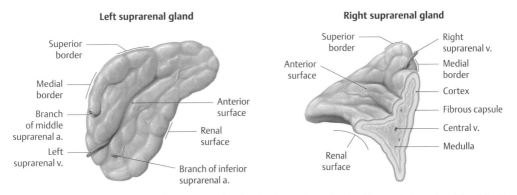

Fig. 18.12   External features of suprarenal glands (anterior view). (From Schuenke M, Schulte E, Schumacher U. THIEME Atlas of Anatomy. Internal Organs. Illustrations by Voll M and Wesker K. © Thieme 2020)

bloodstream. They are readily oxidized to dark brown color by potassium bicarbonate; hence, it forms part of chromatin tissue of the body.

Blood Vessels (Fig. 18.11)

Each gland is supplied by a suprarenal artery, branch of the inferior phrenic artery, a middle suprarenal artery, branch of the abdominal aorta and an inferior suprarenal artery, and branch of the renal artery.

Veins pass inward from cortex to medulla where they come out as a renal vein. Each gland is drained by only one vein. The right suprarenal vein drains into the inferior vena cava, and the left suprarenal vein into the left renal vein.

■ Clinical Notes

1. *Ureteric stone/ureteric colic*: Most ureteric calculi arise for unknown reasons. When impacted, it is characterized by hematuria and agonizing colicky pain (ureteric colic), which classically radiates from loin to groin, scrotum/labium majus. Ureteric stones lead to hydronephrosis and hence need to be removed.

2. *Renal angle*: It is located at the lower border of the 12th rib and outer border of erector spinae. It overlies the kidney; hence, tenderness in kidney is elicited by applying pressure in the area of angle by thumb.

---

19 Diaphragm and Posterior Abdominal Wall

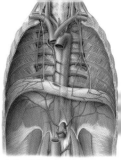

© THIEME Atlas of Anatomy

Learning Objectives

At the end of the dissection of the diaphragm and posterior abdominal wall, students should be able to identify the following:

- Vertebral, costal, and sternal attachments of the diaphragm.
- Shape and extent of the diaphragm.
- Extent and attachments of the crura, arcuate ligaments, and structures passing deep to these ligaments.
- Course and branches of phrenic nerve.
- Abdominal aorta. Note the vertebral levels of its beginning and termination. Trace its various branches (ventral, lateral, and dorsal).
- Inferior vena cava and its tributaries. Note the vertebral levels of its formation, course, and termination.
- Splanchnic nerves. Discuss their formation, course, and termination.
- Celiac and aorticorenal ganglion. Note their location and extent of their branches and contributions to various plexuses.
- Sympathetic chain and trace its various branches and contribution to various autonomic plexus.
- Cisterna chyli and its location. Try to trace the course of the various lymphatic trunks draining into it.
- Various groups of lymph nodes on the posterior abdominal wall.
- Lumbar plexus and its location and formation. Trace its various branches.
- Origin, insertion, and nerve supply of psoas major and minor, quadratus lumborum, and transversus abdominis muscles.
- Common iliac vessels and their branches.
- Formation of azygos system, its tributaries, and area of their drainage.
- Layers of the thoracolumbar fascia, their extent, and attachments.

Dissection and Identification

1. Examine the inferior surface of the diaphragm. Strip the peritoneum from the diaphragm and note the origin of muscle fibers from the xiphoid process, costal margin, tips of the 11th and 12th ribs, and the lumbar vertebrae. Observe that the muscle fibers are inserted into the central tendon.

2. Note that the lumbar part of the diaphragm forms two crura which are attached to the lateral surface of the bodies of the upper three lumbar vertebrae. Observe that the right and left crus are joined by the median arcuate ligament, which passes anterior to the aorta.

3. Lateral to the crura, identify the medial arcuate ligament and lateral arcuate ligament. The medial arcuate ligament is located anterior to the psoas major muscle extending from the body to the transverse process of the L1 vertebra. The lateral arcuate ligament spans over the quadratus lumborum muscle from the transverse process of the L1 vertebra to the 12th rib (**Video 19.1**).

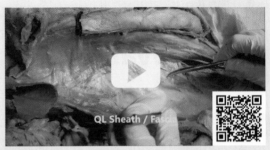

Video 19.1   Posterior abdominal wall.

4. Identify the major openings of the diaphragm: (a) for inferior vena cava located in the tendinous portion of the diaphragm, (b) for the esophageal located in the muscular portion of the diaphragm, and (c) the aortic hiatus located posterior to the median arcuate ligament of the diaphragm.

5. Clean the anterior surface of the abdominal aorta and inferior vena cava. Between the right crus of the diaphragm and the aorta, expose the cisterna chyli and azygos vein. Trace the cisterna chyli upward to the thoracic duct which enters thorax through the aortic hiatus. Follow the azygos vein inferiorly to the posterior surface of inferior vena cava at the level of renal veins and upward to the aortic hiatus through which it enters the thorax.

6. Identify the *sympathetic trunks* which lie on either side of the aorta on the anterior aspect of psoas major muscle. Note, the right sympathetic trunk lies posterior to inferior vena cava.

7. Identify the following autonomic nerve plexuses: celiac plexus, superior mesenteric plexus, inferior mesenteric plexus, renal plexus, suprarenal plexus, and gonadal plexus (testicular plexus or ovarian plexus) around the similar named arteries.

8. The three unpaired branches of aorta, namely, celiac trunk, superior mesenteric artery, and inferior mesenteric artery, and the paired branches to the viscera, namely, middle suprarenal arteries, renal arteries, and gonadal arteries (testicular or ovarian arteries), have already been seen. Follow the course of the gonadal (testicular or ovarian) arteries as they arise from the aorta at the level of the L2 vertebra. As they pass inferiorly to the pelvis, they cross anterior to the ureter and common iliac vessels.

9. Now, identify the parietal branches that pass to the body wall which include: (a) paired inferior phrenic arteries, the first branches of abdominal aorta which pass superolaterally to the diaphragm, (b) four pairs of lumbar arteries which arise from the posterior surface of abdominal aorta and pass laterally on the surfaces of lumbar vertebrae and deep to the psoas muscle, and (c) unpaired middle sacral artery which arises from the posterior surface of the aorta at its bifurcation and passes straight downward into the pelvis.

10. Note that the inferior vena cava is formed by the union of the right common iliac vein and left common iliac vein at the level of the L5 vertebra. The common iliac veins lie posterior to common iliac arteries.

11. Follow the inferior vena cava superiorly till it leaves the abdominal cavity by passing through the hiatus of inferior vena cava located in the tendinous part of the diaphragm.

12. Identify the following veins which are the tributaries of inferior vena cava: renal veins, right suprarenal vein, right gonadal (testicular or ovarian) vein, inferior phrenic veins, and hepatic veins. On the left side of the posterior abdominal wall, identify the left suprarenal vein and left testicular or ovarian vein which joins the left renal vein.

13. Expose the muscles of the posterior abdominal wall by removing the covering fascia. Avoid injury to the nerves which lie deep to the fascia and in front of the muscles. Identify the four muscles, namely, psoas major, iliacus, quadratus lumborum, and transversus abdominis.

14. Note that the psoas major muscle arises from the lumbar vertebra and passes into the pelvis where it joins with the iliacus muscle. On the anterior surface of the psoas major muscle, identify the psoas minor muscle if present. It is absent in about 50% of individuals. Observe the quadratus lumborum muscle attached to the iliac crest inferiorly and to the transverse processes of the lumbar vertebrae and 12th rib superiorly. The transversus abdominis muscle extends laterally from the quadratus lumborum muscle.

15. Identify the nerves arising from the lumbar plexus running along the anterior surface of the muscles of the posterior abdominal wall.

16. Observe the iliohypogastric nerve and ilioinguinal nerve located inferior to the subcostal nerve as they emerge from the lateral border of the psoas major muscle and pass inferiorly and laterally across the quadratus lumborum muscle. Trace the lateral cutaneous nerve of the thigh as it runs across the iliacus muscle. Find the femoral nerve located in the groove between the psoas major muscle and the iliacus muscle, genitofemoral nerves located on the anterior surface of the psoas major muscle, and obturator nerve on the medial side of the psoas major muscle (**Video 19.2**).

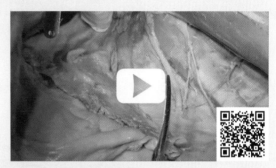

17. Detach and remove the psoas major muscle fibers carefully from the lumbar vertebrae and find the roots, anterior and posterior divisions of the lumbar plexus present among the fibers of the psoas major muscle.

Video 19.2 Lumbar plexus.

Diaphragm

The diaphragm is a large, flat dome-shaped partition between thoracic and abdominal cavities. It serves as a chief muscle of respiration (**Fig. 19.1**). When it contracts, it increases the vertical diameter of the thoracic cavity by flattening its dome. The fibrous central part of diaphragm, the central tendon, is slightly depressed by the weight of the heart which probably leads to the formation of its right and left domes.

Origin: The muscle arises from three sources—sternum, costal cartilage, and lumbar vertebral column (**Fig. 19.1a–c**).

1. The *sternal part* arises by two small fleshy slips from the back of xiphoid process and passes backward.

2. The *costal part* arises by wide slips from the inner surfaces of the lower six costal cartilages on each side, interdigitating with transversus abdominis.

3. The *vertebral part* arises from the lumbar vertebral column by crura and arcuate ligament, medial, and lateral lumbocostal arches and lumbar vertebrae by right and left crura.

Arcuate ligaments (**Fig. 19.2**):

1. The medial arcuate ligament is a tendinous arch in fascia covering psoas major. It is attached to the side of L1 vertebra medially and to the transverse process of L1 vertebra laterally.

2. Lateral arcuate (lateral lumbocostal arch) is a tendinous arch in fascia covering quadratus lumborum. It is attached to the transverse process of L1 vertebrae medially and lower border of the 12th rib laterally.

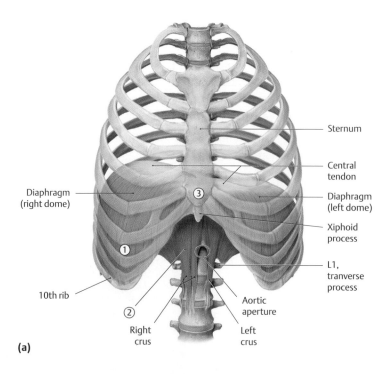

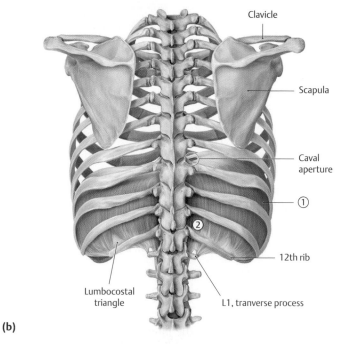

Fig. 19.1 Location of diaphragm. **(a)** Anterior view. 1, Costal part; 2, lumbar part; 3, sternal part. **(b)** Posterior view. (Modified from Schuenke M, Schulte E, Schumacher U. THIEME Atlas of Anatomy. Internal Organs. Illustrations by Voll M and Wesker K. © Thieme 2020)

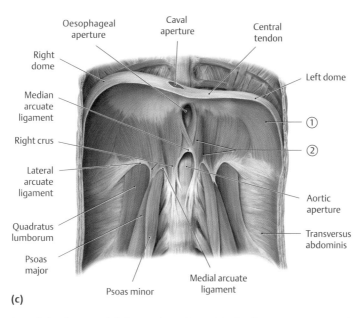

Oesophageal aperture

Caval aperture

Central tendon

Right dome

Left dome

Median arcuate ligament

①

Right crus

②

Lateral arcuate ligament

Aortic aperture

Quadratus lumborum

Transversus abdominis

Psoas major

Psoas minor

Medial arcuate ligament

(c)

Fig. 19.1 Location of diaphragm. **(c)** Coronal section with diaphragm in intermediate position. 1, Costal part; 2, lumbar part. (Modified from Schuenke M, Schulte E, Schumacher U. THIEME Atlas of Anatomy. Internal Organs. Illustrations by Voll M and Wesker K. © Thieme 2020)

Crura of the diaphragm are attached to anterolateral aspects of bodies of upper three lumbar vertebrae and intervening discs; note that the left crus is less in length and attached to the upper two lumbar vertebrae. Medial margins of the two crura form a tendinous arch across the front of the aorta called the median arcuate ligament.

Note, all the three arcuate ligaments, median, medial, and lateral, give rise to the muscle fibers of the diaphragm. Sometimes those arising from lateral ligament may be missing and form vertebrocostal angle. Through this gap, abdominal contents may herniate into the thoracic cavity, called the posterolateral hernia of Bochdalek.

Insertion: All the muscle fibers of the diaphragm converge toward the strong interlacing tendinous bundles called central tendon for insertion (**Fig. 19.2**). The tendon lies below the pericardium with which it is fused. It is trifoliated in shape. Its middle leaflet is triangular, directed toward the xiphoid process. Right and left leaflets are tongue-shaped.

Foramina in the Diaphragm

Major foramina/apertures: Three major openings in the diaphragm are caused by inferior vena cava, esophagus, and abdominal aorta (**Fig. 19.2**):

1. *Vena caval aperture* is quadrilateral and lies at the level of T8 vertebra. It is located in the central tendon 2 to 3 cm to the right of the midline. It provides passage to inferior vena cava. The slender branches of the right phrenic nerve also pass through this opening along the inferior vena cava.

2. *Esophageal hiatus/opening* is elliptical and located in the muscular part of the diaphragm just posterior to the central tendon and to the left of midline at the level of T10 vertebra. It is encircled by the fibers of the right crus. The vagal trunks and the esophageal branches of left gastric vessels also pass through this opening along with esophagus.

3. *Aortic opening* is rounded and lies posterior to the median arcuate ligament at the level of T12 vertebra. The thoracic duct and vena azygos also pass through the opening along with the aorta.

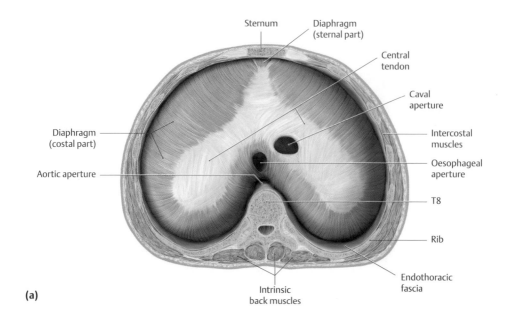

(a)

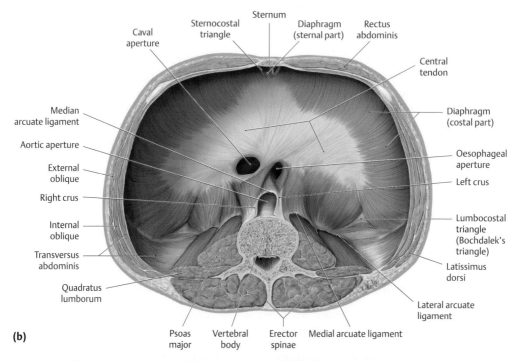

(b)

Fig. 19.2 Diaphragmatic apertures: **(a)** Superior view. **(b)** Inferior view. (From Schuenke M, Schulte E, Schumacher U. THIEME Atlas of Anatomy. General Anatomy and Musculoskeletal System. Illustrations by Voll M and Wesker K. © Thieme 2020)

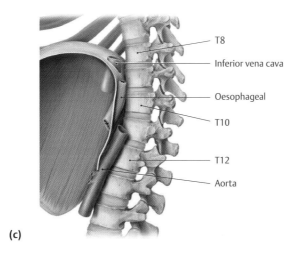

T8

Inferior vena cava

Oesophageal

T10

T12

Aorta

(c)

Fig. 19.2 Diaphragmatic apertures: **(c)** Left lateral view. (From Schuenke M, Schulte E, Schumacher U. THIEME Atlas of Anatomy. General Anatomy and Musculoskeletal System. Illustrations by Voll M and Wesker K. © Thieme 2020)

Minor foramina/openings:

1. Superior epigastric vessels pass through a gap between sterna and costal slips.

2. Musculophrenic vessels pass between the slips from the seventh and eighth ribs.

3. Lower five intercostal nerves pass between the slips from last costal cartilages.

4. Subcostal vessels and nerves pass posterior to the lateral arcuate ligament.

5. Sympathetic trunks pass behind the medial arcuate ligaments.

6. Greater, lesser, and least splanchnic nerves pierce the crus of the corresponding side.

7. Hemiazygos vein pierces the left crus.

8. Left phrenic nerve passes through the muscular part in front of the central tendon.

Nerves and Vessels (Fig. 19.3)

1. *Motor supply* to the diaphragm is by phrenic nerves (C4, C5, and C6). They pierce the diaphragm and ramify on its inferior surface before supplying it.

2. *Sensory supply* to the diaphragm is via phrenic and lower intercostal nerves. The central part of the diaphragm is supplied by the phrenic nerve and the peripheral part by the intercostal nerves.

3. The *main arteries* supplying the diaphragm are the inferior phrenic artery from abdominal aorta and musculophrenic and pericardiacophrenic arteries from the internal thoracic artery. The posterior part of superior surface is supplied by the superior phrenic/phrenic arteries from thoracic aorta.

4. The *venous drainage* is by inferior phrenic veins which accompany the corresponding arteries (**Fig. 19.3**).

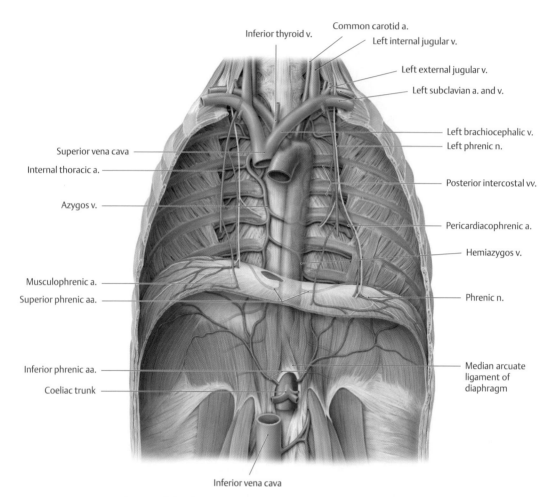

Fig. 19.3 Neurovasculature of diaphragm. (Modified from Schuenke M, Schulte E, Schumacher U. THIEME Atlas of Anatomy. Internal Organs. Illustrations by Voll M and Wesker K. © Thieme 2020)

Posterior Abdominal Wall

Vessels

Abdominal Aorta

The abdominal aorta is a continuation of the thoracic aorta as it passes through the median arcuate ligament of the diaphragm (**Fig. 19.3**). It descends on the vertebral column retroperitoneally and terminates by dividing into left and right common iliac arteries, to the left of the midline at the level of L4 (**Fig. 19.4**). The vertebral bodies (L1–L4), intervertebral discs, and anterior longitudinal ligament lie behind the aorta, while anteriorly from above downward lie the celiac trunk and its branches, lesser sac, the body of the pancreas with splenic vein, the third part of the duodenum, parietal peritoneum, and loops of the small intestine. The main relation to the right of the abdominal aorta is the inferior vena cava, while to the left lie the duodenojejunal junction and inferior mesenteric vein (**Fig. 19.4**).

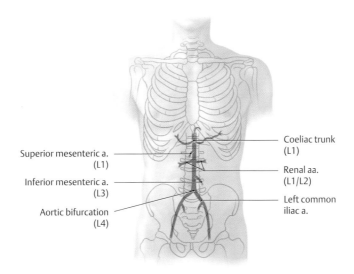

Superior mesenteric a.
(L1)

Inferior mesenteric a.
(L3)

Aortic bifurcation
(L4)

Coeliac trunk
(L1)

Renal aa.
(L1/L2)

Left common
iliac a.

Fig. 19.4 Extent of abdominal aorta. (Modified from Schuenke M, Schulte E, Schumacher U. THIEME Atlas of Anatomy. Internal Organs. Illustrations by Voll M and Wesker K. © Thieme 2020)

Branches (Fig. 19.5)

1. Unpaired ventral branches, namely, celiac trunk, superior mesenteric artery, and inferior mesenteric artery.

2. Paired lateral branches to the structures developed from the intermediate mesoderm, namely, suprarenal glands, kidneys, testes, and ovaries. These branches comprise inferior phrenic arteries, middle suprarenal, renal, and gonadal.

3. Paired posterolateral branches, namely, lumbar arteries to posterior abdominal wall (**Figs. 19.5** and **19.6**).

Unpaired Branches

Celiac Trunk

It arises from the aorta at the level of T12/L1 and after a short course divides into three terminal branches—left gastric, splenic artery, and common hepatic artery:

1. The left gastric artery passes upward to supply the lower esophagus by branches which ascend through the esophageal hiatus in the diaphragm. It then descends in the lesser omentum along the lesser curve of the stomach, which it supplies.

2. The splenic artery passes along the superior border of the pancreas in the posterior wall of the lesser sac to reach the upper pole of the left kidney. Then, it passes to the hilum of the spleen in the lienorenal ligament and divides into the number of branches before entering the spleen. The splenic artery also gives rise to short gastric branches, to the stomach fundus and a left gastroepiploic branch, which passes in the gastrosplenic ligament to reach and supply the greater curvature of the stomach.

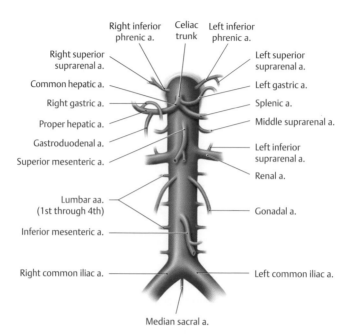

Fig. 19.5 Branches of abdominal aorta. (Modified from Schuenke M, Schulte E, Schumacher U. THIEME Atlas of Anatomy. Internal Organs. Illustrations by Voll M and Wesker K. © Thieme 2020)

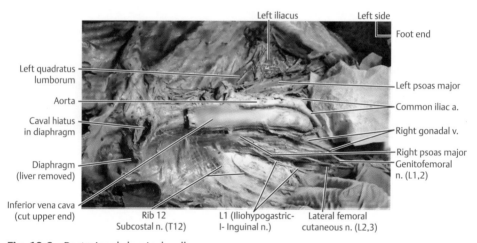

Fig. 19.6 Posterior abdominal wall.

3. The common hepatic artery descends to the right toward the first part of the duodenum in the posterior wall of the lesser sac; then, it ascends in the right free margin of the lesser omentum to reach the porta hepatis in close relation to the portal vein and bile duct. Before reaching the porta hepatis, it divides into right and left hepatic arteries which enter the liver. The right gastric artery gives off the cystic artery. Before ascending into the lesser omentum, the hepatic artery gives rise to gastroduodenal and right gastric branches. The latter passes along the lesser curve of the stomach to supply it. The former passes behind the first part of the duodenum and then branches further into superior pancreaticoduodenal and right gastroepiploic branches. The right gastroepiploic branch runs along the lower part of the greater curvature to supply the stomach.

Table 19.1   Summary of Branches of Abdominal Aorta

Branch from abdominal aorta	Branches	
Inferior phrenic aa. (paired)	Superior suprarenal aa.	
Coeliac trunk	• Left gastric a. • Splenic a. • Common hepatic a.	• Proper hepatic a. • Right gastric a. • Gastroduodenal a.
Middle suprarenal aa. (paired)		
Superior mesenteric a.		
Renal aa. (paired)	Inferior suprarenal aa.	
Lumbar aa. (1st through 4th, paired)		
Testicular/ovarian aa. (paired)		
Inferior mesenteric a.		
Common iliac aa. (paired)	• External iliac a. • Internal iliac a.	
Median sacral a.		

The abdominal aorta gives rise to three major unpaired trunks and the unpaired median sacral artery, as well as six paired branches.

Superior Mesenteric Artery

It arises from the abdominal aorta at the level of L2. For details, see page 176, Chapter 16.

Inferior Mesenteric Artery

It arises from the abdominal aorta at the level of L3. It passes downward and to the left and crosses the left common iliac artery where it changes to the superior rectal artery. For details, see page 178, Chapter 16.

Paired Branches

Inferior phrenic arteries: They arise just above the celiac trunk and pass superolaterally over the crura of the diaphragm. They give off superior suprarenal artery to the corresponding suprarenal gland.

Renal arteries: They arise from abdominal aorta just below the origin of superior mesenteric artery at the level of L2 vertebra. It runs across the crus of the diaphragm and psoas major to enter the hilum of kidney. Before entering the hilum, it gives off inferior suprarenal artery.

Testicular and ovarian arteries: They arise from abdominal aorta below the renal arteries and descend obliquely on the posterior abdominal wall to reach the ovary in the female, or pass through the inguinal canal to reach the testis in males.

Lumbar arteries: The four pairs of the arteries arise from the posterior surface of the abdominal aorta. They pass laterally on the surfaces of lumbar vertebrae and then disappear underneath the psoas major muscle.

Common Iliac Arteries

These are the two terminal branches of aorta. They arise on the anterior surface of the L4 vertebra. Each common iliac artery passes inferolaterally to the sacroiliac joint, where it divides into large external and smaller internal iliac arteries. The left common iliac artery is crossed by superior rectal vessels and some sigmoid arteries, while the right artery lies on the beginning of the inferior vena cava and the right common iliac vein.

External Iliac Arteries

These are the direct continuation of the common iliac arteries. They extend from sacroiliac joint to the midinguinal point. It continues as femoral artery after passing deep to inguinal ligament. Each external iliac artery gives off two branches: (a) a deep circumflex iliac artery and (b) an inferior epigastric artery immediately superior to the inguinal ligament.

The summary of branches of abdominal aorta is given in **Table 19.1**.

■ Clinical Note

Abdominal aortic aneurysm: The atheromatous degeneration of the aorta may cause progressive aortic dilatation called an aneurysm. Aneurysm of the abdominal aorta most commonly occurs below the level of the renal arteries.

Inferior Vena Cava

It is the largest and widest vein in the body. It is formed by the union of right and left common iliac veins in front of the right side of L5 vertebra. It ascends in front of the vertebral column retroperitoneally on the right side of the aorta, grooves the posterior surface of liver and pierces central tendon of diaphragm at the level of T8 vertebra (**Fig. 19.7**), and drains into the right atrium.
Relations:

1. *Anterior* (from above downward): Liver, epiploic foramen, first part of the duodenum and portal vein, head of pancreas and bile duct, horizontal part of duodenum and right gonadal artery, superior mesenteric vessels in the root of mesentery, and right common iliac artery.

2. *Posterior* (from below upward):
   - Right sympathetic chain and right psoas major.
   - Right renal artery, right celiac ganglion and right suprarenal gland, right middle suprarenal vein, and right inferior phrenic artery.

Tributaries: These include common iliac, third and fourth lumbar veins, right testicular or ovarian vein, renal veins, azygos vein, right suprarenal vein, inferior hepatic veins, and hepatic veins (**Fig. 19.8**).

Common Iliac Veins

These veins are on the medial surface of the psoas muscle by the union of the internal and external iliac veins. They end by opening into the inferior vena cava at the level of L5. Each common iliac vein receives an iliolumbar vein. The median sacral vein joins the left common iliac vein.

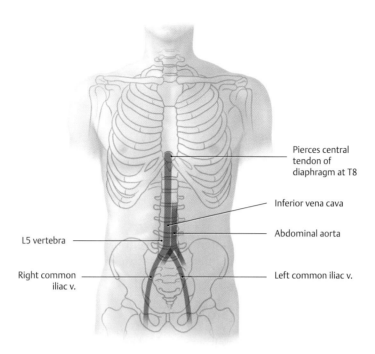

Fig. 19.7 Location of inferior vena cava (anterior view). (From Schuenke M, Schulte E, Schumacher U. THIEME Atlas of Anatomy. Internal Organs. Illustrations by Voll M and Wesker K. © Thieme 2020)

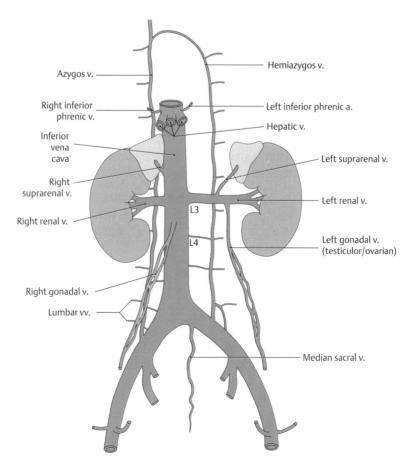

Fig. 19.8 Tributaries of inferior vena cava. (Modified from Schuenke M, Schulte E, Schumacher U. THIEME Atlas of Anatomy. Internal Organs. Illustrations by Voll M and Wesker K. © Thieme 2020)

Summary of Tributaries of Inferior Vena Cava

- Inferior phrenic vv. (paired)
- Hepatic vv.
- Suprarenal vv. (the right vein is a direct tributary)
- Renal vv. (paired)
- Testicular/ovarian vv. (the right vein is a direct tributary)
- Common iliac vv. (paired)
- Median sacral v.

External Iliac Veins

Each external iliac vein unites with the internal iliac vein of the corresponding side to form a common iliac vein. Each vein receives an inferior epigastric and a deep circumflex iliac vein as tributaries.

Azygos and Hemiazygos Veins (Fig. 19.8)

Both azygos and hemiazygos veins lie on either side of thoracic part of vertebral column. Mostly they begin in the abdomen more or less at the same level:

1. Azygos vein begins as a continuation of lumbar azygos vein from the posterior surface of inferior vena cava and ascends into thorax through the right crus of the diaphragm. It lies on the right side of thoracic vertebral column.

2. Hemiazygos vein arises from the posterior surface of the left renal vein and ascends into the thorax through the left crus of the diaphragm. It lies on the left side of thoracic vertebral column.

Note that both these veins may arise from the union of subcostal and ascending lumbar veins on the corresponding side.

Lymph Nodes of the Posterior Abdominal Wall

These are retroperitoneal and situated along the iliac vessels, aorta, and inferior vena cava. They include external iliac nodes, common iliac nodes, and lumbar nodes (**Fig. 19.9**).

1. External iliac nodes (8 to 10 in number) lie along external iliac vessels. Medial nodes receive lymph from lower limb and pelvic viscera, while lateral nodes drain the lymph from the territories of inferior epigastric and deep circumflex iliac vessels. Afferents of external iliac nodes pass to the common iliac nodes.

2. Common iliac nodes (4 to 6 in number) are divided into two groups: medial and lateral. Medial nodes lie in the angle at the bifurcation of aorta, while the lateral nodes lie along the common iliac vessels. The medial nodes drain pelvic viscera, while the lateral nodes drain lower limb and pelvic viscera. The efferents from common iliac nodes pass to the lumbar nodes.

3. Lumbar nodes are scattered along the aorta and inferior vena cava. They drain the lymph from posterior abdominal wall, kidneys, ureters, testes, ovaries, uterus, and uterine tubes. The efferents from lumbar nodes form right and left lumbar lymph trunks which drain into the cisterna chyli.

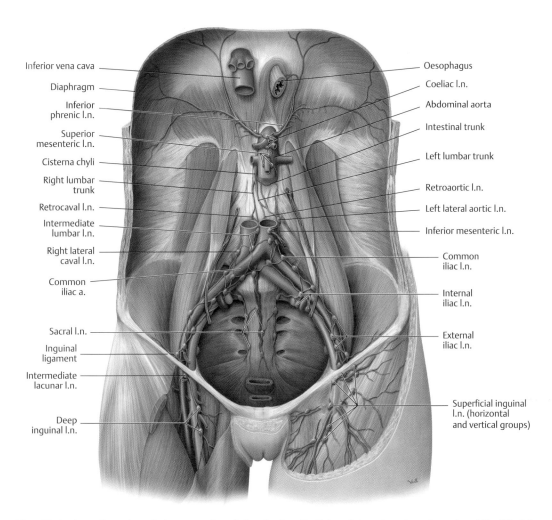

Fig. 19.9   Lymph nodes of the posterior abdominal wall. Abbreviaton: l.n., lymph nodes. (Modified from Schuenke M, Schulte E, Schumacher U. THIEME Atlas of Anatomy. Internal Organs. Illustrations by Voll M and Wesker K. © Thieme 2020)

Cisterna chyli: It is a large (5–7 cm long and 4 mm wide) white lymph sac lying on the upper two lumbar vertebrae between aorta and azygos vein. It continues above through aortic hiatus as the thoracic duct. It receives the following tributaries:

1. Lumbar lymph trunks inferiorly.

2. Intestinal lymph trunk in the middle.

3. Lymph vessels from lower intercostal node superiorly.

Muscles of Posterior Abdominal Wall

The muscles of posterior abdominal wall are psoas major, psoas minor, iliacus, and quadratus lumborum (**Fig. 19.10**). The origin, insertion, nerve supply, and actions of the muscles are shown in **Table 19.2**.

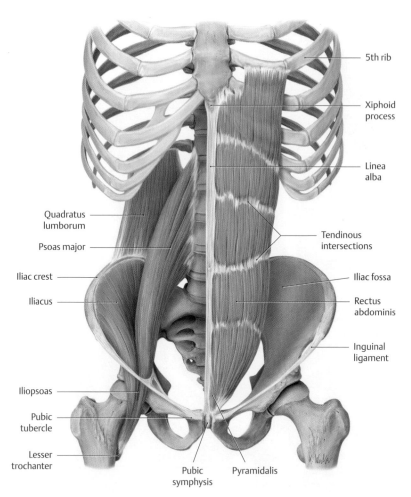

Fig. 19.10   Muscles of posterior abdominal wall (right half). (From Schuenke M, Schulte E, Schumacher U. THIEME Atlas of Anatomy. General Anatomy and Musculoskeletal System. Illustrations by Voll M and Wesker K. © Thieme 2020)

Table 19.2   Origin, insertion, nerve supply, and actions of the posterior abdominal wall muscles.

Muscle	Origin	Insertion	Nerve supply	Actions
Psoas major	Transverse processes of lumbar vertebrae; sides of bodies of T12–L5 vertebrae, and intervening intervertebral discs	Lesser trochanter of femur	Lumbar plexus L2, L3, and L4	Powerful flexion of thigh with trunk
Psoas minor[a]	From T12 and L1 along with psoas major	Iliopubic eminence	Lumbar plexus	No significant action
Iliacus	Upper two-thirds of iliac fossa	Lesser trochanter of femur and shaft inferior to it	Femoral nerve (L2–L4)	Flexion of thigh
Quadratus lumborum	Iliolumbar ligament and posterior part internal lip of iliac crest	Medial half of inferior border of 12th ribs and tips of lumbar transverse processes	Ventral rami of L12 to L4 spinal nerve	Lateral flexion of lumbar vertebral column

[a]Psoas minor muscle lies anterior to the psoas major muscle and is confined to the abdomen only.

Nerves of the Posterior Abdominal Wall

Abdominal Part of Sympathetic Trunk

The thoracic part of sympathetic trunk passes behind the medial arcuate ligament to continue as abdominal part (lumbar part) of the sympathetic trunk. Here, it runs along the medial border of psoas major muscle and becomes continuous with the pelvic part by passing behind the common iliac vessels. There are four ganglia in the lumbar or abdominal part. Only the upper two ganglia receive white rami communicantes from the ventral primary rami of L1 and L2 spinal nerves (**Fig. 19.11**).

Gray rami communicantes to first two or three lumbar spinal nerves which pass along the spinal nerves to be distributed to the sweat glands, cutaneous blood vessels, and arrector pili muscles.

1. Postganglionic fibers pass medially to the aortic plexus.

2. Postganglionic fibers pass in front of common iliac vessels to form hypogastric plexus. The post-ganglionic fibers pass through lumbar splanchnic nerves which arise from the trunk.

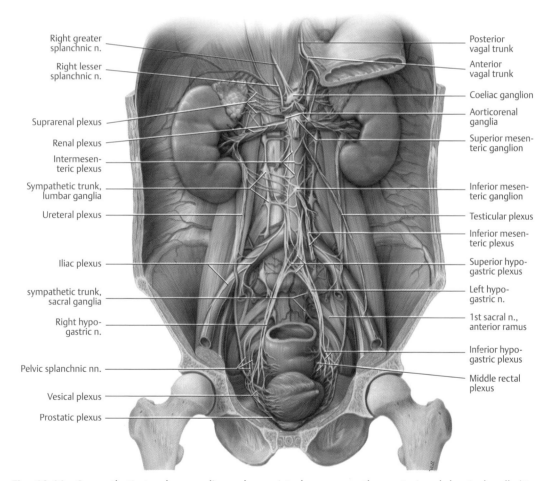

Fig. 19.11 Sympathetic trunks, ganglia, and associated nerves on the posterior abdominal wall. (From Schuenke M, Schulte E, Schumacher U. THIEME Atlas of Anatomy. Internal Organs. Illustrations by Voll M and Wesker K. © Thieme 2020)

Subcostal Nerve

It is the ventral ramus of T12 spinal nerve. First, it runs along the inferior border of the 12th rib and leaves the thorax by passing behind the lateral arcuate ligament to enter the abdomen. It lies on the anterior surface of quadratus lumborum and its lateral border. It pierces transversus abdominis to run in the neurovascular plane of the anterior abdominal wall. It supplies quadratus lumborum, three flat muscles of abdomen, rectus abdominis, and pyramidalis.

Lumbar Plexus (Fig. 19.12)

The lumbar plexus is formed from the ventral primary rami of L1–L4 spinal nerves with a contribution from subcostal nerve. The trunks of the plexus lie within the posterior part of the substance of psoas major. All the branches of lumbar plexus emerge at its lateral border, except obturator, and genitofemoral nerves.

Branches of Lumbar Plexus

1. *Iliohypogastric nerve (T12, L1)* is the main trunk of the first lumbar nerve. It passes inferolaterally between quadratus lumborum and kidney. It supplies the skin of the upper part of the buttock by way of its lateral cutaneous branch and terminates by piercing the external oblique above the superficial inguinal ring, where it supplies the overlying skin of suprapubic region.

2. *Ilioinguinal nerve (L1)* is the collateral branch of the iliohypogastric nerve. The ilioinguinal nerve runs in the neurovascular plane of the abdominal wall to emerge through the superficial inguinal ring to provide a cutaneous supply to the skin of the medial thigh, the root of the penis, and anterior one-third of the scrotum (or labium majus in the female).

3. *Genitofemoral nerve (L1, L2)* emerges from the anterior surface of psoas major. It courses inferiorly on the psoas muscle and divides into genital and femoral components. The genital component enters the spermatic cord and supplies the cremaster (in males) and the femoral component enters into femoral sheath and pierces its anterior wall to supply the skin of the thigh over the femoral triangle.

4. *Lateral cutaneous nerve of the thigh (L2, L3)* emerges from the lateral border of the psoas major above the iliac crest and encircles the iliac fossa to pass under the lateral part of the inguinal ligament to supply the skin on the anterolateral aspect of the thigh.

5. *Femoral nerve (L2–L4 posterior division)* emerges from psoas below the iliac crest (for details, see page 22, Chapter 2).

6. *Obturator nerve (L2–L4 anterior division)* leaves the medial border of psoas at the base of sacrum and enters the pelvis (for details, see page 21, Chapter 2).

Points to note:
- A large part of L4 joins with L5 to contribute to the sacral plexus as the lumbosacral trunk.
- An accessory obturator nerve sometimes arises from L3 and L4 nerves and runs along the medial side of psoas. It gives branches to hip joint and sometimes to pectineus nerve (**Fig. 19.12**).

Lumbar Arteries

1. The upper four pairs arise from the posterior surface of abdominal aorta and curve over the vertebral bodies to pass deep to the sympathetic trunk.

2. The fifth pair may arise from median sacral artery or from iliolumbar artery.

Lumbar Veins

These veins accompany the lumbar arteries:

1. The first and second lumbar veins join the ascending lumbar vein.

2. The third and fourth lumbar veins drain into inferior vena cava.

3. The fifth lumbar vein drains into the iliolumbar vein.

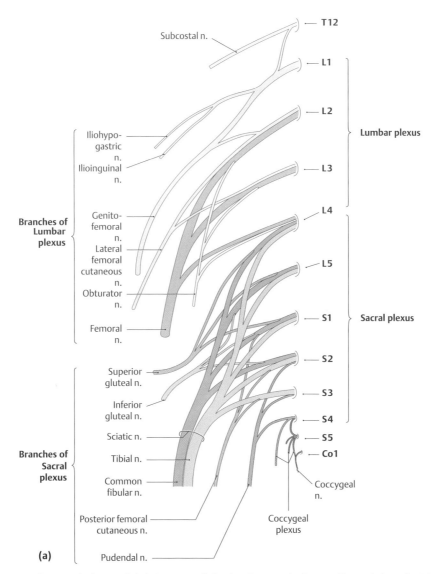

Fig. 19.12 Lumbosacral plexus. **(a)** Structure of the lumbosacral plexus. (From Schuenke M, Schulte E, Schumacher U. THIEME Atlas of Anatomy. General Anatomy and Musculoskeletal System. Illustrations by Voll M and Wesker K. © Thieme 2020). *(Continued)*

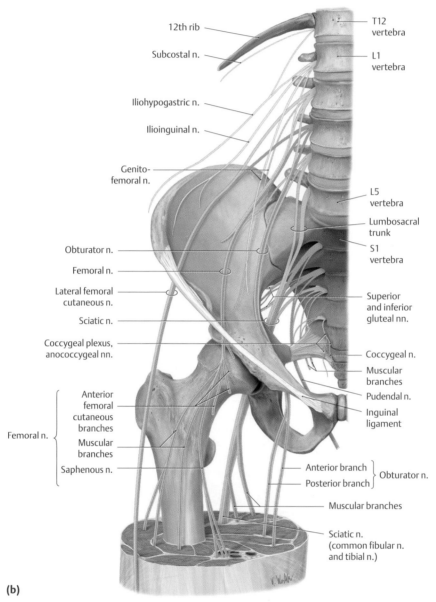

(b)

Fig. 19.12 *(Continued)* Lumbosacral plexus. **(b)** Course of the lumbosacral plexus. (From Schuenke M, Schulte E, Schumacher U. THIEME Atlas of Anatomy. General Anatomy and Musculoskeletal System. Illustrations by Voll M and Wesker K. © Thieme 2020)

▌ Clinical Notes

1. *Paralysis of diaphragm*: It occurs due to injury of phrenic nerve either in the neck or in the thorax, and involves only hemidiaphragm. This can be detected by X-ray screening, as the paralyzed hemidiaphragm moves paradoxically during respiration.

2. *Posterolateral hernia of diaphragm (hernia of Bochdalek)*: It is the commonest congenital hernia of diaphragm. In this, abdominal viscera are pushed into thoracic cavity through a gap between costal and vertebral origins of the diaphragm called vertebrocostal triangle or foramen of Bochdalek.

3. *Aortic aneurysm*: It commonly occurs below the origin of renal artery due to atherosclerosis. Clinically, it presents a pulsatile, nontender, palpable mass below the umbilicus. Rupture of aortic aneurysm is fatal unless promptly repaired by surgeons.

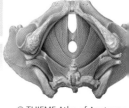
The term *pelvis* is derived from Latin, and it literally means basin. The bony pelvis consists of four bones: two hip bones, sacrum, and coccyx. These bones are united by four joints: two synovial sacroiliac joints posterosuperiorly and two fibrocartilaginous joints—the pubic symphysis antero-inferiorly and the sacrococcygeal joint posteriorly (**Fig. 20.1**).

In the erect posture, the upper margin of the pubic symphysis and the anterior superior iliac spines lie in the same coronal plane. The articulated pelvis is placed in the anatomical position with these three points touching a vertical surface.

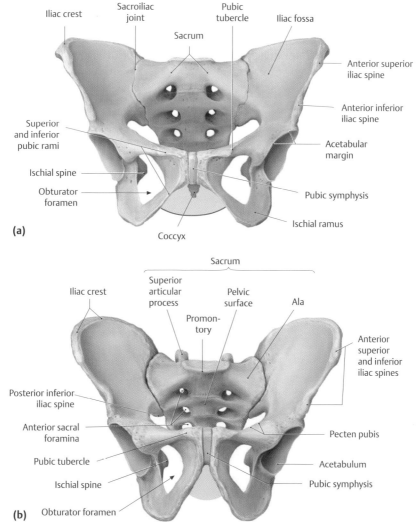

Fig. 20.1 Pelvis (anterior view): **(a)** Female pelvis. **(b)** Male pelvis. (From Schuenke M, Schulte E, Schumacher U. THIEME Atlas of Anatomy. General Anatomy and Musculoskeletal System. Illustrations by Voll M and Wesker K. © Thieme 2020)

Parts

The pelvis is divided into two parts, *greater pelvis* and *lesser pelvis*, by the *plane of superior aperture of the lesser pelvis/pelvic inlet*. It is an oblique plane that passes from the sacral promontory to the upper surface of the pubic symphysis. The part anterosuperior to this plane is the greater pelvis. It is formed by the iliac fossae and is part of the posterior wall of the abdomen. The part posteroinferior to the plane is called lesser pelvis. In clinical practice, the term "pelvis" is usually applied to the lesser pelvis. The plane of pelvic inlet is bounded posteriorly by the anterior margin of sacral promontory, on either side by arcuate line, and anteriorly by the upper margin of pubic symphysis (**Fig. 20.2**).

Lesser Pelvis

The pelvic brim (also termed the "linea terminalis") separates the pelvis into the false pelvis (above) and the true pelvis (below). The true pelvis (pelvic cavity) lies between the inlet and outlet. The pelvic outlet is bounded by the coccyx posteriorly, sacrotuberous ligament posterolaterally, the ischial tuberosities laterally, and the pubic arch anteriorly.

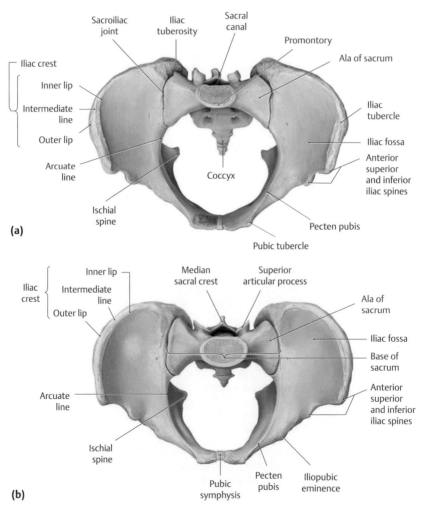

Fig. 20.2 Pelvis (superior view): **(a)** Female pelvis. **(b)** Male pelvis. (From Schuenke M, Schulte E, Schumacher U. THIEME Atlas of Anatomy. General Anatomy and Musculoskeletal System. Illustrations by Voll M and Wesker K. © Thieme 2020)

Walls of the Pelvis

In the sagittal section, the cavity of pelvis is C-shaped with long posterosuperior wall and short anteroinferior wall (**Fig. 20.3**).

1. Posterosuperior wall is long and formed by the sacrum and coccyx.

2. Anteroinferior wall is short and formed by the bodies of pubic bones and pubic symphysis.

3. Anterolateral wall is formed by ischiopubic rami surrounding the obturator foramen and pelvic surface of hip bone below the pelvic inlet. The obturator foramen is filled by obturator membrane except anteroinferiorly to form obturator canal.

4. Posterolateral wall is a gap between the hip bone, sacrum, and coccyx. This gap is divided by sacrotuberous and sacrospinous ligaments into greater and lesser sciatic foramen.

The walls of pelvis are lined by muscles, namely, piriformis on sacrum, obturator internus on the anterolateral wall, and coccygeus on sacrospinous ligament. All these structures are covered by the pelvic fascia.

Inferior Aperture of Pelvis/Pelvic Outlet

It is a diamond-shaped aperture bounded anterolaterally by ischial and inferior pubic rami and posterolaterally by sacrotuberous ligaments. The angles of this aperture are formed as under: anterior angle by pubic symphysis, posterior angle by coccyx, and lateral angles by ischial tuberosities. These are actually the boundaries of perineum.

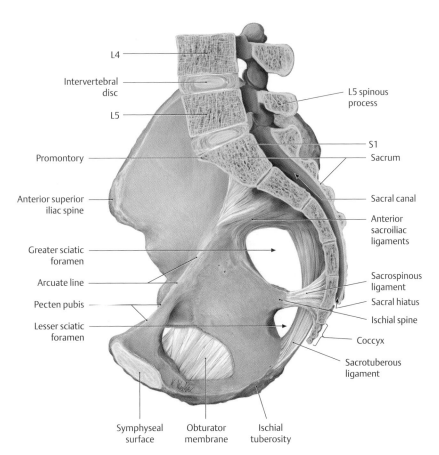

Fig. 20.3 Wall of the pelvis. (From Schuenke M, Schulte E, Schumacher U. THIEME Atlas of Anatomy. General Anatomy and Musculoskeletal System. Illustrations by Voll M and Wesker K. © Thieme 2020)

Joints of Pelvis

The joints of pelvis comprise pubic symphysis, right and left sacroiliac joints, and sacrococcygeal joint.

1. The pubic symphysis is a secondary cartilaginous joint between the bodies of pubic bones.

2. The sacroiliac joint is a synovial joint between the auricular surfaces of sacrum and ilium.

3. The sacrococcygeal joint is a secondary cartilaginous joint between the apex of sacrum and base of coccyx.

Pelvic Diaphragm/Pelvic Floor

It is the muscular partition between the pelvis and perineum. The pelvic floor supports the viscera and produces a sphincter action on the rectum and vagina to produce increased intra-abdominal pressure during straining, namely defecation and micturition. The rectum and urethra (and also the vagina in female) traverse the pelvic floor to gain access to the exterior. The pelvic floor is formed by levator ani and coccygeus muscles (**Fig. 20.4**).

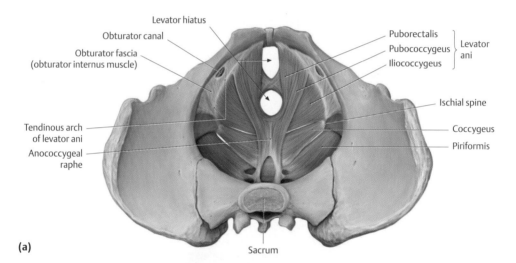

(a)

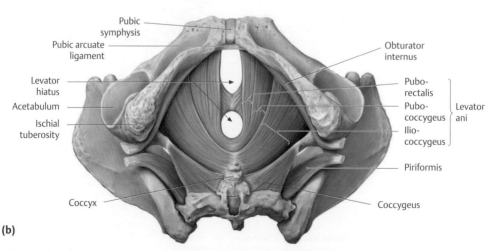

(b)

Fig. 20.4   Pelvic floor: **(a)** Superior view. **(b)** Inferior view. (From Schuenke M, Schulte E, Schumacher U. THIEME Atlas of Anatomy. General Anatomy and Musculoskeletal System. Illustrations by Voll M and Wesker K. © Thieme 2020)

1. *Levator ani*: It slopes downward in the median plane and fuses with each other to form gutter-shaped pelvic floor. The levator ani muscle arises from the posterior aspect of the body of pubis, fascia overlying the obturator internus on the side wall of the pelvis, and the ischial spine. From this broad origin, fibers sweep backward toward the midline to end as follows:

   - Anterior fibers (*sphincter vaginae* or levator prostatae) surround the vagina in the female (sphincter vaginae) and prostate in the male (levator prostatae) and insert into the perineal body. It is a fibromuscular node lying anterior to the anal canal.
   - Intermediate fibers (*puborectalis*) surround the anorectal junction and insert into the anococcygeal median raphe, a fibrous raphe extending between anorectal junction and tip of coccyx.
   - Posterior fibers (*iliococcygeus*) insert into the lateral aspect of the coccyx and anococcygeal raphe.

2. *Coccygeus*: It is a small triangular muscle. It arises from the ischial spine and inserts into the last piece of sacrum and upper two pieces of coccyx.

Differences between Male and Female Pelvis

The female pelvis differs from that of the male for the purpose of childbearing and childbirth (**Fig. 20.5**). The major differences between the male and female pelvis are:

1. Pelvic inlet is transversely oval in the female. In the male, the sacral promontory is more prominent, producing a heart-shaped inlet.

2. Pelvic outlet is wider in females as the ischial tuberosities are everted.

3. Pelvic cavity is more spacious in the female than in the male, that is, roomy and shallow in female and long and narrow in male.

4. False pelvis is shallow in the female.

5. Subpubic angle is wider (90–100 degrees) in female and narrow (70 degrees) in male.

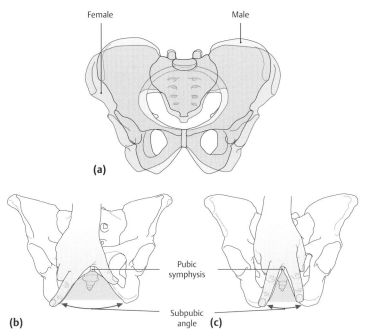

Fig. 20.5 Differences between male and female pelvis. **(a)** Male and female pelvis superimposed. **(b)** Female pelvis. **(c)** Male pelvis. (From Schuenke M, Schulte E, Schumacher U. THIEME Atlas of Anatomy. General Anatomy and Musculoskeletal System. Illustrations by Voll M and Wesker K. © Thieme 2020)

Pelvic Viscera

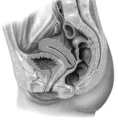

© THIEME Atlas of Anatomy

The pelvic viscera comprise urinary bladder, prostate in male, uterus in female, rectum, and pelvic part of sigmoid colon.

Urinary Bladder, Prostate, and Urethra

Learning Objectives

At the end of the dissection of urinary bladder, prostate, and urethra, students should be able to identify the following:

- Retropubic space (space of Retzius) and note its limits and contents. Identify the attachments of puboprostatic/pubovesical ligaments.
- Peritoneal reflections in the male pelvis. Note the location and limits of rectovesical pouch.
- Extent, course, and relations of pelvic part of the ureter.
- Neck, apex, base, borders, surfaces, and ligaments (supports) of urinary bladder.
- Bladder trigone, ureteric orifices, uvula, interureteric fold, and internal urethral orifice in the interior of the bladder.
- Structural differences between mucosa lining of trigone of bladder and rest of the bladder.
- Ductus deferens, seminal vesicles, ejaculatory ducts, and prostate gland in the male pelvis.
- Size, shape, apex, surfaces, capsules, and relations of the prostate gland.
- Urinary bladder, seminal vesicle, rectovesical septum, prostate gland, ejaculatory duct, median lobe of prostate, and prostatic utricle.
- Prostatic, membranous, and spongy parts of urethra, bulbourethral glands, intrabulbar and navicular fossae in the sagittal section of male pelvis.
- Prostatic urethra and note its length, shape, and internal features, namely, urethral crest, prostatic sinuses, colliculus seminalis, openings of prostatic utricle, and ejaculatory ducts.
- Superior and inferior vesical arteries, arteries of ductus deferens, and urethral arteries.

Dissection and Identification

1. Trace the reflection of peritoneum in the true pelvis and examine the pelvic viscera in situ.

2. Identify the urinary bladder as it lies behind the pubic symphysis. Follow the peritoneal covering of the urinary bladder from its superior surface to upper part of its posterior surface. In males, note that it is then reflected onto the anterior surface of the rectum, forming the rectovesical pouch (**Fig. 21.1**). In females, observe that the uterus lies between the urinary bladder and rectum. The peritoneum from the urinary bladder passes onto the anterior surface of uterus thereby forming *uterovesical pouch* and then over the fundus of the uterus to its posterior surface down till the upper part of vagina. Now it is reflected onto the anterior aspect of rectum to form *rectouterine pouch* (**Fig. 21.2**).

3. Trace the lateral reflections of the peritoneum from the rectum onto the lateral wall of the pelvis. Identify the *paravesical fossae* and *pararectal fossae* lined by peritoneum on either side of the urinary bladder and rectum, respectively (**Video 21.1**).

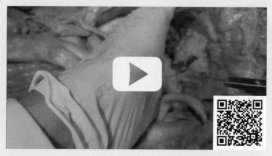

Video 21.1   Urinary bladder: Parts, ligaments, and vessels.

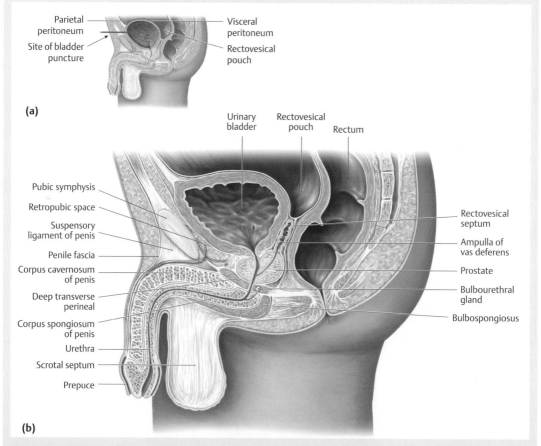

(a)

(b)

Fig. 21.1   Sagittal section of male pelvis. **(a)** Peritoneal covering. **(b)** Right male hemipelvis. (Modified from Schuenke M, Schulte E, Schumacher U. THIEME Atlas of Anatomy. Internal Organs. Illustrations by Voll M and Wesker K. © Thieme 2020)

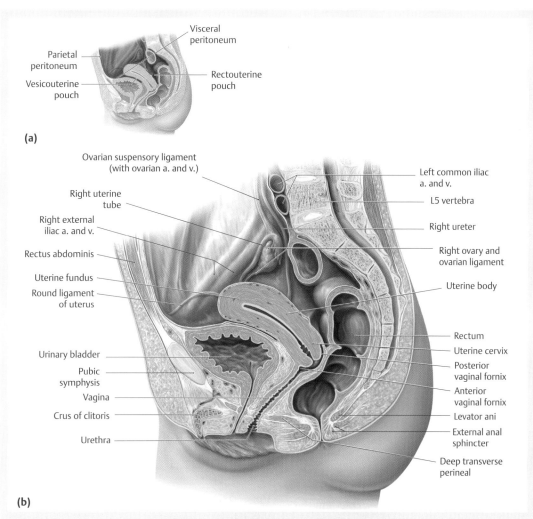

Fig. 21.2 Sagittal section of female pelvis. **(a)** Peritoneal covering. **(b)** Right female hemipelvis. (From Schuenke M, Schulte E, Schumacher U. THIEME Atlas of Anatomy. General Anatomy and Musculoskeletal System. Illustrations by Voll M and Wesker K. © Thieme 2020)

4. Remove the peritoneum from the superior surface of the urinary bladder. Note that the most anterior and superior part of the bladder is the apex. The median umbilical ligament, a remnant of the urachus, extends from the apex of the bladder to the umbilicus. The posterior surface of the bladder is the base of the urinary bladder. Posterior to the base, identify the ampullae of ductus deferens and, more lateral to them, the seminal vesicles.

5. Identify the ureter in the abdominal cavity once again. Trace the ureters down to the pelvis in front of the common iliac arteries. Follow them further down into the pelvis first laterally in front of internal iliac artery and then medially to the superolateral angles of the bladder.

6. Pull the apex of the bladder posteriorly. On the internal surface of the bladder, note the retropubic space (space of Retzius) located between the pubic symphysis and bladder and expose the pubovesical/puboprostatic ligaments (**Video 21.2**).

7. Make incisions through the bladder wall along the junction of superior and inferolateral surface on either side extending backward till the superolateral angles of the base. Fold back the superior wall of the bladder and examine the interior of the bladder. Identify the trigone, a smooth triangular area bounded superolaterally by the openings of the ureters and inferiorly by the internal urethral orifice. Observe the bulge, uvula vesicae, caused by the middle lobe of

prostate just posterior to the internal urethral orifice. Note that the remainder of the internal surface of the bladder has thick mucosal folds.

8. To facilitate the study of the pelvic organs, hemisect the pelvis. Cut through the pubic symphysis and extend it across the urinary bladder through the internal urethral orifice, then through the uterus and vagina or between the ductus deferens and divide the rectum longitudinally. Cut the soft tissues of the pelvis and perineum with a knife or scalpel and extend the incisions through the sacrum and lumbar vertebra with a saw.

9. Separate the halves of the pelvis, wash out the rectum, and examine the cut surfaces of the tissues and organs.

10. Inferior to the bladder, identify the pyramidal-shaped firm structure, prostate gland which surrounds the urethra. The apex of the prostate rests on the urogenital diaphragm. The base of the prostate contacts with the bladder. Clean the fascia around the prostate and note the plexus of veins, prostatic venous plexus, which surrounds the prostate gland.

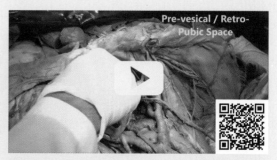

Video 21.2 Urinary bladder, UV junction, and trigone.

11. Examine the prostatic part of the urethra which begins at the internal urethral orifice and runs inferiorly through the prostate gland to the level of the urogenital diaphragm. On the posterior wall of the prostatic urethra, identify the elevation called the seminal colliculus, which lies on the median posterior ridge, urethral crest which extends the whole length of the prostatic urethra with a groove on either side of it, and the prostatic sinus. On the anterior surface of the seminal colliculus, identify the opening of the prostatic utricle, a blind median pouch which extends posterosuperiorly into the prostate. On either side of the opening of utricle, identify the openings of the two ejaculatory ducts. Note that the ejaculatory ducts are formed by the union of ductus deferens with the duct of seminal vesicle (**Videos 21.3** and **21.4**).

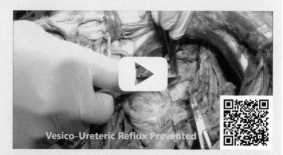

Video 21.3 Bladder neck, trigone, and prostatic urethra.

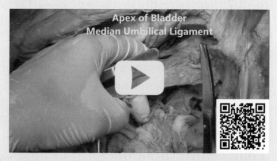

Video 21.4 Pelvic part of ureter, bladder of urinary relations, and trigone of urinary bladder.

Urinary Bladder

The urinary bladder is a muscular reservoir of urine. When empty, it lies in the anteroinferior part of the pelvis behind the pubis, covered superiorly by peritoneum (**Figs. 21.1** and **21.2**). It has a capacity of approximately 220 mL (120–320 mL).

The empty bladder is pyramidal in shape. The apex of the pyramid points forward and is continuous with a fibrous cord, the median umbilical ligament (obliterated urachus) which passes upward to the umbilicus. The base (posterior surface) is triangular in the male; its upper part is separated from rectum by rectovesical pouch and lower part is related to seminal vesicles and vasa deferentia. In females, it is related to uterine cavity and the vagina. The seminal vesicles are separated by the vas deferens. The rectum lies behind. In females, the vagina intervenes between the bladder and rectum. The inferolateral surfaces are related inferiorly to the pelvic floor and anteriorly to the retropubic pad of fat and pubic bones. The superior surface is completely covered by peritoneum in males, while in females it is not completely covered by peritoneum because a small area posteriorly is related to the supravaginal part of the cervix. The peritoneum from superior surface is reflected on the isthmus of uterus to form the vesicouterine pouch. The neck fuses with the prostate in males, whereas it lies directly on the pelvic fascia in females. The pelvic fascia is thickened in the form of puboprostatic ligaments (in males) and pubovesical ligaments (in females) to hold the neck of the bladder in position.

Interior of Bladder

In empty bladder, the mucous membrane of the bladder is thrown into folds, except in the region of small triangular area over the base (called trigone), where it is smooth (**Fig. 21.3**). The superolateral angles of the trigone mark the openings of the ureteric orifices, while internal urethral orifice forms the inferior angle of the trigone. In males, it is guarded by a small elevation called *uvula vesicae* produced by the median lobe.

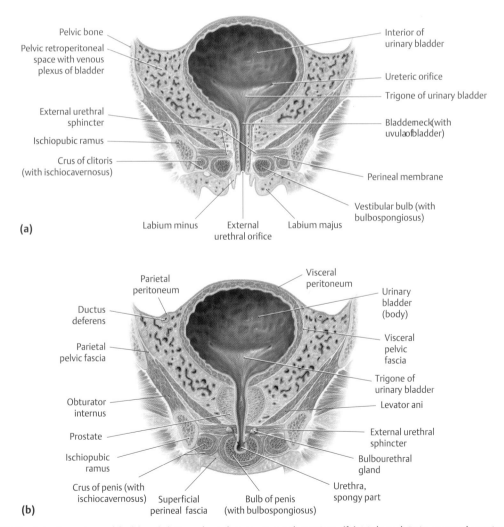

Fig. 21.3 Interior urinary bladder. **(a)** Female pelvis in coronal section. **(b)** Male pelvis in coronal section. (Modified from Schuenke M, Schulte E, Schumacher U. THIEME Atlas of Anatomy. Internal Organs. Illustrations by Voll M and Wesker K. © Thieme 2020) *(Continued)*

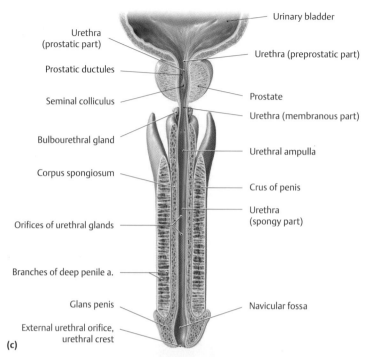

Urinary bladder

Urethra (prostatic part)

Urethra (preprostatic part)

Prostatic ductules

Seminal colliculus

Prostate

Urethra (membranous part)

Bulbourethral gland

Corpus spongiosum

Urethral ampulla

Crus of penis

Urethra (spongy part)

Orifices of urethral glands

Branches of deep penile a.

Glans penis

Navicular fossa

External urethral orifice, urethral crest

(c)

Fig. 21.3 *(Continued)* **(c)** Male urethra in longitudinal section. (Modified from Schuenke M, Schulte E, Schumacher U. THIEME Atlas of Anatomy. Internal Organs. Illustrations by Voll M and Wesker K. © Thieme 2020)

Male Genital Organs

The male genital organs to be studied in pelvis include ductus deferens, seminal vesicles, ejaculatory ducts, prostate, and urethra.

Ductus Deferens

This thick-walled muscular duct begins at the caudal end of epididymis. Its course in spermatic cord and inguinal canal up to the deep inguinal ring has already been traced.

At deep inguinal ring, it leaves the spermatic cord and hooks around the lateral aspect of the inferior epigastric artery. Then, it passes backward and medially across the external iliac vessels to enter the lesser pelvis.

In the *lesser pelvis*, it runs downward and backward on the lateral pelvic wall, deep to the peritoneum across the obturator nerve and vessels. It then crosses the ureter near the posterolateral angle of the bladder and turns medially on the base of the bladder superior to the seminal vesicle and bonds inferiorly medial to the vesicle. Here, it expands to form ampulla. Now it approaches the opposite duct and reaches the base of the prostate (**Fig. 21.4**).

At the base of the prostate, it is joined by the duct of the seminal vesicle to form the ejaculatory duct.

Seminal Vesicles

These are sacculated tubes which are folded upon themselves to form piriform structures (**Fig. 21.4**). They are situated between the bladder and the rectum. Each vesicle is about 15 cm long and is directed upward and laterally. The duct of the seminal vesicle joins the ductus deferens to form the ejaculatory duct.

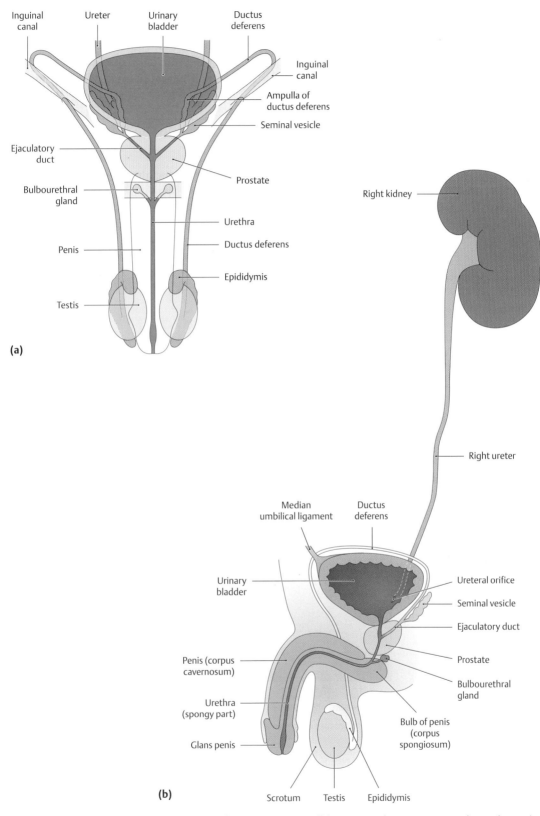

Fig. 21.4 Male genital organs. **(a)** Seminiferous structures. **(b)** Urogenital system. Note: The male urethra serves as a common passage for urine and semen. (Modified from Schuenke M, Schulte E, Schumacher U. THIEME Atlas of Anatomy. Internal Organs. Illustrations by Voll M and Wesker K. © Thieme 2020)

Ejaculatory Ducts

They are formed posterior to the neck of the urinary bladder close to the median plane. Each duct enters the upper posterior half of the prostate, passes along the side of prostatic utricle to open into the prostatic urethra on the seminal colliculus (verumontanum) at the side of the opening of prostatic utricle.

Prostate

The prostate gland resembles a compressed inverted cone, measuring about 3.5 cm transversely at the base and 3 cm vertically from the base to the apex. It weighs about 8 g and shows firmness in its consistency. Its firmness is due to the presence of a dense fibromuscular stroma in which the glandular elements are embedded. It is situated below the neck of the urinary bladder (**Fig. 21.5**).

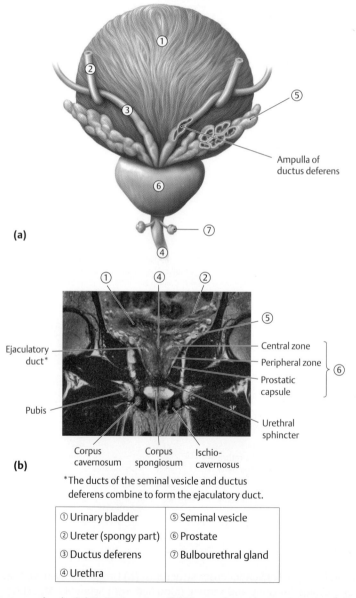

(a)

Ampulla of ductus deferens

Ejaculatory duct*

Central zone
Peripheral zone
Prostatic capsule

Pubis

Urethral sphincter

Corpus cavernosum   Corpus spongiosum   Ischio-cavernosus

(b)

*The ducts of the seminal vesicle and ductus deferens combine to form the ejaculatory duct.

① Urinary bladder	⑤ Seminal vesicle
② Ureter (spongy part)	⑥ Prostate
③ Ductus deferens	⑦ Bulbourethral gland
④ Urethra	

Fig. 21.5 Accessory sex glands. **(a)** Posterior view. **(b)** Magnetic resonance imaging (MRI). Coronal section (anterior view). (From Schuenke M, Schulte E, Schumacher U. THIEME Atlas of Anatomy. Internal Organs. Illustrations by Voll M and Wesker K. © Thieme 2020)

The gland comprises an apex directed downward, a base directed upward, and anterior, posterior, and two inferolateral surfaces.

The anterior surface is separated from pubic symphysis by retropubic space (space of Retzius), while posterior surface is separated from rectum by fascia of Denonvilliers.

Lobes and Zones of the Prostate (Fig. 21.6)

Lobes: Anatomically, the gland comprises anterior, posterior, middle, and lateral lobes. The anterior lobe is small and lies in front of the ejaculatory duct connecting two lateral lobes. Posterior

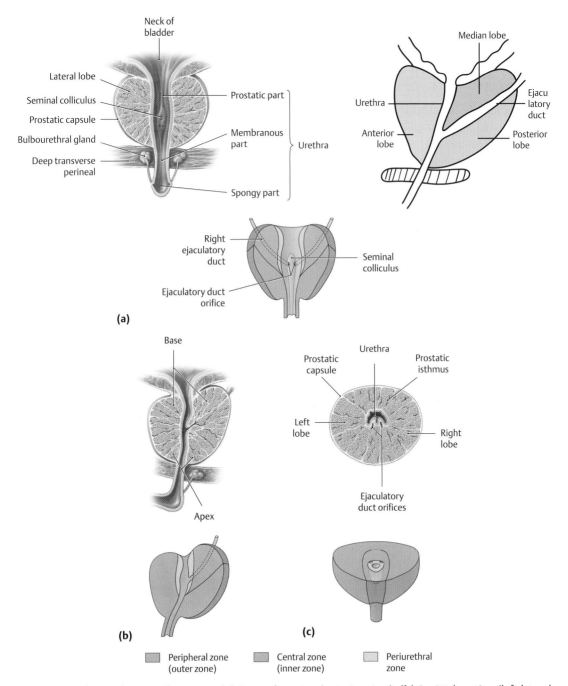

Fig. 21.6 Lobes and zones of prostate. **(a)** Coronal section (anterior view). **(b)** Sagittal section (left lateral view). **(c)** Transverse section (superior view). (Modified from Schuenke M, Schulte E, Schumacher U. THIEME Atlas of Anatomy. Internal Organs. Illustrations by Voll M and Wesker K. © Thieme 2020)

lobe lies behind the median lobe and ejaculatory ducts. The lateral lobes are present one on each side of urethra. The median lobe lies behind the upper part of the urethra in front of ejaculatory ducts just behind the neck of the urinary bladder. Superiorly, it bulges upward into the inferior part of the trigone of the bladder to produce a small elevation called the uvula of the bladder. The prostate gland is traversed by urethra and ejaculatory ducts and contains a small blind saccule in its posterior lobe called prostatic utricle which opens into the middle of the urethral crest.

Zones: The clinicians, especially urologists and sonographers, divide the prostate into peripheral, central, and periurethral zones. The central zone corresponds to the middle lobe (**Fig. 21.6**).

Capsules of Prostate

The prostate gland is enclosed in two capsules, true and false.

True capsule: It is formed by condensation of the peripheral part of the gland and hence is fibromuscular in structure.

False capsule: It lies outside the true capsule and is formed by the endopelvic fascia. Anteriorly, it is continuous with the puboprostatic ligaments. Posteriorly, it is avascular and is formed by the rectovesical fascia of Denonvilliers.

Puboprostatic and Pubovesical Ligaments

They are formed by the condensation of fibroelastic pelvic fascia and contain few smooth muscle fibers. They are arranged in two pairs: medial and lateral. They pass from back of the bodies of the pubic bones to the anterior aspect of the sheath of the prostate gland and the neck of the bladder in males or to the neck of the bladder and adjoining urethra in females.

These ligaments play an important role in maintaining the position of the urinary bladder, prostate, and urethra.

Blood Vessels

The blood to the prostate gland is supplied by inferior vesical, middle rectal, and internal pudendal arteries.

The veins draining the gland form rich plexus around the sides and base of the gland called prostatic venous plexus. It is continuous above with vesical venous plexus. The prostatic venous plexus communicates with vertebral venous plexus through valveless vesical and internal iliac veins, thus providing a venous route of spread of cancer of prostate into the vertebral column.

▮ Clinical Notes

1. *Benign prostatic hypertrophy* (BPH) often occurs above 50 years of age due to the formation of adenoma in its median lobe; hence, it is also called senile enlargement of the prostate. It causes increased frequency, urgency, and difficulty in micturition.

2. *Prostatic cancer* usually occurs above 60 years of age and involves the posterior lobe of the gland. It causes pain in perineum, urinary obstruction, and difficulty in micturition.

3. *Trabeculated bladder* is a condition in which muscular fasciculi in the bladder wall increase in size and interlace in all directions, producing an open weave appearance. It occurs due to continuous distention of bladder caused by chronic obstruction to the outflow of urine by an enlarged prostate.

Urethra

Male Urethra

The male urethra is approximately 18 to 20 cm long and extends from internal urethral orifice to the external urethral meatus on the tip of glans penis. It is divided into three parts: prostatic, membranous, and spongy (penile) (**Fig. 21.3c**).

1. *Prostatic urethra* (3 cm) bears a midline longitudinal elevation (urethral crest) on its posterior wall. On either side of the crest, a shallow depression, the prostatic sinus, is pierced by 15 to 20 prostatic ducts. The prostatic utricle is a 5-mm blind sac which opens into an eminence in the middle of the crest—the verumontanum. The ejaculatory ducts open on either side of the utricle opening.

2. *Membranous urethra* (2 cm) lies in the urogenital diaphragm and is surrounded by the external urethral sphincter (sphincter urethrae muscle).

3. *Spongy penile urethra* (15 cm) traverses the corpus spongiosum of the penis to the external urethral meatus. It presents a dilatation in the bulb of penis to form intrabulbar fossa and in the glans penis to form the navicular fossa.

Female Urethra

It is only 4 cm long, that is, equal to the length of prostatic part of male urethra. It extends from internal urethral orifice of bladder to the vestibule of vagina where it opens above the vaginal orifice. It is wider and more dilatable than male urethra. It is embedded in the anterior wall of the vagina (**Fig. 21.3a**).

▌Clinical Note

Rupture of urethra: It usually occurs in males during instrumentation or catheterization, the commonest site being the bulb of urethra. It causes extravasation of urine in superficial perineal pouch which may extend into spaces of scrotum, penis, and lower part of anterior abdominal wall deep to Scarpa fascia. The rupture of urethra is rare in females.

Rectum and Anal Canal

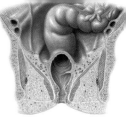

© THIEME Atlas of Anatomy

Learning Objectives

At the end of the dissection of rectum and anal canal, students should be able to identify the following:

- Location, extent, and peritoneal relations of rectum.
- Anorectal junction, rectal ampulla, and flexures of rectum.
- Structures related to rectum in the male and the female.
- Transverse rectal folds and anorectal ring in the interior of the rectum.
- Muscular and fascial supports of the rectum: levator ani, puborectalis, and rectourethralis.
- Waldeyer fascia, lateral ligaments, and rectovesical fascia (Denonvilliers fascia).
- Superior, middle, and inferior rectal vessels and their relative distribution in the rectal wall.
- Location, length, flexures, and relations of anal canal.
- Anal columns, valves, and sinuses on its internal aspect and their clinical significance.

Dissection and Identification

1. Examine the rectum, as it begins as a continuation of sigmoid colon in front of the body of the third sacral vertebra. Observe that it follows the curve of the sacrum and coccyx in the sagittal plane. Confirm that only the anterior and lateral surface of the rectum is covered by peritoneum and is reflected forward from the junction of middle and lower third of rectum. It is continuous distally with the anal canal at the rectoanal junction (**Fig. 22.1**).

2. Observe the interior of the rectum and try to identify three transverse rectal folds (valves of Houston), which project into its lumen.

3. Find the superior rectal artery and trace it to the posterior surface of the upper part of the rectum. Follow its branches to the posterolateral surfaces of the rectum.

4. Examine the lining of the anal canal and note the vertical anal columns. At the distal end of the anal columns, identify anal valves, which are semilunar-shaped folds of mucous membrane that span between adjacent columns. They enclose small pockets of mucous membrane—anal sinuses.

5. Identify the pectinate line, which runs along the bases of the anal valves. This line serves as an important anatomic landmark to delineate the blood supply and innervation of the anal canal. Inferior to the pectinate line, identify the area of pecten and the white line (Hilton white line), which separates the mucosa from the cutaneous portion of the anal canal.

6. Observe that the anal canal contains two muscular sphincters: the internal and external anal sphincters. Identify the external anal sphincter muscle, which is composed of striated muscle. The involuntary internal anal sphincter is composed of thick circular layers of smooth muscle which is continuous with the smooth muscle of the anal canal.

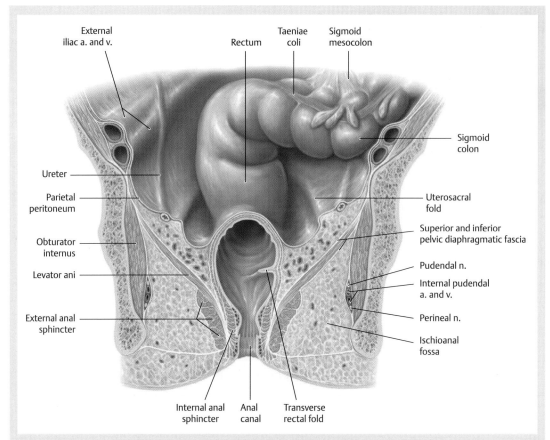

Fig. 22.1 Rectal and anal canal in situ. (From Schuenke M, Schulte E, Schumacher U. THIEME Atlas of Anatomy. Internal Organs. Illustrations by Voll M and Wesker K. © Thieme 2020)

Rectum

It is the distal part of the large intestine. It measures 10 to 15 cm in length. It commences in front of the third sacral vertebra as a continuation of the sigmoid colon and follows the curve of the sacrum anteriorly (sacral flexure). It runs backward abruptly in front of the coccyx (perineal flexure) (**Fig. 22.2**).

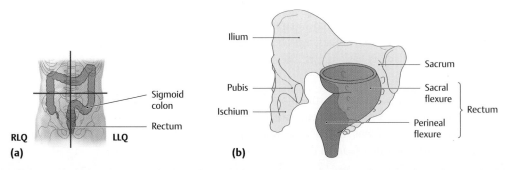

Fig. 22.2 Location of rectum and anal canal. **(a)** Anterior view. **(b)** Left anterolateral view. (Based on Schuenke M, Schulte E, Schumacher U. THIEME Atlas of Anatomy. Internal Organs. Illustrations by Voll M and Wesker K. © Thieme 2020)

The mucosa of the rectum is thrown into three transverse/horizontal folds, namely, superior, middle, and inverse transverse rectal folds, which project into the lumen of rectum. These are called the valves of Houston (**Fig. 22.3**). The rectum lacks haustrations, taeniae coli, and appendices epiploicae. The taeniae coli fan out over the rectum to form anterior and posterior bands. It is slightly dilated at its lower end—the ampulla—and is supported laterally by the levator ani.

Relations (Video 22.1)

The peritoneum covers the upper two-thirds of the rectum anteriorly but only the upper third laterally. In males, it is reflected on to the urinary bladder to form rectovesical pouch. In females, it is reflected onto the uterus forming rectouterine pouch (pouch of Douglas). In males, rectum is separated from prostate by a tough fascial sheet called rectovesical fascia/fascia of Denonvilliers.

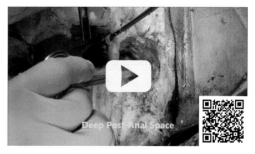

Video 22.1 Ampulla of ductus deferens, seminal vesicle, rectum, and pelvic vessels.

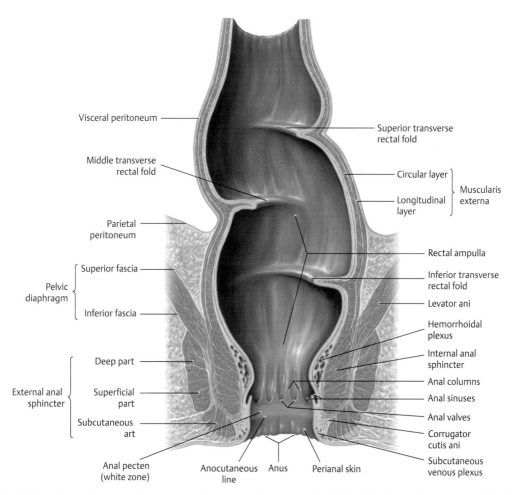

Fig. 22.3 Coronal section of rectum and anal canal (anterior view). (Modified from Schuenke M, Schulte E, Schumacher U. THIEME Atlas of Anatomy. Internal Organs. Illustrations by Voll M and Wesker K. © Thieme 2020)

Visceral Relations

1. In males, the upper two-thirds are related anteriorly to coils of small intestine and sigmoid colon lying in the rectovesical pouch, while the lower one-third is related to the base of the urinary bladder, seminal vesicle, vas deferens, and prostate.

2. In females, the upper two-thirds are related anteriorly to coils of small intestine and sigmoid colon lying in the rectouterine pouch, while the lower one-third is related to the lower part of the vagina.

3. Posteriorly, both in males and females, it is related to lower three pieces of sacrum, coccyx, and anococcygeal raphe. It is also related to:

   a. Median sacral, superior rectal, and lower lateral sacral arteries.

   b. Sympathetic chain with ganglion impar.

   c. Anterior primary rami of S3, S4, S5, and Col and pelvic splanchnic nerves.

Vessels and Nerves

The rectum is supplied by superior, middle, and median sacral arteries. Internal rectal venous plexus forms in the submucosa, whereas external rectal venous plexus forms outside the muscle coat of rectal wall. The two plexus are in communication with each other.
The rectal venous plexus drainage takes place as under:

1. From upper part via superior rectal vein into portal system.

2. From middle part via middle rectal vein into internal iliac vein.

3. From lower part via inferior rectal vein into internal pudendal vein.

The nerve supply is provided by sympathetic (L1, L2) and parasympathetic (S2, S3, S4) nerves through superior rectal and inferior hypogastric plexus.

Anal Canal

The anal canal extends from anorectal junction to the anus. It is directed downward and backward (i.e., angled posteroinferiorly). The anorectal junction is slung by the puborectalis component of the levator ani which pulls it forward. The anus opens onto the surface of perineum about 4 cm below and in front of the coccyx (**Fig. 22.4**).

Interior of anal canal: Developmentally, the midpoint of the anal canal is represented by the dentate/ pectinate line. This is the site at which the ectodermal proctodeum meets endodermal anorectal

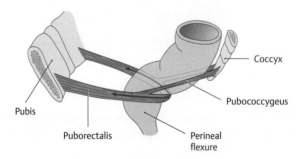

Fig. 22.4 Muscular sling of puborectalis. (From Schuenke M, Schulte E, Schumacher U. THIEME Atlas of Anatomy. Internal Organs. Illustrations by Voll M and Wesker K. © Thieme 2020)

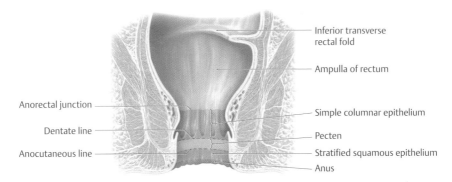

Inferior transverse rectal fold

Ampulla of rectum

Anorectal junction

Simple columnar epithelium

Dentate line

Pecten

Anocutaneous line

Stratified squamous epithelium

Anus

Fig. 22.5 Interior of anal canal. (From Schuenke M, Schulte E, Schumacher U. THIEME Atlas of Anatomy. Internal Organs. Illustrations by Voll M and Wesker K. © Thieme 2020)

canal. This developmental implication is reflected by the following characteristics seen in the interior of the anal canal (**Fig. 22.5**; **Video 22.2**):

1. The epithelium of the upper half of the anal canal is simple columnar. In contrast, the epithelium of the lower half of the anal canal is stratified squamous. The mucosa of the upper half canal is thrown into vertical columns (*columns of Morgagni*). At the bases of the columns are valve-like/crescenteric fold mucous membrane called *valves of ball.*

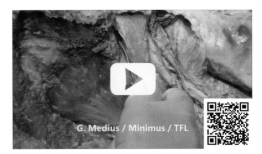

G. Medius / Minimus / TFL

Video 22.2 Ischioanal fossa, Alcock's canal, and sciatic foramen.

2. The blood supply to the upper half of anal canal is derived from the superior rectal artery, a continuation of inferior mesenteric artery, whereas the lower half of anal canal is supplied by the inferior rectal artery, a branch of the internal iliac artery. The upper half of anal canal is drained by superior rectal vein into the portal venous system, while venous blood from lower half is drained by inferior rectal veins into the portacaval system. The anal canal is an important site of portosystemic anastomosis.

3. The upper anal canal is insensitive to pain as it is supplied by autonomic nerves. The lower anal canal is sensitive to pain as it is supplied by somatic nerves (inferior rectal nerve).

4. The lymph from the upper anal canal drains upward along the superior rectal vessels to the internal iliac nodes, whereas lymph from the lower anal canal drains into the inguinal nodes.

5. The pectinate line acts as a watershed line of the anal canal.

Anal Sphincters

1. The internal anal sphincter is formed by the thickening of circular muscle coat. It is involuntary and surrounds the upper three-fourths of the anal canal.

2. The external anal sphincter is formed by striate muscle and surrounds the whole of the anal canal (**Fig. 22.3**).

From above downward, it is divided into deep, superficial, and subcutaneous parts. The latter lies below the level of internal sphincter. It is voluntary in control. It is considered to be a simple, functional, and anatomical entity.

▌Clinical Notes

1. *Rectal prolapse*: It can be incomplete if there is protrusion of rectal mucosa only through anus and complete (procidentia) if whole thickness of rectal wall protrudes through the anus. It occurs in debilitate diseases due to weakness of rectal support.

2. *Hemorrhoids (piles)*: The internal or true piles are the saccular dilatation of the internal rectal venous plexus and occur above the pectinate line. They are usually located at the 3, 7, and 11 o'clock positions of the anal canal and bleed profusely during strain or defecation. They are painless. The external piles occur below the pectinate line, due to dilatation of inferior rectal vein. They are painful and do not bleed on strain or defecation.

Uterus, Vagina, and Ovary

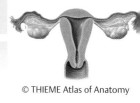

© THIEME Atlas of Anatomy

At the end of the dissection of uterus, vagina, and ovary, students should be able to identify the following:

- The peritoneal reflections in the female pelvis and see the location of rectouterine and uterovesical pouches.
- Ovarian fossa in the lateral pelvic walls and structures forming the boundaries of ovarian fossa.
- Size, location, ligaments, surfaces, relations, and blood vessels of ovaries.
- Parts of uterine tube and note their length.
- Round and broad ligaments of uterus. Parts of the broad ligament and structures present within it.
- Parts (fundus, body, isthmus, cervix) of uterus and note the flexures (anteversion and anteflexion), surfaces and relations, nerve supply, and lymphatic drainage of uterus.
- Supravaginal and vaginal parts of cervix, cervical canal, internal os, and external os.
- Relationship of the ureter with uterine artery and the cervix.
- Transverse cervical and uterosacral ligaments.
- Location of vagina in pelvis. Note length, fornices, walls, and their relations.
- Urethra in a sagittal section of female pelvis. Note its length and differences from male urethra.

Dissection and Identification

1. In sagittal section of the female pelvis, examine the pear-shaped, muscular uterus. Identify parts of the uterus. The part above the opening of the uterine tube is fundus and the main part below the fundus is body. The most inferior cylindrical-shaped part is cervix and in nulliparous the junction between the cervix and uterus is indicated by a shallow groove on the external surface known as isthmus of the uterus. Note that the inferior one-third of the cervix is surrounded by the fornices of vagina. Also, identify the external os at the lower end of the cervical canal and the internal os at its upper end.

2. Note that the uterus is normally bent forward at right angle to the vagina (anteverted position) and is also usually flexed forward at the junction of cervix and body (anteflexed position).

3. On the cut surface of the uterine wall, identify the three layers: (a) perimetrium, which represents the peritoneal covering of the uterus; (b) myometrium, which is the thick, muscular wall of the uterus; and (c) endometrium, which is the mucosal lining of the uterine cavity.

4. Identify the fold of the peritoneum on either side of the uterus, called the broad ligament extending from the lateral border of the uterus to the floor and lateral walls of the pelvis.

5. Note the superolateral termination of the broad ligament that attaches onto the lateral pelvic wall. The broad ligament is the suspensory ligament of the ovary, which runs from the ovary to the lateral pelvic wall. It conveys the ovarian artery, ovarian vein, lymphatic vessels, and nerve plexuses to oviduct and ovary.

6. Identify two more folds of the peritoneum: (a) the mesosalpinx, which lies between the oviduct and the ovary; and (b) the mesovarium, which lies posterior to the mesosalpinx and connects the posterior aspect of the broad ligament to the ovary.

7. Inferiorly to the mesosalpinx is the mesometrium that forms the largest part of the broad ligament and spans between the uterus and the lateral wall of the pelvis.

8. Identify the fallopian tube which is a narrow tube, 9 to 10 cm long, occupying the superior free border of the broad ligament. Note that it is divided into four parts: (a) infundibulum, the funnel-shaped distal end; (b) ampulla, the longest, most convoluted, and widest part of the tube; (c) isthmus, the narrowest, shortest part of the tube; and (d) intramural segment, which pierces the uterine wall and connects the lumen of the tube with the uterine cavity.

9. At the distal end of the infundibulum, identify the opening called the abdominal ostium of the oviduct, which is surrounded by the finger-like processes, fimbriae.

10. Identify the vagina, the elastic fibromuscular canal, about 7 to 9 cm long, extending from the cervix of the uterus to the vestibule of the vagina.

11. As seen earlier, the cervix projects into the lumen of the vagina. Surrounding the cervix are the fornices of the vagina. The posterior fornix of the vagina is located between the posterior wall of the vagina and the cervix. It is clinically important because it is closely associated with the rectouterine pouch (pouch of Douglas) which is the lowest point of the peritoneal cavity in females. The anterior fornix of the vagina is located between the anterior wall of the vagina and the cervix. It is not covered by the peritoneum.

12. Identify the ovaries that usually are present in shallow depressions, called ovarian fossae, on the posterolateral wall of the pelvis between the ureter posteromedially, the external iliac vein laterally, the obturator nerve posterolaterally, and uterine tube in the free margin of broad ligament anteriorly. Observe that the distal end of the uterine tube curves around the lateral end of the ovary and is attached to it by one or more of the fimbriae. Note again that the ovary is an oval organ attached to the broad ligament by the mesovarium. It is also attached via the suspensory ligament of the ovary to the lateral pelvic wall and by the ovarian ligament to the uterus.

Uterus (Video 23.1)

The uterus is a thick-walled muscular organ with a narrow lumen. It is piriform in shape and measures approximately 8 cm in length in an adult nulliparous female. It comprises a fundus (part lying above the entrance of fallopian tubes), body, and cervix. The cervix protrudes into the anterior wall of the vagina and is consequently divided into supravaginal part and vaginal parts. The cavity of the cervix communicates with the cavity of the body at the internal os and with that of the vagina at the external os.

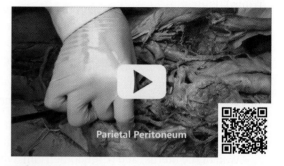

Video 23.1   Layers of uterine wall.

The fallopian tubes lie in the free upper edges of the broad ligaments and serve to transmit ova from the surface of the ovary to the uterus. Each tube comprises an infundibulum, ampulla, isthmus, and interstitial part. The uterus is made up

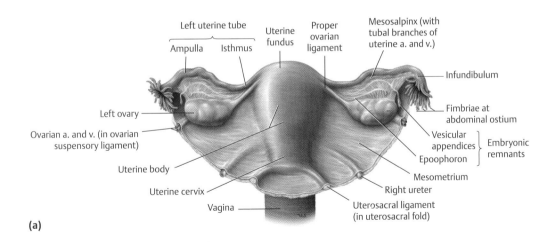

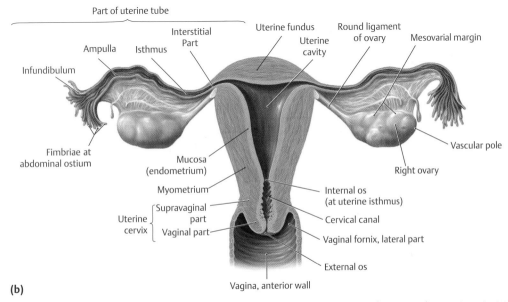

Fig. 23.1 Uterus and uterine tubes. **(a)** Posterosuperior view. **(b)** Coronal section (posterior view with uterus straightened). *Removed*: Mesometrium. (From Schuenke M, Schulte E, Schumacher U. THIEME Atlas of Anatomy. Internal Organs. Illustrations by Voll M and Wesker K. © Thieme 2020)

of a thick muscular layer (myometrium) and lined internally by a mucous membrane (endometrium). Endometrium undergoes massive cyclical changes during menstruation. Externally, it is covered by peritoneum (perimetrium) (**Fig. 23.1**).

Position and Axes of Uterus

In majority of cases, the uterus is anteverted, that is, the axis of cervix is bent forward on the axis of vagina at right angle (i.e., 90 degrees), and anteflexed, that is, the axis of the body of uterus is bent forward at isthmus, making an angle of 170 degrees between the long axis of the body and the cervix (**Fig. 23.2**). In some cases, uterus is retroverted. The isthmus is the zone of narrowing between the body of uterus and cervix.

Relations

Anteriorly, the body of uterus is related to rectovesical pouch and posteriorly to rectouterine pouch. Laterally, it is related to broad ligament. Supravaginal portion of cervix is related anteriorly to bladder, posteriorly to rectouterine pouch, and on each side to ureter and uterine artery.

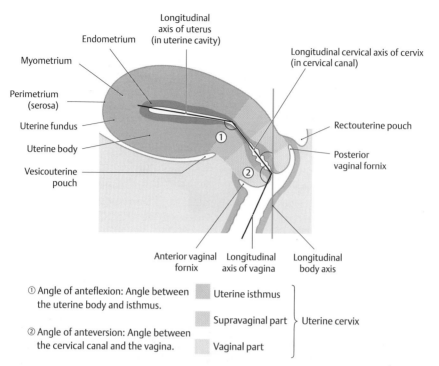

Fig. 23.2   Position and axes of uterus. (Modified from Schuenke M, Schulte E, Schumacher U. THIEME Atlas of Anatomy. Internal Organs. Illustrations by Voll M and Wesker K. © Thieme 2020)

Supports of Uterus

The supports of uterus are divided into primary and secondary. The main primary supports comprise pelvic diaphragm, perineal body, and transverse cervical ligaments (ligaments of Mackenrodt). The main secondary support is broad ligament.

Broad ligament is a fold of peritoneum extending from the side of uterus to the lateral wall of pelvis. It contains uterine tube, round ligament of uterus, ligament of ovary and ovarian arteries, and remnants of mesonephric duct (via epoophoron and paroophoron).

Vessels and Nerves

The arterial supply is predominantly from the uterine artery, a branch of the internal iliac artery. It runs in the broad ligament and the level of the internal os and crosses the ureter above at right angle to reach and supply the uterus before anastomosing with ovarian artery, a branch of the abdominal aorta. The venous drainage occurs through uterine (mainly) and ovarian veins (**Fig. 23.3**; **Videos 23.2 and 23.3**).

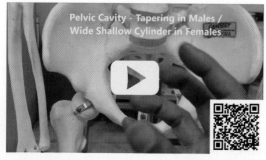

Video 23.2   Female pelvic organs with endopelvic fascia and pelvic vessels.

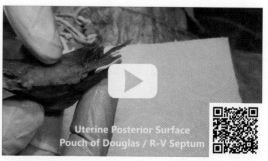

Video 23.3   Bony pelvis male vs. female: obstetric fractures.

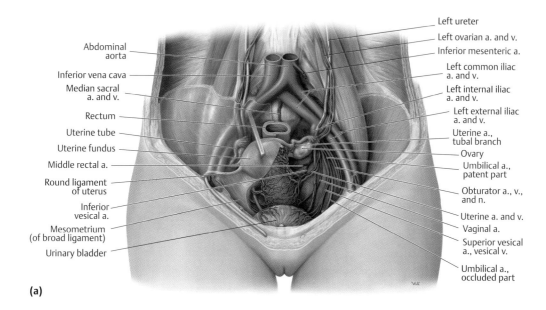

Left ureter
Left ovarian a. and v.
Inferior mesenteric a.
Left common iliac a. and v.
Left internal iliac a. and v.
Left external iliac a. and v.
Uterine a., tubal branch
Ovary
Umbilical a., patent part
Obturator a., v., and n.
Uterine a. and v.
Vaginal a.
Superior vesical a., vesical v.
Umbilical a., occluded part

Abdominal aorta
Inferior vena cava
Median sacral a. and v.
Rectum
Uterine tube
Uterine fundus
Middle rectal a.
Round ligament of uterus
Inferior vesical a.
Mesometrium (of broad ligament)
Urinary bladder

(a)

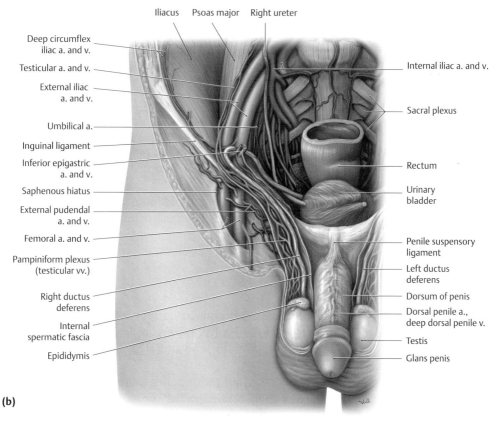

Iliacus   Psoas major   Right ureter

Deep circumflex iliac a. and v.
Testicular a. and v.
External iliac a. and v.
Umbilical a.
Inguinal ligament
Inferior epigastric a. and v.
Saphenous hiatus
External pudendal a. and v.
Femoral a. and v.
Pampiniform plexus (testicular vv.)
Right ductus deferens
Internal spermatic fascia
Epididymis

Internal iliac a. and v.
Sacral plexus
Rectum
Urinary bladder
Penile suspensory ligament
Left ductus deferens
Dorsum of penis
Dorsal penile a., deep dorsal penile v.
Testis
Glans penis

(b)

Fig. 23.3 Blood vessels and genital organs. **(a)** Female pelvis. *Removed:* Peritoneum (left side). *Displaced:* Uterus. **(b)** Male pelvis. Opened: Inguinal canal and coverings of the spermatic cord. (Modified from Schuenke M, Schulte E, Schumacher U. THIEME Atlas of Anatomy. Internal Organs. Illustrations by Voll M and Wesker K. © Thieme 2020)

The lymphatics from the fundus accompany the ovarian artery and drain into the para-aortic nodes. Lymphatics from the body and cervix drain to the internal and external iliac lymph nodes. Few lymph vessels from lateral angle (cornua) of uterus run along the round ligaments of uterus and drain into superficial inguinal lymph nodes (**Fig. 23.4**).

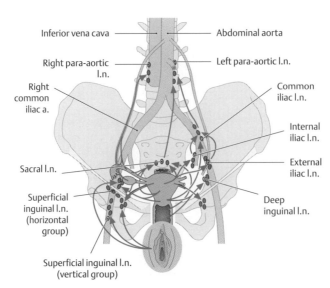

Fig. 23.4 Lymphatic drainage of the female genitalia. (From Schuenke M, Schulte E, Schumacher U. THIEME Atlas of Anatomy. Internal Organs. Illustrations by Voll M and Wesker K. © Thieme 2020)

The sympathetic (T12, L1) and parasympathetic (S2, S3, S4) innervations are derived through inferior hypogastric and ovarian plexuses.

Uterine Tubes

Each tube is about 10 cm and lies on the upper free margin of the broad ligament. Proximally, it opens into uterine cavity at its lateral angle (uterine ostium) and distally into peritoneal cavity (abdominal ostium) (**Fig. 23.1**).

From lateral to medial, it comprises infundibulum, ampulla, isthmus, and interstitial parts. The finger-like projections from the infundibulum around the abdominal ostium are called fimbriae. The fertilization most commonly occurs in the ampullary part.

Vagina

The vagina is an organ of copulation in females. It is a muscular tube which passes upward and backward from the vaginal orifice in the vestibule of vulva. The cervix projects into the upper part of its anterior wall of vagina, creating anterior, posterior, and lateral fornices, the posterior fornix being the deepest (**Fig. 23.5**).

Its anterior wall measures about 3 cm in length, while the posterior wall measures 10 cm in length. The diameter of the vagina gradually increases from below upward. The lumen is circular at the upper end like a transverse slit in the middle part and is H-shaped in the lower part.

In a virgin, the lower end of vagina is partially closed by a thin annular fold of mucous membrane (hymen). In nonvirgin women, the hymen is ruptured and is represented by rounded elevations around the vaginal orifice, the caruncula hymenalis.

Anterior wall is in contact with the base of the bladder and terminal parts of the ureters. Posterior wall in its upper part is covered by peritoneum which reflected on the anterior aspect of rectum to form rectouterine pouch (pouch of Douglas). The lower part of the posterior wall is separated from rectum only by loose areolar tissue. Laterally from above downward, the vagina is related to cardinal ligaments, ureter, pubococcygeus, and urogenital diaphragm.

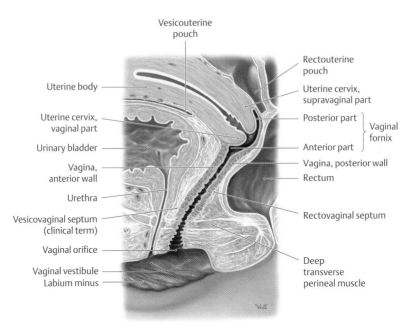

Fig. 23.5 Location of vagina (midsagittal section, left lateral view). (Modified from Schuenke M, Schulte E, Schumacher U. THIEME Atlas of Anatomy. Internal Organs. Illustrations by Voll M and Wesker K. © Thieme 2020)

Vessels of Vagina

The vagina is highly vascular. It is supplied on either side by vaginal artery (corresponding to inferior vesical artery in males), a branch of internal iliac artery, and supplemented by the branches of uterine, middle rectal, and arteries of the bulb of vestibule (**Fig. 23.3a**).

Lymph vessels from upper part drain into external iliac nodes, from middle part into internal iliac, and from lower part into superficial inguinal lymph nodes (**Fig. 23.4**).

Ovary

The ovaries (female gonads) are pinkish, white, ovoid structures measuring about 3 cm in length, 1.5 cm in width, and 1 cm in thickness (**Figs. 23.6** and **23.7**).

The ovary lies in the ovarian fossa on side wall of the pelvis. It is secured in this position by two structures: the broad ligament which attaches the ovary posteriorly by the mesovarium (**Fig. 23.6**) and the round ligament of ovary which secures the ovary to the cornu of the uterus.

The two ovaries between them produce one ovum per menstrual cycle. Each ovary contains a number of primordial follicles, which develop in early fetal life and await full development to release ova. In addition to the production of ova, the ovaries are also responsible for the production of sex hormones, namely, progesterone and estrogen.

Vessels

The ovary is supplied by ovarian artery (a branch of the abdominal aorta) (**Fig. 23.3a**). Venous drainage is into inferior vena cava on the right side and into the left renal vein on the left side.

Lymph vessels from the ovary drain into the para-aortic nodes.

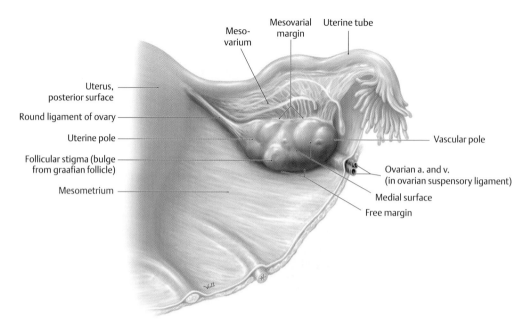

Fig. 23.6 Ovary (posterior view of right kidney). (Modified from Schuenke M, Schulte E, Schumacher U. THIEME Atlas of Anatomy. Internal Organs. Illustrations by Voll M and Wesker K. © Thieme 2020)

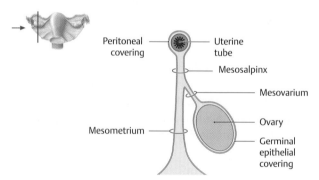

Fig. 23.7 Mesenteries of female genital organs. (Modified from Schuenke M, Schulte E, Schumacher U. THIEME Atlas of Anatomy. Internal Organs. Illustrations by Voll M and Wesker K. © Thieme 2020)

▌Clinical Notes

1. *Cervical carcinoma* is very common (11%) in females between 45 and 55 years of age. It is squamous cell carcinoma.

2. *Uterine prolapse* often occurs in multiparous elderly females due to weakness of pelvic diaphragm. It may occur in young females if there is a rupture of perineal body.

3. *Ovarian cyst*: The developmental arrest of ovarian follicles leads to formation of one or more ovarian cysts.

4. *Corpectomy* and *colporrhaphy* are done to drain fluid or pus from rectouterine pouch of Douglas.

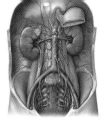

© THIEME Atlas of Anatomy

Introduction

The pelvic wall is made up of bones and ligaments. It is clothed by muscles which are covered by pelvic fascia and parietal peritoneum. The anterior pelvic wall is short and formed by bodies of pubic bones, pubic rami, and pubic symphysis. The posterior pelvic wall is formed by sacrum and coccyx. It is clothed by piriformis muscle.

The lateral pelvic wall is formed by the pelvic surface of hip bone surrounding obturator foramen and closed by obturator membrane. It is clothed by obturator internus muscle with it covering obturator fascia.

Dissection and Identification

1. Pull the pelvic viscera away from the pelvic walls and remove the peritoneum and underlying fat from the lateral pelvic wall to expose the pelvic vessels and nerves and pelvic part of the ureter (**Video 24.1**).

2. Follow the internal iliac vessels, and their branches and tributaries. To study the internal iliac artery and its branches, it is recommended that the internal iliac vein and its tributaries be identified and removed.

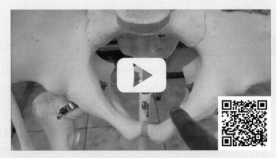

Video 24.1   Bony pelvis inlet–outlet and diameters.

3. Retract the internal iliac artery to identify its anterior and posterior divisions. Next, identify the branches of the posterior division of the internal iliac artery: iliolumbar artery which supplies the iliacus muscle, lateral sacral artery as it passes along the lateral border of the sacrum, and superior gluteal artery which passes through the greater sciatic foramen to enter the gluteal region.

4. Now, identify the branches of the anterior division of the internal iliac artery. Trace the obturator artery accompanied by the obturator nerve as they cross the lateral wall of pelvis and enter the obturator canal. Find the superior vesical arteries to the apex and superior wall of the bladder. Follow the uterine artery (in female cadaver) as it crosses in the parametrium, superior to the ureter. As the uterine artery reaches the isthmus of the uterus, it gives off the vaginal artery, which supplies the superior part of the vagina.

5. Trace the other branches of internal iliac artery, that is, inferior vesical artery which supplies the posterolateral wall of the bladder, middle rectal artery to rectum, and internal pudendal artery as it leaves pelvis through the greater sciatic foramen. Inferior gluteal artery also passes through the greater sciatic foramen into the gluteal region.

6. Identify pelvic part of the ureter and follow its course in the pelvis. Observe that it crosses the pelvic brim, passes inferior and posterior to the uterine artery, and continues anteriorly to the posterior wall of the urinary bladder.

7. Find sympathetic trunks as they enter the pelvis in front of the ala of sacrum and lumbosacral trunk from the lumbar plexus which descends into the pelvis medially to the psoas major muscle. Attempt to identify the pelvic splanchnic (parasympathetic) nerves that arise from the ventral primary rami of S2–S4 and that pass to the pelvic viscera. The sacral splanchnic (sympathetic) nerves arise from the sacral ganglia of the pelvic portion of sympathetic trunk.

8. Define the attachment of piriformis muscle to the sacrum and follow it to the greater sciatic foramen. On one side of the hemisected pelvis, remove the viscera to examine the muscles that form the pelvic diaphragm (levator ani and coccygeus), which separates the pelvis from the perineum.

9. Identify the ischial spines and locate the tendinous arch of the obturator internus fascia, which runs from the ischial spines to the lower border of the obturator canal. Trace the origin of levator ani from the back of the pubis to the ischial spine and between these two points from the tendinous arch of obturator fascia. Observe that the levator ani muscle is composed of three parts: puborectalis, which attaches to the pubic rami and encircles the rectum, pubococcygeus, which attaches to the pubic rami and the coccyx, and iliococcygeus muscle, which originates from the tendinous arch of the obturator internus fascia. These three muscles are

often difficult to separate from one another in the cadaver and are usually identified as the levator ani muscle.

10. The coccygeus muscle attaches to the anterior surface of the sacrospinous ligament and has a fibrous appearance.

Vertebropelvic Ligaments

They comprise iliolumbar, sacrotuberous, and sacrospinous ligaments.

1. The *iliolumbar ligament* is a strong triangular ligament which unites thick transverse process of L5 vertebra to the inner lip of iliac crest posteriorly; its lower fibers, which descend to the lateral part of the sacrum, form the lateral lumbosacral ligament (**Fig. 24.1**).

2. The *sacrotuberous ligament* is a strong broadband of the fibrous tissue with narrowing in the middle end. The wide upper end is attached from above downward to the posterior superior iliac spine, posterior inferior iliac spine, lower part of the posterior surface, and lateral border of the sacrum and adjoining upper part of the coccyx. Its relatively less broad lower end is attached to the medial margin of the ischial tuberosity. Some of the fibers from the lower end are continued on to the ramus of the ischium to form falciform process. The sacrotuberous ligament forms boundaries of both sciatic foramina (greater and lesser) and perineum.

3. The *sacrospinous ligament* is a triangular sheet of fibrous tissue. Its apex is attached laterally to the ischial spine and the base is attached medially to the lateral margin of the last piece of sacrum and coccyx.

The medial part of sacrospinous ligaments is covered by sacrotuberous ligament. The perineal branch of S4 spinal nerve and perforating cutaneous nerve intervene between them.

The sacrotuberous and sacrospinous ligaments help convert the greater and lesser sciatic notches of the hip bone into greater and lesser sciatic foramina (**Fig. 24.2**)–the two important exits from the pelvis.

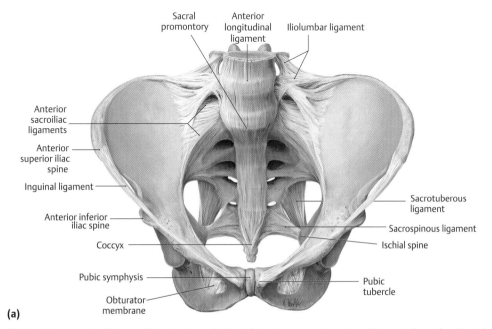

Fig. 24.1 Ligaments of the pelvis (male pelvis). **(a)** Anterosuperior view. (From Schuenke M, Schulte E, Schumacher U. THIEME Atlas of Anatomy. General Anatomy and Musculoskeletal System. Illustrations by Voll M and Wesker K. © Thieme 2020) *(Continued)*

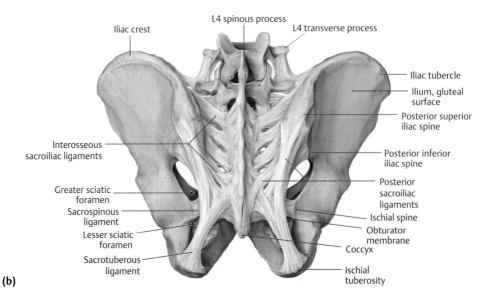

(b)

Fig. 24.1 *(Continued)* **(b)** Posterior view. (From Schuenke M, Schulte E, Schumacher U. THIEME Atlas of Anatomy. General Anatomy and Musculoskeletal System. Illustrations by Voll M and Wesker K. © Thieme 2020)

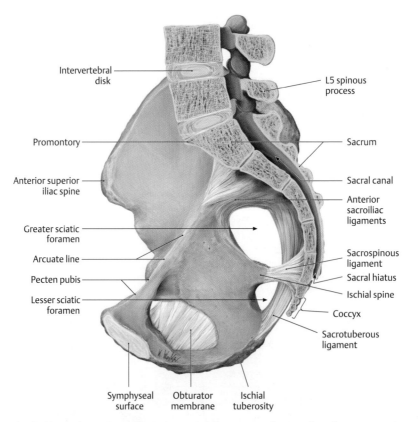

Fig. 24.2 Right half of the pelvis showing sacrotuberous and sacroiliac ligaments. (From Schuenke M, Schulte E, Schumacher U. THIEME Atlas of Anatomy. General Anatomy and Musculoskeletal System. Illustrations by Voll M and Wesker K. © Thieme 2020)

Obturator membrane: It is a sheet of fibrous tissue which covers the obturator foramen completely except for a small area anteriorly for the passage of obturator nerve and vessels from pelvis to the thigh.

Pelvic Fascia

The pelvic fascia is a thin fascia lining the pelvic muscles, viscera, and neurovascular structures. It is dense over nonexpansile structures, while it is loose over mobile structures. It does not extend over bare area of bones and fuses with peritoneum at the margins of muscles. The part lining the pelvic walls is called parietal pelvic fascia and that surrounding the pelvic viscera is called visceral pelvic fascia.

Parietal fascia of lateral pelvic wall comprises obturator fascia and fascia over piriformis.

Parietal fascia of pelvic floor comprises superior and inferior layers of pelvic diaphragm.

The pelvic fascia condenses to form ligaments of prostate, bladder, rectum, and uterus.

Pelvic Peritoneum

It passes over the superior surfaces of the pelvic viscera and dips between them to form pouches. The layout of peritoneum in pelvis is well appreciated by tracing it within the pelvis in sagittal section (**Figs. 24.1** and **24.2**).

Muscles of Pelvic Wall

The muscles of pelvic wall comprise obturator internus, piriformis, levator ani, and coccygeus. The piriformis is a triangular muscle lying one on either side on the front of the posterior pelvic wall. It passes through greater sciatic notch to reach gluteal region for insertion on the greater trochanter.

The obturator internus is a thick fan-shaped muscle which covers the lateral pelvic wall. Its tendon passes through lesser sciatic foramen for insertion on the greater trochanter.

Levator ani and coccygeus form the pelvic floor. The levator ani is divided into two parts: the anterior pubococcygeus and posterior iliococcygeus. The origin, insertion, nerve supply, and actions of these muscles are given in **Table 24.1** and are shown in **Fig. 24.3**.

Table 24.1   Origin, insertion, nerve supply, and actions of muscles of the pelvis

Muscle	Origin	Insertion	Nerve supply	Actions
Piriformis	By three digitation from the front of three pieces of sacrum	Tip of greater trochanter	Sacral plexus (S1, S2)	Lateral rotation of thigh
Obturator internus	1. Obturator membrane 2. Inner surface of hip bone below the pelvic brim	Medial surface of greater trochanter	Nerve to obturator internus (L5, S1, S2) from sacral plexus	Lateral rotation of thigh
Levator ani 1. Pubococcygeus (from levator prostate or sphincter vaginae) 2. Iliococcygeus	1. Body of pubis 2. Anterior part of the tendinous arch of pelvis fascia 3. Posterior part of the tendinous arch of pelvic fascia 4. Ischial spine	Perineal body walls of prostate or vagina, rectum, and anal canal 1. Anococcygeal raphe 2. Tip of coccyx	1. Nerve to levator ani (S4 nerve) 2. Inferior rectal nerve or peroneal branch of pudendal nerve (S2, S3)	1. Form large part of pelvic diaphragm 2. Supports pelvic viscera 3. Resists increase in intra-abdominal pressure
Coccygeus	Ischial spine	1. Side of coccyx 2. S4 vertebra	Branches of S4 and S3 nerves	1. Form small posterior part of pelvic diaphragm 2. Pulls coccyx forward

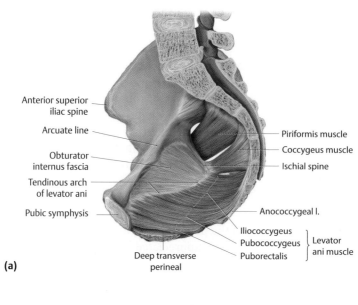

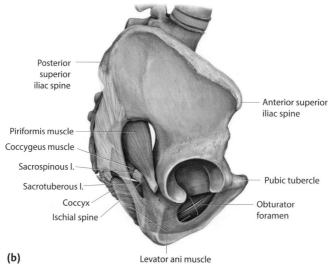

Fig. 24.3 Muscles of pelvic wall. **(a)** inner view. **(b)** outer view. (From Schuenke M, Schulte E, Schumacher U. THIEME Atlas of Anatomy. General Anatomy and Musculoskeletal System. Illustrations by Voll M and Wesker K. © Thieme 2020)

Nerves of Pelvis

The nerves of pelvis comprise lumbosacral trunk, sacral plexus, coccygeal plexus, and autonomic nerves of the pelvis (**Fig. 19.11**, **Figs. 24.4** and **24.5**).

Lumbosacral trunk: It is a thick cord formed by the entire ventral ramus of L5 and descending part of the ventral rami of L4. It descends obliquely over the lateral part of the sacrum to enter the pelvis posterior to pelvic fascia.

Sacral plexus: The sacral plexus is formed by the ventral rami of L4 and L5. It lies on the pelvic surface of piriformis deep to pelvic fascia (lumbosacral trunk) and S1–S3 nerves.

1. The superior gluteal vessels separate lumbosacral trunk from S1 ramus.

2. The inferior gluteal vessels separate S1 and S2 rami.

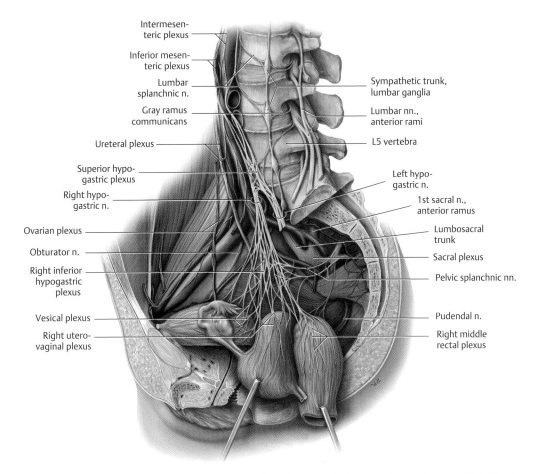

Fig. 24.4 Innervation of female pelvis. (From Schuenke M, Schulte E, Schumacher U. THIEME Atlas of Anatomy. Internal Organs. Illustrations by Voll M and Wesker K. © Thieme 2020)

Branches

From both dorsal and ventral divisions:

1. Sciatic nerve (L4, L5, and S1, S2, S3).
2. Posterior cutaneous nerve of thigh (S1, S2, S3).

From dorsal divisions:

1. Superior gluteal nerve (L4, L5, S1).
2. Inferior gluteal nerve (L5, S1, S2).
3. Nerve to piriformis (S1, S2).
4. Perforating cutaneous nerve (S2, S3).

Branches from ventral divisions:

1. Nerve to quadratus femoris (L4, L5, S1).
2. Nerve to obturator internus (L5, S1, S2).
3. Pudendal nerve (S2, S3, S4).
4. Muscular branches to levator ani, coccygeus, and sphincter ani externus.
5. Pelvic splanchnic nerves (S2, S3, S4).

The terminal branches of the plexus comprise sciatic and pudendal nerves.

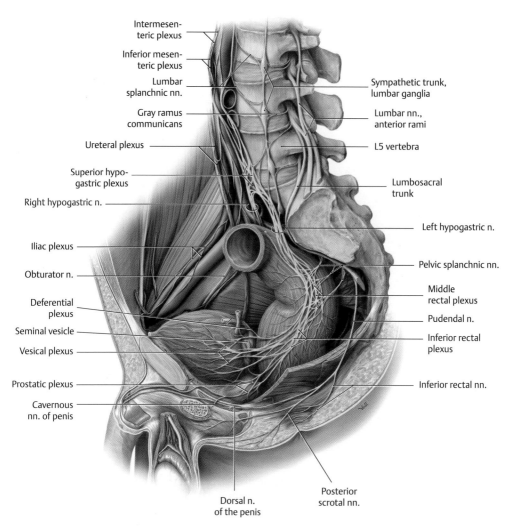

Fig. 24.5 Innervation of male pelvis. (From Schuenke M, Schulte E, Schumacher U. THIEME Atlas of Anatomy. Internal Organs. Illustrations by Voll M and Wesker K. © Thieme 2020)

Autonomic Nerves (Refer to Fig. 19.11)

Sympathetic trunks: The right and left trunks descend in the pelvis on either side between the bodies of the sacral vertebrae and the pelvic sacral foramina. The distal parts of the trunks converge and unite in the median to form *ganglion impar* on the coccyx. They lie posterior to the pelvic fascia (**Fig. 24.3**).

There are four sacral ganglia on each trunk and the common ganglion impar branches:

1. Gray rami communicantes to all the sacral and coccygeal ventral rami.

2. Small branches to the median sacral artery.

3. Sacral splanchnic nerves to the inferior hypogastric plexus from the upper ganglia and to the rectum from the lower ganglia.

4. Twigs to the coccygeal body from ganglion impar.

Inferior Hypogastric Plexus

They are located on either side of the rectum and made up of sympathetic and parasympathetic fibers. The superior hypogastric plexus (presacral nerve) descends into the pelvis and divides into right and left inferior hypogastric plexus. Each of these plexuses surrounds the corresponding internal iliac artery and receives small branches from the upper sacral ganglia of the sympathetic trunk. The plexus divides into subsidiary plexuses, namely, rectal, vesical, uterine, and vaginal plexuses to supply the pelvic organs. The small ganglia are present in these plexuses and their extensions.

Visceral Plexus

These are extensions of the inferior hypogastric plexuses on the walls of the pelvic viscera (vide supra).

1. Rectal plexus surrounds the middle rectal artery. It receives a contribution from the inferior mesenteric plexus. It supplies pelvic parts of sigmoid colon and rectum.

2. The vesical plexus is continuous on the vas deferens, seminal vesicle, and prostate which it supplies, respectively.

3. Prostatic plexus surround the prostate which it supplies and sends cavernous nerves to the penis.

4. Uterine and vaginal plexuses accompany the corresponding arteries, respectively. The vaginal plexus supplies the vagina and urethra, and sends cavernous nerves to the bulbs of the vestibule and to the clitoris.

Blood Vessels of the Pelvis (Fig. 24.6)

Arteries of the Pelvis

The arteries of pelvis comprise superior rectal artery, median sacral artery and internal iliac artery.

Superior Rectal Artery

It is the continuation of inferior mesenteric artery at the middle of left common iliac artery. It descends with medial limb of sigmoid colon and divides into two branches on the third piece of sacrum. It supplies rectum and upper half of the anal canal (**Fig. 24.6**).

Median Sacral Artery

This small artery arises from back of the caudal part of the aorta. Just above the bifurcation, it descends in the median plane sequentially on to vertebral column, sacrum, and end in the coccygeal body on the front of coccyx. It gives off the fifth lumbar artery and supplies a little bit to the rectum.

Internal Iliac Artery

It is the smallest terminal branch of common iliac artery. It courses from its origin in front of sacroiliac joint to the upper margin of greater sciatic notch; here, it divides into anterior and posterior trunks.

Branches from anterior division:

1. *Umbilical artery*: It passes anteroinferiorly between the bladder and lateral pelvic wall. Its proximal part remains patent and gives rise to the superior vesical artery which supplies bladder, ureter, and ductus deferens. Its distal part gets obliterated and runs up to umbilicus to form medial umbilical ligament.

2. *Obturator artery*: It runs with the obturator nerve on the pelvic wall and then passes through the obturator canal to enter the thigh.

3. *Inferior vesical artery*: It passes forward and supplies the bladder; it also gives off a branch to the vas deferens called artery of vas deferens (in males).

4. *Middle rectal artery*: It passes medially to rectum where it anastomoses with the superior and inferior rectal arteries to supply the rectum.

5. *Internal pudendal artery*: It predominantly supplies the peritoneum. It exits the pelvis briefly through the greater sciatic foramen, but then re-enters below piriformis through the lesser sciatic foramen into the pudendal canal together with the pudendal nerve.

6. *Uterine artery*: It passes medially on the pelvic floor in the root of the broad ligament and then passes over the ureter into lateral fornix of the vagina to ascend in the lateral aspect of the uterus between the layers of the broad ligament.

7. *Inferior gluteal artery*: It passes out of the pelvis through the greater sciatic foramen to the gluteal region which it supplies.

8. *Vaginal artery*: It replaces the inferior vesical artery in females and supplies vagina, bladder, and pelvic parts of urethra.

All the branches of anterior division are visceral branches except inferior gluteal and obturator arteries, which are parietal branches.

Branches of posterior division:

1. *Superior gluteal artery*: It passes backward between lumbosacral trunk and the ventral ramus of S1. Above piriformis, it leaves the pelvis through the greater sciatic foramen to enter gluteal region.

2. *Iliolumbar artery*: It ascends upward across the ala of sacrum deep to psoas major and divides into iliac and lumbar arteries.

3. *Lateral sacral arteries*: They are usually two on each side and descend in front of pelvic foramina.

Veins of Pelvis (Fig. 24.6)

The veins of pelvis comprise internal iliac, superior rectal, median sacral, and ovarian veins:

1. The internal iliac vein lies posterosuperior to the corresponding artery and its tributaries correspond to the branches of internal iliac artery except umbilical and iliolumbar veins, which drain into liver and common iliac vein, respectively.

2. The median sacral vein runs along the median sacral artery to open into left common iliac vein.

3. The superior rectal vein runs upward along the superior rectal artery to continue as inferior mesenteric vein at common iliac artery.

4. The ovarian vein is formed by the condensation of pampiniform plexus of veins around ovary and passes through inguinal canal to drain into inferior vena cava on the right side and left renal vein on the left side.

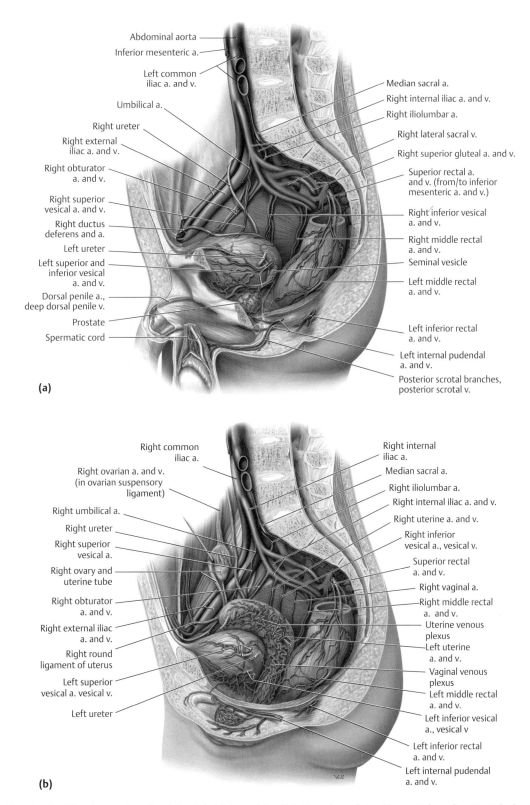

Fig. 24.6 Blood vessels of pelvis. **(a)** Male pelvis. **(b)** Female pelvis. (From Schuenke M, Schulte E, Schumacher U. THIEME Atlas of Anatomy. Internal Organs. Illustrations by Voll M and Wesker K. © Thieme 2020)

Lymph Nodes and Lymph Vessels of Pelvis

They are described with individual organs and shown in **Figs. 24.7–24.10**.

- *Lymphatic drainage of Rectum:* From upper part into inferior mesenteric lymph nodes and from inferior half into internal iliac lymph nodes (**Fig. 24.7**).
- *Lymphatic drainage of bladder and urethra:* It occurs into common iliac, external iliac, internal iliac, and inguinal lymph nodes (**Fig. 24.8**).
- *Lymphatic drainage of male genitalia:* It occurs into paraaortic, external iliac, and sacral lymph nodes (**Fig. 24.9**).
- *Lymphatic drainage of female genitalia:* It occurs into paraaortic, common iliac, external iliac, internal iliac and inguinal lymph nodes (**Fig. 24.10**).

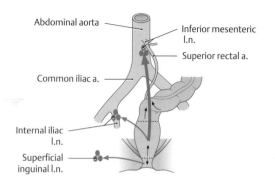

Fig. 24.7 Lymphatic drainage of rectum. (From Schuenke M, Schulte E, Schumacher U. THIEME Atlas of Anatomy. Internal Organs. Illustrations by Voll M and Wesker K. © Thieme 2020)

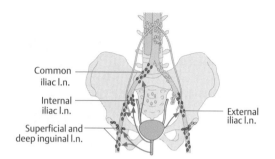

Fig. 24.8 Lymphatic drainage of bladder and urethra. (From Schuenke M, Schulte E, Schumacher U. THIEME Atlas of Anatomy. Internal Organs. Illustrations by Voll M and Wesker K. © Thieme 2020)

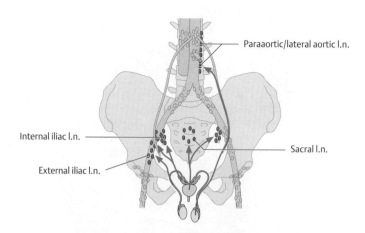

Fig. 24.9 Lymphatic drainage of male genitalia. (From Schuenke M, Schulte E, Schumacher U. THIEME Atlas of Anatomy. Internal Organs. Illustrations by Voll M and Wesker K. © Thieme 2020)

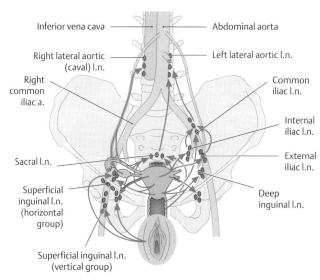

Fig. 24.10 Lymphatic drainage of female genitalia. (From Schuenke M, Schulte E, Schumacher U. THIEME Atlas of Anatomy. Internal Organs. Illustrations by Voll M and Wesker K. © Thieme 2020)

▌ Clinical Note

Osteomalacia of bony pelvis: The Osteomalacia is insufficient mineralization of bone due to vitamin D deficiency or defect in phosphate metabolism (**Fig. 24.11**). This leads to softening of pelvic bones. Its lateral walls are pushed inwards and anterior wall is pushed wall forwards, giving a '*trifoliate*' shape to pelvis. This leads to difficult childbirth.

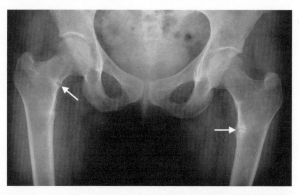

Fig. 24.11   X-ray pelvis AP view: Osteomalacia. Note the typical looser transformation zones ("bone softening') along the medial femoral neck on both sides (*arrows*).

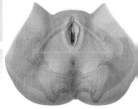

Learning Objectives

At the end of the dissection of the perineum, students should be able to identify the following:

- Boundaries of perineum, anal, and urogenital triangles.
- Pubic symphysis, ischiopubic rami, ischial tuberosities, and coccyx by palpitation.
- Boundaries, contents, and recesses of the ischiorectal/ischioanal fossa.
- Pudendal nerve and internal pudendal vessels in the pudendal canal.
- Membranous layer of superficial fascia and its attachment sites.
- Boundaries and contents of superficial perineal pouch.
- Attachments of perineal membrane and structures piercing the perineal membrane in males and females.
- Transverse perineal and arcuate pubic ligaments. Trace the dorsal nerves and deep dorsal vein of penis.
- Boundaries of the deep perineal pouch. Urethra/vagina sphincter urethrae and bulbourethral glands and other contents of this pouch.
- Location of perineal body and muscles attached to it.
- Course of branches of the pudendal nerve and internal pudendal artery from the pudendal canal to the perineum.

Introduction

The perineum lies below the pelvic diaphragm. It consists of all the structures that fill the inferior aperture of the pelvis. In the lithotomy position, the perineum is diamond-shaped. It is bounded anteriorly by scrotum (in males)/mons pubis (in females), posteriorly by buttocks, and on either side by upper medial aspect of the thigh. Note that the perineum is almost completely hidden by above structures in the erect position (**Fig. 25.1**).

1. Perineum extends anteroposteriorly from inferior margin of pubic symphysis to the tip of coccyx. Its lateral boundary on each side from before backward is formed by ischiopubic ramus, ischial tuberosity, and sacrotuberous ligament.

2. Perineum is divided into anterior and posterior triangular areas by an imaginary transverse line passing through ischial tuberosities immediately in front of anus. The anterior area is called the urogenital region and the posterior area is called the anal region.

3. The urogenital region contains urethra enclosed in the root of penis and scrotum in males, while in females it contains urethral and vaginal orifices, clitoris, labia minora, and labia majora.

4. The anal region transmits anal canal.

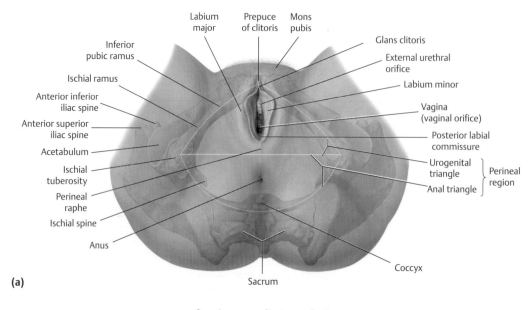

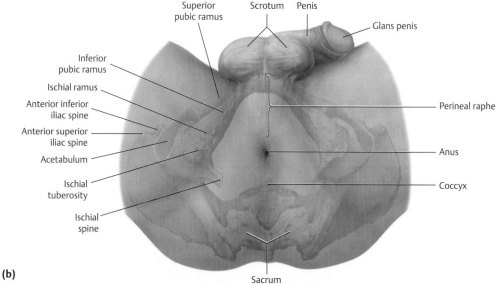

Fig. 25.1   Perineal region. **(a)** Female. **(b)** Male. (From Schuenke M, Schulte E, Schumacher U. THIEME Atlas of Anatomy. General Anatomy and Musculoskeletal System. Illustrations by Voll M and Wesker K. © Thieme 2020)

Urogenital Region

Superficial structures: The superficial structures in the urogenital region comprise external genital organs of males and females. The external genital organs of males are already studied in Chapter 11. The following account deals with female external genital organs. In the deeper plane, urogenital region contains superficial and deep perineal spaces/pouches.

Female External Genital Organs

The female external genital organs together are referred to as vulva or pudendum femininum. The female external genitalia comprise mons pubis, labia majora, labia minora, clitoris, vestibule of vagina, and urethral orifices (**Fig. 25.2**).

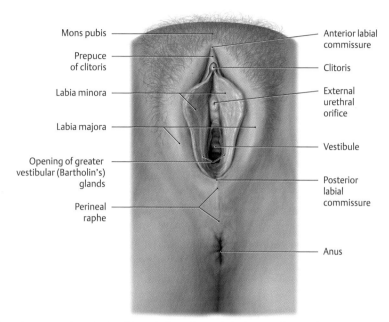

Mons pubis

Prepuce
of clitoris

Labia minora

Labia majora

Opening of greater
vestibular (Bartholin's)
glands

Perineal
raphe

Anterior labial
commissure

Clitoris

External
urethral
orifice

Vestibule

Posterior
labial
commissure

Anus

Fig. 25.2   Female external genitalia. (From Schuenke M, Schulte E, Schumacher U. THIEME Atlas of Anatomy. General Anatomy and Musculoskeletal System. Illustrations by Voll M and Wesker K. © Thieme 2020)

1. The mons pubis is the fatty protuberance over the pubic symphysis and pubic bones. The overlying skin is hairy. The hairs are turned outward and cease abruptly at a horizontal line where mons pubis meets the anterior abdominal wall. The mons acts as a cushion during coitus.

2. The labia minora are smooth, pink lip-like folds that extend posteriorly from mons and lie internal to the labia majora. Anteriorly, the labia minora split to enclose the clitoris.

3. The clitoris corresponds to the penis in male but is not traversed by urethra. It has similar structure, in that it is made up of three masses of erectile tissue: the bulb (corresponding to the penile bulb) and right and left crura covered by similar but smaller muscles than those in the male.

4. The vestibule of vagina is the area enclosed by the labia minora; it contains orifices of urethra, vagina, and ducts of greater vestibular glands.

5. The vaginal orifice is located in the posterior part of the vestibule of the vagina. It is partly closed by a membrane called hymen in virgin. In sexually active women, hymen gets ruptured and is seen as rounded tags on the margin of vaginal orifice called carunculae hymenales.

6. The urethral orifice lies just anterior to vaginal orifice. Its margins are raised and palpable.

Dissection and Identification

1. In a male cadaver, pass a lubricated metal bougie gently through the spongy part of the urethra in a plane parallel to the perineum. Keep the tip of bougie along the floor of urethra to avoid rupture of navicular fossa in the roof of the urethra. Keep palpating the tip as it advances through corpus spongiosum, until it gets arrested in the intrabulbar fossa midway between the scrotum and anus. Now withdraw the bougie a little and carry the handle in midline toward the thighs while applying slight pressure on the tip with a finger on the perineum. The tip now enters into the membranous part of the urethra and then enters into urinary bladder. Note that the bougie can be readily palpated in the spongy urethra and membranous parts by a finger in the rectum, but not in the prostatic part.

2. In a female cadaver, first identify the urethral orifice and then pass a bougie through it into urethra and the urinary bladder. Note that the bougie is easily palpable through the anterior vaginal wall. Introduce a speculum in the vagina to expose the cervix and a sulcus separating it from the vaginal wall called vaginal fornices.

3. Give a transverse incision in the skin between the ischial tuberosities, just anterior to the anus. In a male cadaver, cut the skin between the scrotum and coccyx, encircling the anus. In a female cadaver, make a similar cut encircling the pudendal cleft. Elevate skin flaps and identify the radiating strands of involuntary muscle fibers (corrugator cutis ani) passing outward from the anus (**Fig. 25.3**).

4. Now define superficial perineal space by inserting a finger downward and backward deep to the membranous layer of the superficial fascia (Scarpa fascia) of the anterior abdominal wall. In a female, remove fat from labium majus and expose the membranous layer. Cut this membrane to explore the posterior part of this space. Note its posterior limit where the membranous layer passes superiorly to fuse with the perineal membrane. In a male, expose the

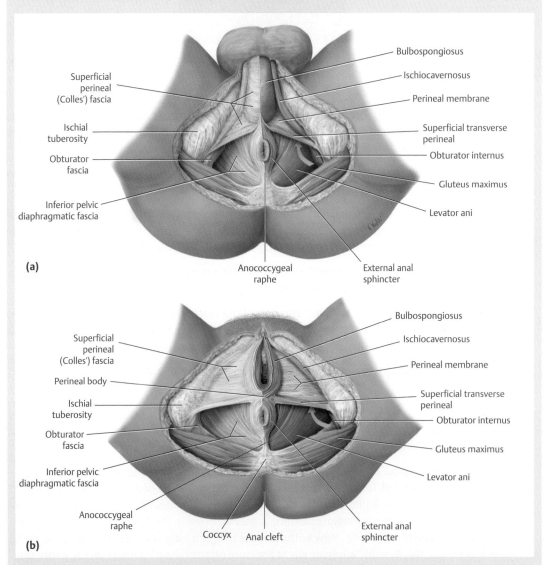

Fig. 25.3 Muscles of pelvic floor. **(a)** Male. **(b)** Female. (From Schuenke M, Schulte E, Schumacher U. THIEME Atlas of Anatomy. General Anatomy and Musculoskeletal System. Illustrations by Voll M and Wesker K. © Thieme 2020)

membranous layer in the perineum. Make an incision in it and explore one side of the superficial perineal space by pushing a finger into it through an incision.

5. Now divide the membranous layer in the median plane behind the scrotum in a male (or the frenulum of the labia in a female). Extend the incision posterolaterally to each ischial tuberosity from the perineal body. Reflect the fascia carefully without damaging the scrotal (labial) nerves and vessels which lie just deep to it. Note the sites of attachments of the fascia.

6. Remove the fascia from external anal sphincter, anococcygeal body, anal margins, and perineal body. Identify inferior rectal vessels and nerve in the ischiorectal fossa. Find the perineal branch of the fourth sacral nerve on the surface of levator ani, coming from the side of the coccyx.

7. If the gluteal region is not dissected, expose the lower border of gluteus maximus by incising superficial fascia from a point 2 cm superior to the tip of coccyx to the lateral side of ischial tuberosity. Note the small gluteal branches of posterior cutaneous nerve of thigh curving around the lower border of the muscle lateral to the ischial tuberosity (**Fig. 25.4**; **Video 25.1**).

8. Identify sacrotuberous ligament deep to the lower border of gluteus maximus. Expose the posterior scrotal (labial) nerves and vessels near the lateral part of the posterior margin of the perineal membrane and trace them into the superficial perineal space.

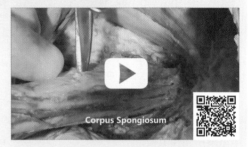

Video 25.1 Neurovascular structures of male perineum.

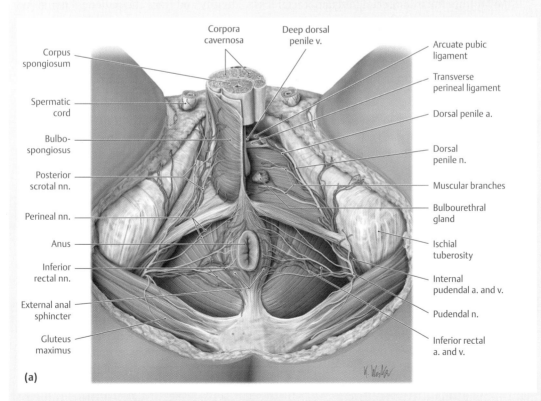

(a)

Fig. 25.4 Neurovasculature of perineum. **(a)** Male perineum. (From Schuenke M, Schulte E, Schumacher U. THIEME Atlas of Anatomy. General Anatomy and Musculoskeletal System. Illustrations by Voll M and Wesker K. © Thieme 2020) *(Continued)*

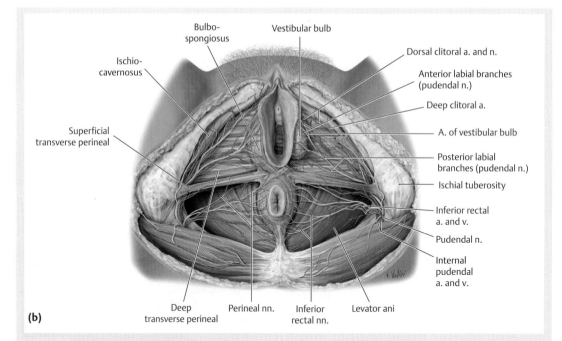

(b)

Fig. 25.4 Neurovasculature of perineum *Continued.* **(b)** Female perineum. (From Schuenke M, Schulte E, Schumacher U. THIEME Atlas of Anatomy. General Anatomy and Musculoskeletal System. Illustrations by Voll M and Wesker K. © Thieme 2020)

9. Trace the inferior rectal nerve and vessels to the lateral wall of the ischiorectal fossa. Remove the fat from the ischiorectal fossa/anorectal fossa. Identify and trace the pudendal nerve and vessels in the pudendal canal on the lateral wall.

10. Trace the posterior scrotal (labial) nerves and vessels from superficial perineal space to the scrotum (labia majora). Find perineal branch of posterior branch of posterior cutaneous nerve of the thigh 2 to 3 cm in front of ischial tuberosity. Trace its branches to the scrotum (labium majus).

11. Expose the structures in the superficial perineal pouch. Find ischiocavernosus muscle covering lower surface of each crus of penis/clitoris along the margin of pubic arch. Note that bulbospongiosus muscles in the male passes anterosuperiorly around either side of the bulb of penis from a median, ventral raphe which begins posteriorly at the perineal body. Note that in a female these muscles are small and course from perineal body, around the sides of the vestibule, to the crura of clitoris. Identify superficial transverse perineal muscles between the posterior ends of the two muscles described earlier.

12. Pass an index finger in the ischiorectal fossa and push it gently forward. Note it passes above the urogenital diaphragm, lateral to the levator ani. Palpate the urogenital diaphragm between the thumb and index finger.

13. Cut posterior scrotal (labial) nerves and vessels and turn them aside. Separate superficial perineal muscles to expose the part of perineal membrane between them. Cut transverse perineal muscles from the central perineal body and reflect them laterally. Expose deep branches of perineal nerve deep to them. In a male, separate two bulbospongiosus muscles along the raphe. Turn them away from the corpus spongiosum and trace the course of their fibers. In a female, elevate bulbospongiosus muscles from underlying erectile tissue on either side of the vaginal orifice. Detach the ischiocavernosus muscles from the crura of penis/clitoris and see their attachments (**Fig. 25.5**).

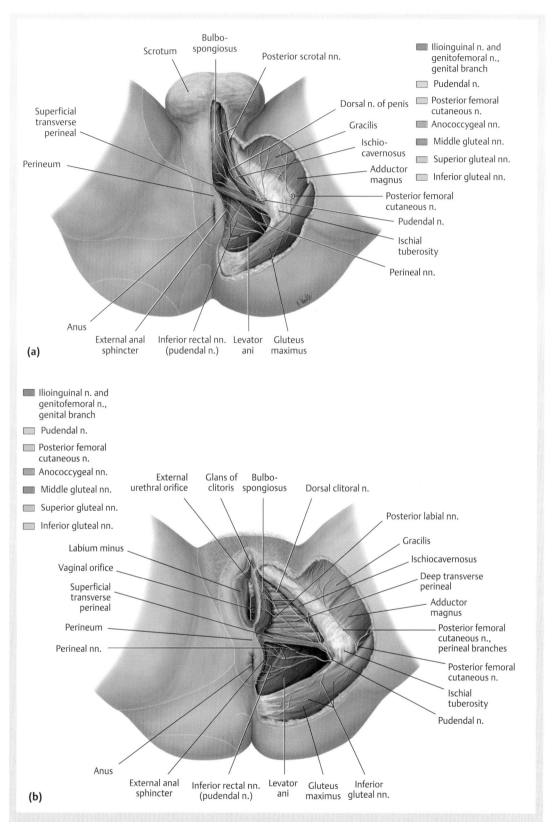

Fig. 25.5 Deep dissection of perineum. **(a)** Male perineum and genitalia. **(b)** Female perineum and genitalia. (From Schuenke M, Schulte E, Schumacher U. THIEME Atlas of Anatomy. General Anatomy and Musculoskeletal System. Illustrations by Voll M and Wesker K. © Thieme 2020)

14. Remove the superficial perineal muscles and detach one crura of penis/clitoris from the ischiopubic ramus. Turn it forward to the deep artery and vein on its upper surface. Trace the dorsal nerve and artery of clitoris. They lie close to the deep artery, passing lateral to the deep dorsal vein. Trace this vein proximally to where it passes into the pelvis between the pubic symphysis and anterior margin of perineal membrane/arcuate ligament.

15. In a male, detach the bulb of penis from central perineal body and turn it forward; you will see urethra and artery of bulb piercing the perineal membrane to enter the bulb. In a female, elevate the posterior end of bulb of vestibular glands lying at the side of urethra. Trace it forward to its duct. Identify the artery to the bulb. Cut the artery and turn the bulb forward, to expose the perineal membrane as much as possible.

16. Detach the perineal membrane from the pubic arch on the side. Turn the membrane medially to expose a thin sheet of muscle, sphincter urethrae anteriorly and deep transverse perineal muscles posteriorly. Individual differentiation of muscles is difficult.

17. Trace internal pudendal artery along the dorsal nerve of penis/clitoris forward into the deep perineal pouch and through the perineal membrane to its branches, deep and dorsal arteries of penis or clitoris. Identify and trace the artery of the bulb.

18. Look for the bulbourethral gland posterolateral to the urethra on the superior surface of the deep transverse perineal muscle in a male.

19. Remove the muscles exposed in the deep perineal space and superficial fascia of the urogenital diaphragm. Clear the fat and fascia to expose the perineal surface of levator ani. Note the free medial border of the anterior part of this muscle, which is separated from the muscle of the opposite side by a gap in front of the attachment of its most medial fibers to the central perineal body. Note the urethra passing through this gap in a male, and the urethra and vagina in a female. Identify the fibers which turn around the posterior vaginal wall and form a sphincter. In a male, the prostate is sandwiched between the medial margins of the levator ani and form levator prostate.

20. Trace the posterior fibers of levator ani to the sides of anal canal, passing deep to the external sphincter. Identify the attachment of levator ani to the fascia covering the obturator muscle.

21. Pass a finger between the bladder and pubis until it is held by the pubovesical or puboprostatic ligaments. Note the presence of loose areolar connective tissue around the side of the bladder.

22. Put one finger in the ischiorectal fossa and another in the pelvic cavity. Note that these two fingers are separated from each other by levator ani muscle and its fascia.

23. As far as possible, explore the relationship of pelvic cavity with ischiorectal fossa.

Fasciae and Perineal Pouches/Spaces in the Urogenital Region

The urogenital region contains two spaces: one above the perineal membrane called deep perineal pouch and one below this membrane called superficial perineal pouch (**Fig. 25.6**).

Perineal Membrane

It is a triangular fascial sheet which stretches between the two ischiopubic rami. Its narrow anterior margin thickens to form transverse perineal ligament and is continuous with the fascia forming the superior boundary of the deep perineal space. Its wide posterior margin splits into two

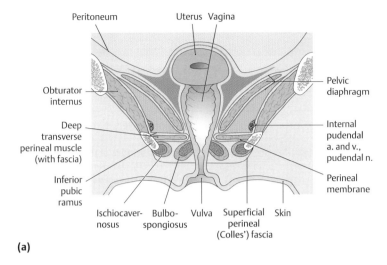

(a)

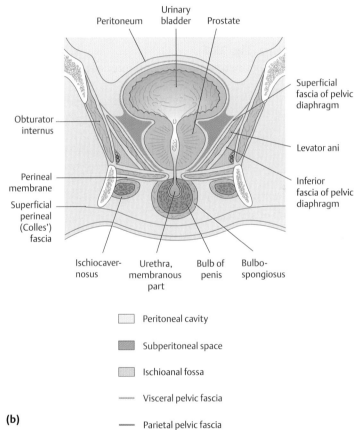

Peritoneal cavity

Subperitoneal space

Ischioanal fossa

Visceral pelvic fascia

Parietal pelvic fascia

(b)

Fig. 25.6 Coronal section of pelvis and urogenital triangle. **(a)** Female. **(b)** Male. (From Schuenke M, Schulte E, Schumacher U. THIEME Atlas of Anatomy. General Anatomy and Musculoskeletal System. Illustrations by Voll M and Wesker K. © Thieme 2020)

layers. The upper layer is continuous with the fascia forming the superior boundary of deep perineal space and inferior layer is continuous with the Colles fascia forming the inferior boundary of the superficial perineal space. In the midline, posterior margin is fixed to the perineal body.

The perineal membrane is pierced by urethra in males and urethra and vagina in females. In addition, it is also pierced by a number of nerves and vessels supplying structures in the urogenital region. The details are given in **Table 25.1**.

Table 25.1   Structures piercing the perineal membrane

In males	In females
Urethra and ducts of the bulbourethral glands	Urethra and vagina
Artery to the bulb of penis	Artery to the bulb of vestibule
Dorsal artery of the penis	Dorsal artery of the clitoris
Deep arteries of the penis	Deep arteries of the clitoris
Posterior scrotal nerves and vessels	Posterior labial nerves and vessels
Muscular branches of the perineal nerve	Muscular branches of the perineal nerve

Perineal Body (Central Tendon of Perineum)

The perineal body (also called "central tendon of perineum") is a wedge-shaped mass/node of fibromuscular tissue situated in median plane about 1.25 cm (1/2 inch) in front of anus and close to bulb of penis/vestibule of vagina (**Fig. 25.3**).

The following 10 muscles of the perineum converge and interlace in the perineal body:

1. Two superficial transverse perinei.

2. Two deep transverse perinei.

3. Two bulbospongiosus.

4. Two levator ani.

5. One sphincter ani externus.

6. One longitudinal muscle coat of anal canal.

Superficial Perineal Space/Pouch

It is located below the perineal membrane in urogenital region (**Fig. 25.6**).

Boundaries.

Superficial: Colles fascia.

Deep: Perineal membrane.

Lateral (on each side): Ischiopubic rami.

Posterior: Closed by fusion of perineal membrane with Colles fascia.

Anterior: Continuous with spaces of scrotum, penis, and anterior abdominal wall in males and spaces of labia majora and clitoris and anterior abdominal wall in females.

Contents of superficial perineal pouch are given in **Table 25.2**.

Table 25.2   Contents of superficial perineal pouch

In males	In females
Root of penis (two crura and one bulb) 1. Bulb of penis covered by the bulbospongiosus muscles 2. Crura of penis covered by the ischiocavernosus muscle	Root of clitoris (two crura and two bulbs of vestibules) 1. Bulbs of vestibule covered by the bulbospongiosus muscles 2. Crura of clitoris covered by the ischiocavernosus muscles
Superficial transverse perinei	Superficial transverse perinei
Ducts of bulbourethral glands	Greater vestibular glands (Bartholin glands) and their ducts
Urethra (within the bulb of penis)	Urethra
Branches of the internal pudendal artery 1. Perineal artery 2. Dorsal artery of penis 3. Deep artery of penis	Branches of the internal pudendal artery 1. Perineal artery 2. Dorsal artery of clitoris 3. Deep artery of clitoris
Branches of the perineal nerve 1. Posterior scrotal nerve 2. Nerve to bulb 3. Perineal branch of posterior cutaneous nerve of the thigh	Branches of the perineal nerve 1. Posterior labial nerve 2. Nerve to vestibule 3. Perineal branch of posterior cutaneous nerve of the thigh

Deep Perineal Space/Pouch

It is located above the perineal membrane in the urogenital region. It is tightly filled with musculature to make it a rigid structure called urogenital diaphragm. This diaphragm closes the urogenital region of the inferior aperture of pelvis below the pelvic diaphragm.

Boundaries.

Superficial: Perineal membrane.

Deep: Superior fascia of urogenital diaphragm.

Lateral (on each side): Ischiopubic rami.

Anterior: Closed by the fusion of perineal membrane with superior fascia of urogenital diaphragm.

Contents of deep perineal space are given in **Table 25.3**.

Table 25.3   Contents of deep perineal pouch

In males	In females
1. Urethra 2. Muscles 3. Sphincter urethra 4. Deep transverse perineal	1. Urethra 2. Vagina muscles 3. Sphincter urethra 4. Deep transverse perineal
Nerves 1. Dorsal nerve of penis 2. Muscular branches of perineal nerve	Nerves 1. Dorsal nerve of clitoris 2. Muscular branches of perineal nerve
Arteries 1. Artery of penis 2. Stems of branches of arteries to penis	Arteries 1. Artery of clitoris 2. Stems of branches of arteries to clitoris
Bulbourethral glands	No glands

Pudendal Nerve

It provides principal innervations to the perineum. It arises from the sacral plexus (ventral rami of S2, S3, and S4) in the pelvis and leaves the pelvis through the lower part of the greater sciatic foramen. After crossing ischial spine, it enters the pelvis through lesser sciatic foramen and runs in the pudendal canal after giving off the inferior rectal nerve. In the canal, it divides into perineal nerve and the dorsal nerve of penis (clitoris).

The perineal nerve passes with the internal pudendal artery to the posterior margin of the deep perineal space. Here, it gives off two posterior scrotal or labial nerves, and divides into small terminal branches, which enter the superficial and deep perineal spaces to supply the muscles within them and the bulb of the penis or bulb of the vestibule.

The dorsal nerve of penis or clitoris runs in the pudendal canal and in the deep perineal space close to the pubic arch. It gives a branch to the crus of the penis or clitoris; it passes through the gap between pubic ligament and transverse perineal ligament to reach the dorsum of penis/clitoris where it runs with the dorsal artery of the penis or clitoris and supplies the skin, body, and the glans of penis. The pudendal nerve also carries autonomic nerve fibers to the erectile tissue of the penis or clitoris.

Internal Pudendal Artery

It arises in the pelvis from the anterior division of internal iliac artery. It leaves the pelvis through the greater sciatic foramen to enter the ischiorectal fossa in the pudendal canal (Alcock canal). Now it enters into the deep perineal space at the posterior border of the perineal membrane and runs forward with the dorsal nerve of the penis or clitoris after giving rise to dorsal and deep arteries of the penis or clitoris.

The branches of internal pudendal artery comprise inferior rectal, perineal, posterior scrotal or labial, artery to bulb, dorsal and deep arteries of the penis.

Anal Region

It contains anal canal in the middle and an ischiorectal/ischioanal fossa on each side. The fossa is widest and deepest posteriorly and narrow and shallow anteriorly.

Anal Canal

The anal canal (4 cm long) extends posteroinferiorly from the lower end of rectum to the anus. (It is described in detail on pages 247–252, Chapter 22.)

Ischiorectal Fossa

This wedge-shaped space lateral to anal canal and levator ani is filled with fat. The two fossae help in dilatation of anal canal during defecation.

Boundaries.

Base: Formed by the perineal skin.

Medial wall (slopes upward and laterally): Fascia covering the external anal sphincter and levator ani.

Lateral wall (vertical): Formed by fascia covering the obturator internus and ischial tuberosity below it.

Posterior wall: Formed by sacrotuberous ligament.

Apex: Here, obturator fascia meets the inferior fascia of pelvic diaphragm.

Note that posteriorly the fossa is continuous with lesser sciatic foramen above the sacrotuberous ligament and form posterior recess.

Anteriorly, it is continuous with the narrow space which extends forward between the levator ani and obturator internus above the urogenital diaphragm (anterior recess).

Behind the anal canal, right and left fossae communicate with each other (horseshoe-shaped recess).

Contents:

1. Ischiorectal pad of fat.

2. Inferior rectal nerves and vessels, running from lateral to medial side.

3. Posterior scrotal/labial nerves and vessels cross the anterolateral part of fossa to enter deep perineal space.

4. Perineal branch of S4 nerve entering the posterior angle of fossa and running over levator ani to reach sphincter ani externus which it supplies.

5. Pudendal canal and its contents lie along lateral wall.

Pudendal Canal

1. It is a fascial canal in the lateral wall of the ischiorectal fossa 1.25 cm (1 inch) above the ischial tuberosity.

2. It is formed either by splitting of obturator fascia or by separation between fascia lunata and obturator fascia.

3. It extends from lesser sciatic foramen to the deep perineal branch.

Contents:

1. Pudendal nerve.

2. Internal pudendal vessels.

▎Clinical Notes

1. *Ischiorectal abscess*: The infections in the ischiorectal pad of fat are fairly common either as a result of small tears in anal mucous membrane or from disease of perianal skin. Formation of abscess is a natural consequence. If abscess forms, it may either burst medially into the anal canal or through perianal skin of base or both. In the latter, a track may form connecting perianal skin and anal canal (fistula-in-ano).

   The infections readily pass from one fossa to the other and form horseshoe-shaped abscess.

2. *Rupture of urethra*: The rupture of bulbous and membranous parts of urethra is not uncommon during instrumentation. If bulbous part of urethra ruptures, extravasation of urine occurs in the superficial perineal pouch and can spread to scrotum, penis, and lower anterior abdominal wall. If the membranous part of urethra ruptures, the extravasation of urine takes place in the extraperitoneal space of the anterior abdominal wall.

3. *Rupture of perineal body*: It may occur due to difficult childbirth or inadvertently during episiotomy. The perineal body plays a key role in maintaining the integrity of pelvic diaphragm which supports pelvic viscera, namely, uterus, bladder, and rectum. Its rupture often leads to prolapse of uterus and other pelvic organs (vide supra).

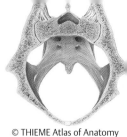
Introduction

The pelvis is formed by sacrum, coccyx, and hip bones. The sacrum is joined to the coccyx by the sacrococcygeal joint. It is wedged between two hip bones posteroinferiorly. On each side, sacrum articulates with ilium to form sacroiliac joint. The hip bones are joined anteriorly by pubic symphysis. The sacrum is joined to the lumbar vertebral column superiorly by lumbosacral joints.

Note that strictly speaking there are only four joints in the pelvis, namely, right and left sacroiliac joints, pubic symphysis, and sacrococcygeal joints.

Surface Landmarks

With the help of articulated bony pelvis, renew the following bony features in the gluteal region:

1. Palpate the pubic symphysis in the midline at the lower limit of the anterior abdominal wall.
2. Posterior superior iliac spine lies deep to skin dimple at the level of S2 spine.
3. Skin dimple marking the position of posterior superior iliac spine lies at the level of the middle of the sacroiliac joint.
4. Palpate the iliac crest forming the lower limit of the flank and back of the trunk.
5. Posterior inferior iliac spine marks the posterior and most superficial part of the sacroiliac joint.
6. Coccyx can be palpated with deep pressure just behind the anal orifice.
7. Greater and lesser sciatic notches, and ischial spine separating these two notches.
8. Crest on the dorsal surface of the sacrum. Note tubercles on median and lateral sacral crests.

Dissection and Identification

1. Remove the thoracolumbar fascia and erector spinae muscle from the dorsal aspect of the sacrum and fifth lumbar vertebra.

2. Now identify the ventral sacroiliac ligament on the pelvic surface of the sacroiliac joint and see its thinness.

3. Make a cut in the ligament and open the joint cavity by bending the sacrum backward.

4. Identify cartilage-covered articular surfaces that are irregular and closely fitted.

5. Now remove the dorsal sacroiliac ligament to expose the interosseous sacroiliac ligament.

6. Now separate the sacrum from ilium by dividing the interosseous ligament.

Lumbosacral Joints

The sacrum articulates superiorly with lumbar vertebral column. The lumbosacral joints are formed between the fifth lumbar vertebra and sacrum. They include two zygapophyseal joints between the inferior articular surfaces of L5 and S1 vertebrae and a secondary cartilaginous joint (symphysis) between the bodies of L5 and S1.

These joints are similar to those between the other vertebrae except that the anterior part of intervertebral disc between the two bones is thicker than the posterior part. As a result, there is considerable angulation posteriorly between the adjacent surfaces of L5 and S1 vertebrae. For this reason, the body of L5 vertebra has a tendency to slip forward on S1 vertebra. However, the stability of this joint is maintained by (a) widely spaced articular process and (b) strong iliolumbar and lumbosacral ligaments which extend from transverse process of L5 vertebra to ilium and sacrum, respectively.

Sacroiliac Joint

It is a synovial joint between the L-shaped articular surfaces on the lateral surface of sacrum and a similar facet on the ilium. The joint surfaces are irregular and interlock to resist any movements. The articular surfaces are firmly coapted (**Fig. 26.1**).

Note that the sacroiliac joints are strong synovial joints and transmit the weight of the body to the hip bones. These joints also transmit forces from lower limbs to the vertebral column. The sacroiliac joint on each side is stabilized by the following three ligaments:

1. *Ventral sacroiliac ligament*: It is a thin ribbon-like band of transverse fibers which stretch between the margins of articular surfaces anteroinferiorly. The main role of this ligament is to close the abdominopelvic surface of the joint.

2. *Interosseous sacroiliac ligament*: It is the largest and strongest ligament of the three. It unites the wide rough areas that adjoin the concave margins of the articular surfaces of ilium and sacrum. It fills the gap between the two bones.

3. *Dorsal sacroiliac ligament*: It covers the interosseous sacroiliac ligament superiorly and gets fused with it. It consists of two parts:
   • A short transverse band of fibers which pass from ilium to the first and second tubercles of lateral sacral crest.
   • A long, more or less vertical band which passes from third and fourth tubercles of lateral sacral crest to medial edge of the sacrotuberous ligament with which it blends.

   Note that the abdominal surface of the joint is very close to obturator and femoral nerves, while its pelvic surface is crossed by lumbosacral trunk and first sacral ventral ramus. These nerves are likely to be involved in diseases of the sacroiliac joint and thereby give rise to pain which is felt at the sites of their cutaneous distribution.

4. *Pubic symphysis*: It is a secondary cartilaginous joint between the two pubic bones. The articular surfaces are crossed by hyaline cartilage and linked with each other across the midline by a disc

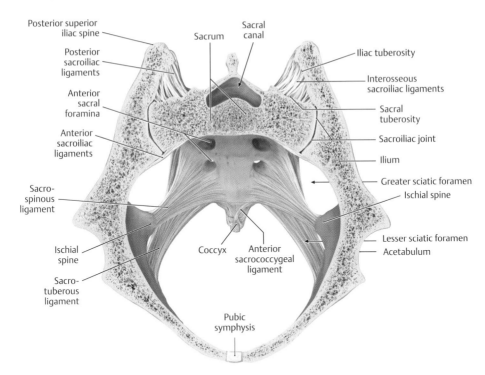

Fig. 26.1 Oblique section through true pelvis to show ligaments of sacroiliac joints. (From Schuenke M, Schulte E, Schumacher U. THIEME Atlas of Anatomy. General Anatomy and Musculoskeletal System. Illustrations by Voll M and Wesker K. © Thieme 2020)

of fibrocartilage. The disc is surrounded by ligaments. The two ligaments associated with it are as follows:

- *Superior pubic ligament*: It is very strong and located above the joint. It is fused superficially with abdominal aponeurosis.
- *Inferior pubic ligament*: It is located below the joint. It is a curved band which rounds off the apex of pubic arch and extends along the inferior pubic rami. It is also called arcuate ligament.

Note that the deep dorsal vein of penis/clitoris enters the pelvis between the arcuate and transverse perineal ligaments.

5. *Sacrococcygeal joint*: It is a secondary cartilaginous joint between the sacrum and coccyx. The articular surfaces are united by an intervertebral disc. Stability to this joint is provided by ventral and dorsal sacrococcygeal ligaments and intercorneal ligaments.

▌ Clinical Notes

1. *Spondylolisthesis* is the forward slipping of L5 vertebra on the superior surface of S1 vertebra. It occurs when inferior articular process, laminae, and spine of L5 vertebrae get separated from the rest of the vertebra. Clinically, it presents as backache and pain radiating along the sciatic nerve.

2. *Sacroiliac arthritis*: Being weight-bearing joints, degenerative changes are likely to occur in these joints which may cause pain and discomfort in sacroiliac regions.

3. *Coccydynia* is a name given to painful coccyx. Normally, the coccyx moves a little backward during defecation and parturition, but in multiparous and weak women, it may become mobile and cause pain during sitting on a hard surface.

Appendix

Cross-Sectional Anatomy of Abdomen and Pelvis

Nowadays the cross-sectional anatomy is also taught to first year medical students as an adjunct information to improve their *spatial anatomical knowledge*. This is essential to improve their ability to accurately interpret the CT and MRI scans which are commonly used these days by clinicians to make proper diagnosis of various diseases.

The anatomical cross sections are cut at right angle to the main axis and the cut surface is viewed in two dimensions. This provides an essential view of depth of viscera in two dimensions/2D-view.

The brain intuitively creates a 3D view of these sections (**Fig. 17.12**, page 196, Chapter 17). Actually, the serial cross sections are cut at different vertebral levels corresponding to those of CT and MRI scans.

The cadaveric cross-sectional prosections can be used for teaching cross-sectional anatomy. Further, students can go to the museum and learn this from mounted cross sections from different regions of the body.

Clinical Correlation

The CT and MRI scans of abdomen and pelvis are routinely done these days to diagnose the pathology and abnormalities associated with various viscera.

Index

A

Abdomen, 97. *See also* Bones of abdomen and pelvis
Abdominal aorta, 216–217, 217f
Abdominal aortic aneurysm, 220
Abdominal cavity, 97, 139
    abdominal viscera disposition, 142f
    dissection and identification of, 140–141
Abdominal part of esophagus, 154
Abductor brevis, 21f
Acquired posterior dislocation, 82
Adductor canal, 26
Anal canal, 286
    anal sphincters, 251
    dissection and identification of, 247–248
    interior of, 250–251, 251f
    location of, 248f
Anal region
    anal canal, 286
    ischiorectal fossa, 286–287
    pudendal canal, 287
Ankle joint
    dissection and identification of, 89–90
    ligaments, 90, 91f, 92f
    movements, 90
    type of, 90
Ankle sprains, 93
Anterior abdominal wall, 103
    arteries of, 119–120
    cutaneous nerves in, 110
    cutaneous vessels of, 110–111
    dissection and identification of, 106–108
    inner aspect of lower part of, 140f
    muscles of, 111, 112f, 113f
        fascia transversalis, 115
        inguinal canal, 116–117, 117f, 118f
        origin, insertion, nerve supply, and actions of, 114, 114t
        rectus abdominis, 114f
        rectus sheath, 115–116, 116f
        spermatic cord, 119
    nerves of, 119
    regions of, 104–106, 106f
    superficial fascia in, 109–110
    superficial veins, 111
    surface landmarks of, 104
Anterior compartment of leg
    dissection and identification of, 46–49
    muscles of, 51f
        to superior extensor retinaculum, 50
    superficial cutaneous veins and nerves of, 47f
    surface landmarks of, 45
Anterior (extensor) compartment of thigh
    arteries of, 22–23
    dissection and identification of, 15–21
    location of, 13
    muscles of, 22t
    nerves of, 23–24
    surface landmarks of, 14–15

Anterior thigh
    muscle, 16
    neurovascular structure of, 20f
Anterior tibial compartment syndrome, 54
Anterior transverse arch, 75
Aortic aneurysm, 228
Appendicitis, 186
Arches of foot
    bony components of, 74–75
    classification of, 74
    factors maintaining, 76, 76t
    functions of, 74
Azygos veins, 222

B

Back, neurovasculature of, 136f
Back of leg. *See* Calf
Back of thigh, 37, 38f
Barium meal x-ray abdomen, 172
Benign prostatic hypertrophy (BPH), 244
Biliary apparatus, 192–193, 193f
Bones of abdomen and pelvis
    coccyx, 100f, 101f, 102
    hip bone, 102
    lower ribs and costal cartilages, 97
    lumbar vertebrae, 97–98, 99f
    sacrum, 98, 100f, 101f, 102
Bones of lower limb, 2–11, 3f
    femur, 2
        lower end of, 5
        right, 5f
    fibula, 6f, 7
    foot bones, 7
        metatarsals, 8
        phalanges, 9
        right foot, 9f
        tarsal bones, 8
    hip bone, 2
    patella (knee cap), 7, 8f
    tibia (shin bone)
        characteristic features of, 5–7
        and fibula, 6f

C

Calcaneus, 8, 10f, 11f
Calf, 55
    deep neurovascular structures on, 58f
    superficial neurovascular structures on, 57f
Calot triangle (cystohepatic triangle), 196
Carcinoma head of pancreas, 171
Celiac trunk, 152f, 153f, 159, 217–218
Central tendon of perineum. *See* Perineal body
Cervical carcinoma, 260
Cholelithiasis, 196
Cirrhosis of liver, 192, 196
Claw toes, 96
Club foot. *See* Talipes equinovarus
Coccydynia, 291

Coccyx, 100*f*, 101*f*, 102
Common iliac arteries, 220
Common iliac veins, 220
Condyles, medial and lateral, 5
Congenital dislocation, 82
Cruciate anastomosis, arteries participating in, 36
Cryptorchidism, 134
Cuneiforms, 9

D
Deep circumflex iliac artery, 120
Deep perineal space/pouch, 285
Diaphragm
    dissection and identification of, 209–211
    foramina in, 213–215
    location of, 212*f*, 213*f*
    nerves and vessels of, 215, 216*f*
    origin of, 211
Direct inguinal hernia, 121
Dorsalis pedis artery, branches of, 52
Dorsiflexion, 90
Ductus deferens, 124*f*
Duodenal cap, 172*f*
Duodenal ulcers, 171
Duodenum, 153*f*, 163
    functions of, 164
    interior of, 166, 166*f*
    parts of, 164–166, 165*f*

E
Epididymis, 124*f*, 128
Epiploic foramen, 151
Esophageal varices, 161
Eversion, 96
External iliac arteries, 220
Extracapsular ligaments, 85

F
Fascia transversalis, 115
Female genitalia
    lymphatic drainage of, 273*f*
Femoral artery, 22–23, 27
Femoral hernia, 27
Femoral nerve, 18*f*, 23
Femoral pulse, 27
Femoral triangle, 19*f*
Foot dorsum
    dissection of, 49*f*
    tendon, 48
Foot drop, 54
Foot, joints of. *See* Joints of foot
Foot region, 2
Fracture of neck of femur, 82

G
Gallbladder, 152*f*
    bile duct, 194–195, 195*f*
    cystic duct, 193–194
    location of, 194*f*
Gallstones. *See* Cholelithiasis
Gastric ulcers, 161
Gluteal region, 1
    cutaneous nerves of, 31*f*
    dissection and identification of, 30–34, 33*f*
    intramuscular injections in, 36
    location of, 29

    muscles of
        bony attachments to, 32*f*
        nerve supply and, 35–36, 35*t*
        priformis muscle, 34*f*
        surface landmarks of, 29, 30*f*
Gluteus maximus—left, 33*f*
Greater sciatic foramen, structures passing through, 35

H
Hemiazygos veins, 222
Hemorrhoids (piles), 252
Hepatitis, 192
Hip bone, 4*f*, 102
Hip joint, 77
    articular capsule, 79, 80*f*
    articular surfaces of, 79, 79*f*
    dislocation of, 82
    dissection and identification of, 78
    ligaments of, 78*f*, 80
    movements, 80, 82
    relations of, 80, 81*f*
Hydrocele, 134

I
Iliofemoral ligament, 80
Ilium, 2
Indirect inguinal hernia, 121
Inferior epigastric artery, 120
Inferior hypogastric plexus, 269
Inferior mesenteric artery, 178–179, 179*f*, 219
Inferior mesenteric vein, 180
Inferior vena cava, 220, 221*f*
Inguinal canal, 116–117, 117*f*, 118*f*, 119
Inguinal hernia, 120–121, 120*f*
Intermittent claudication, 54
Internal hernia, 150
Internal pudendal artery, 286
Intracapsular ligaments, 85, 88*f*
Intramuscular injections, 36
Inversion, 96
Ischiofemoral ligament, 80
Ischiorectal abscess, 287
Ischiorectal fossa, 286–287
Ischium, 2

J
Jejunum and ileum, 175, 175*f*
Joints of foot
    calcaneocuboid joint, 95, 95*f*
    dissection and identification of, 93
    movements, 96
    subtalar joint, 94, 94*f*
    talocalcaneonavicular joint, 94
    transverse talar joint, 95, 95*f*
Joints of lower limb
    ankle joint
        dissection and identification of, 89–90
        ligaments, 90, 91*f*, 92*f*
        movements, 90
        type of, 90
    classification of, 77, 77*t*
    hip joint, 77
        articular capsule, 79, 80*f*
        articular surfaces of, 79, 79*f*
        dislocation of, 82

dissection and identification of, 78
   ligaments of, 78*f,* 80
   movements, 80, 82
   relations of, 80, 81*f*
  knee joint
   articular surfaces of, 85
   blood and nerve supply of, 89
   bursae around, 87
   dissection and identification of, 82–83
   ligaments, 85, 86*f*
   meniscal tear, 89
   movements, 87, 89
   opened joint capsule, 84*f*
   types, 85

K
Kidneys
  blood and nerve supply of, 206
  coverings of, 200–201, 202*f*
  dissection and identification of, 197–198
  hilum, 199
  relations of, 201–203, 202*f,* 203*f*
  structure of, 203–204, 204*f*
  and suprarenal glands in situ, 199*f*
  ureter, 205
  vessels of, 204
Knee joint
  articular surfaces of, 85
  blood and nerve supply of, 89
  bursae around, 87
  dissection and identification of, 82–83
  ligaments, 85, 86*f*
  meniscal tear, 89
  movements, 87, 89
  opened joint capsule, 84*f*
  types, 85

L
Large intestine, 180
  ascending colon, 183
  blood supply of, 184–185, 185*f*
  cardinal features of, 182–183, 182*f*
  cecum, 183
  descending colon, 183
  dissection and identification of, 181
  location and parts of, 181*f*
  sigmoid colon (pelvic colon), 183
  transverse colon, 183
  vermiform appendix, 184
Lateral compartment of leg
  dissection and identification of, 52
  muscles of, 53–54, 53*f,* 54*t*
  surface landmarks of, 45
Lateral longitudinal arch, 75
Leg, 45, 46*f*
Lesser pelvis, 230–233
Lesser sciatic foramen, structures passing through, 36
Ligament of head of femur, 80
Liver, 152*f*
  blood supply of, 192
  dissection and identification of, 187
  lobes of, 189–191, 189*f,* 190*f*
  location of, 188, 189*f*
  peritoneal relations, 190*f,* 191
  in situ, 188

Loin
  definition of, 135
  dissection and identification of, 135
  lumbar triangle (of Petit), 137
  thoracolumbar fascia, 137–138, 137*f*
Loss of inversion and eversion, 96
Lower limb
  bones of. *See* Bones of lower limb
  parts of, 1, 3*f*
Lower ribs and costal cartilages, 97
Lumbar arteries, 226
Lumbar hernia, 138
Lumbar plexus, 226, 226*f,* 227–228*f*
Lumbar triangle, neurovasculature of, 136*f*
Lumbar veins, 227
Lumbar vertebrae, 97–98, 99*f*
Lumbosacral joints, 290

M
Male and female pelvis, 233, 233*f*
Male external genital organs
  dissection and identification of, 123–125
  ductus deferens, 124*f*
  epididymis, 124*f,* 128
  penis, 124*f,* 131*f,* 132*f*
   arterial supply to, 132
   body, 130
   ligaments supporting, 130
   lymphatic drainage of, 134
   nerve supply of, 134
   neurovasculature of, 133*f*
   root, 130
   venous drainage of, 134
  scrotum, 124*f,* 126
   neurovasculature of, 133*f*
  spermatic cord, 124*f,* 125*f*
  testis, 124*f,* 126–129
   blood vessels of, 128
   descent of, 129
   dissection and identification of, 130
   nerve supply of, 128
Male genitalia, lymphatic drainage of, 272*f*
Meckel diverticulum, 186
Medial compartment of thigh
  arteries of, 22–23
  dissection and identification of, 21
  muscles of, 22*t*
  nerves of, 23–24
Medial longitudinal arch, 74
Medial meniscus, 85
Meniscal tear, 89
Metatarsals, 8
Micronodular cirrhosis of liver, 151
Moren Baker cyst, 44
Muscular sling of puborectalis, 250*f*
Musculophrenic artery, 120

N
Navicular bones, 9

O
Obturator nerve, muscles supplied by
  adductor canal, 26
  by anterior division, 24
  femoral canal, 25–26
  femoral sheath, 25

femoral triangle, 24–25, 24f
    by posterior division, 24
Osteomalacia of bony pelvis, 273
Ovarian cyst, 260
Ovaries
    dissection and identification of, 254
    location of, 259, 260f
    vessels of, 259

P

Pancreas, 153f, 166, 168f
    ducts of, 168
    and duodenum, 167
    relations, 168
    in situ, 167
    structure, 168
    vessels and lymph nodes, 169
Paralysis of diaphragm, 228
Parasympathetic innervation, 134
Parietal peritoneum, 97
Pelvic abscess, 150
Pelvic diaphragm/pelvic floor, 232–233, 232f
Pelvic floor, muscles of, 278
Pelvic viscera, 235
    dissection and identification of, 236–238
    male genital organs, 241f
        ductus deferens, 240
        ejaculatory ducts, 242
        seminal vesicles, 240
    prostate, 242–244
    urethra, 237f, 245
        male, 240f, 245
    urinary bladder, 236f, 237f, 238–240
Pelvic wall, 261
    autonomic nerves, 268–269
    dissection and identification of, 262–263
    muscles of, 265–266, 266f
    pelvic fascia, 265
    vertebropelvic ligaments, 263–264, 263f, 264f
Pelvis, 289
    blood vessels of, 269–271, 271f
    bones of, 229. *See also* Bones of abdomen and
        pelvis
    dissection and identification of, 289–290
    joints of, 232
    lumbosacral joints, 290
    lymph nodes and lymph vessels of, 272–273f
    male and female, 233, 233f
    nerves of, 266–268, 267f, 268f
    or pelvic outlet, inferior aperture of, 231
    parts of, 230, 230f
    sacroiliac joint, 290–291
    surface landmarks of, 289
    and urogenital triangle, 283f
    walls of, 231, 231f
Penis, 124f, 131f, 132f
    arterial supply to, 132
    body, 130
    ligaments supporting, 130
    lymphatic drainage of, 134
    nerve supply of, 134
    neurovasculature of, 133f
    root, 130
    venous drainage of, 134
Perineal body, 284, 287
Perineal membrane, 282–283, 284t

Perineal region, 276f
Perineum, 275
    deep dissection of, 281f
    neurovasculature of, 279f, 280f
Peripheral heart, 62
Peritoneal cavity, 143
Peritoneal folds and pouches
    greater omentum, 144–145
    lesser omentum, 145
    mesentery, 145–146
    mesoappendix, 146
    sigmoid mesocolon, 147
    transverse mesocolon, 146
Peritoneal recess and pouches
    epiploic/omental foramen (foramen of Winslow),
        149
    hepatorenal pouch (Morison's pouch), 149–150
    lesser sac (omental bursa), 147–149
    rectouterine pouch (pouch of Douglas), 150
Peritoneum
    parietal, 142
    visceral, 143
Peritonitis, 150
Peroneus brevis, 54
Peroneus longus, 54
Pes cavus, 76
Pes planus (flat foot), 76
Phalanges, 9
Piriformis muscle, 34f
Plantar flexion, 90
Popliteal aneurysm, 44
Popliteal artery, 44
Popliteal fossa, 37
    boundaries of, 42
    contents of, 42
    dissection and identification of, 40–41, 41f
    nerve, artery, and lymph nodes in, 43–44
Popliteal lymph nodes, 44
Porta hepatis, 188
Portal hypertension, 171
Portal vein, 169–171, 171f
Portosystemic (portacaval) anastomosis, 170–171
Posterior abdominal wall
    lymph nodes of, 222–223, 223f
    muscles of, 223, 224f
    nerves of, 225–228
    origin, insertion, nerve supply, and actions of,
        224t
    paired branches, 219–223
    unpaired branches, 217–218, 218f
    vessels, 216–217
Posterior compartment of leg
    deep neurovascular structures on, 58f
    dissection and identification of, 55–58
    muscles of, 59–60t, 59–62, 61f
        deep, 62f
        for dorsiflexion of foot, 60
        for eversion of foot, 60
        for inversion of foot, 60
        for plantar flexion of foot, 60
        plantaris and soleus, 61f
        on upper part of medial surface of tibia, 60
    subdivisions of, 56f
    superficial neurovascular structures on, 57f
    surface landmarks of, 45
Posterior compartment of thigh

dissection and identification of, 37–39, 38f
hamstring muscles of, 39–40, 39f
iliotibial tract, 40
popliteal fossa. *See* Popliteal fossa
surface landmarks of, 37
Posterior transverse arch, 75
Posterolateral hernia of diaphragm (diaphragm of Bochdalek), 228
Pott fracture, 93
Profunda femoris artery, 23
Prostate, 242
blood vessels of, 244
capsules of, 244
lobes and zones of, 243–244, 243f
puboprostatic and pubovesical ligaments, 244
Prostatic cancer, 244
Pubis, 2
Pubofemoral ligament, 80
Pudendal canal, 287
Pudendal nerve, 286

Q
Quadriceps tendon right knee, 83f

R
Rectal prolapse, 252
Rectum, 249f
dissection and identification of, 247–248
location of, 248f
lymphatic drainage of, 272f
mucosa of, 249
relations of, 249–250
vessels and nerves of, 250
Rectus abdominis, 114f
Rectus sheath, 115–116, 116f
Renal angle, 208
Renal/ureteric colic, 138
Right femur, 5f
Right hip bone, 4f
Right lower limb, superficial cutaneous vein and nerves of, 17f

S
Sacroiliac arthritis, 291
Sacrum, 98, 100f, 101f, 102
Sciatic nerve, 36
Scrotum, 124f, 126, 133f
Small intestine, 173
blood supply of
inferior mesenteric artery, 178–179, 179f
superior mesenteric artery, 176–178, 177f, 178f
superior mesenteric vein, 178, 178f
branches, 180
general features, 174–176
inferior mesenteric vein, 180
lymph nodes of mesentery of, 180
Sole of foot
definition of, 63
dissection and identification of, 63–66
deep, 67f
superficial, 64f, 65f
layers of, 67f
muscles of, 63, 68–72
bony attachments of, 72, 72f
dorsalis pedis artery, 72

first muscular layer, 68, 68f
fourth muscular layer, 71, 71f
second muscular layer, 69, 69f
third muscular layer, 70, 70f
nerves of
lateral plantar, 74
medial plantar, 73, 73f
skin of, 63
Spermatic cord, 119, 124f, 125f
Spleen, 153f
blood supply, 161
external features, 159–160, 160f
structure and function of, 161
Splenomegaly, 161
Spondylolisthesis, 291
Stomach, 152f, 154, 156f, 172f
blood vessels and nerves of, 157, 158f
curvatures, 155
external features, 155
interior of, 159
orifices, 155
peritoneal relations, 157
subdivisions, 156–157
surfaces, 156
visceral relations, 157
Subcostal nerve, 226
Subphrenic abscess, 150
Subsartorial canal. *See* Adductor canal
Superficial perineal space/pouch, 284, 285t
Superior epigastric artery, 120
Superior mesenteric artery, 176–178, 177f, 219
Superior mesenteric vein, 178, 178f
Suprarenal (adrenal) glands, 206–208, 207f
Sympathetic innervation, 134
Sympathetic trunk, abdominal part of, 225, 225f

T
Tail bone. *See* Coccyx
Talipes equinovarus, 76
Talus, 8, 10f, 11f
Tarsal bones, 8
Testis, 124f, 126–129
blood vessels of, 128
descent of, 129
dissection and identification of, 130
nerve supply of, 128
Thigh, 1, 13
ascia lata, 20f
back of, 37
proximal part of front of, 18f
transverse section of, 14f
Tibial nerve, 43
Trabeculated bladder, 244
Trendelenburg sign, 36
Triceps surae dissection, 59f
Trochanteric anastomosis, 36
Typhoid ulcers, 186

U
Umbilical hernia, 120
Undescended testis, 134
Ureteric stone/ureteric colic, 208
Urethra
female, 237f, 245
lymphatic drainage of, 272f
male, 240f, 245

rupture of, 245, 287
Urinary bladder, 236f, 237f, 238
    female, 237f
    interior of, 239, 239f, 240f
    lymphatic drainage of, 272f
Urogenital region
    dissection and identification of, 277–282
    fasciae and perineal pouches/spaces in, 282–286
    female external genital organs, 276–277
    superficial structures in, 276
Urogenital triangle and pelvis, 283f
Uterine prolapse, 260
Uterus
    dissection and identification of, 253–254

    position and axes of, 255
    relations, 255
    supports of, 256
    and uterine tubes, 254, 255f, 258
    vessels and nerves of, 256–258, 257f

V

Vagina
    dissection and identification of, 254
    location of, 258, 259f
    vessels of, 259
Varicocele, 134
Visceral peritoneum, 97
Visceral plexus, 269